CW00792711

On Asthma

Henry Hyde Salter

Nabu Public Domain Reprints:

You are holding a reproduction of an original work published before 1923 that is in the public domain in the United States of America, and possibly other countries. You may freely copy and distribute this work as no entity (individual or corporate) has a copyright on the body of the work. This book may contain prior copyright references, and library stamps (as most of these works were scanned from library copies). These have been scanned and retained as part of the historical artifact.

This book may have occasional imperfections such as missing or blurred pages, poor pictures, errant marks, etc. that were either part of the original artifact, or were introduced by the scanning process. We believe this work is culturally important, and despite the imperfections, have elected to bring it back into print as part of our continuing commitment to the preservation of printed works worldwide. We appreciate your understanding of the imperfections in the preservation process, and hope you enjoy this valuable book.

ON

ASTHMA:

ITS PATHOLOGY AND TREATMENT.

BY

HENRY HYDE SALTER, M.D., F.R.S.

FELLOW OF THE ROYAL COLLEGE OF PHYSICIANS;

ASSISTANT-PHYSICIAN TO CHARING CROSS HOSPITAL, AND LECTURER ON
PHYSIOLOGY AND PATHOLOGY AT THE CHARING CROSS
HOSPITAL MEDICAL SCHOOL.

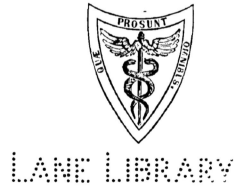

LANE LIBRARY

PHILADELPHIA:
BLANCHARD AND LEA.
1864.

TO MY RELATIVE,

THOMAS BELL, ESQ., F.R.S.

PRESIDENT OF THE LINNEAN SOCIETY,

𝔗𝔥𝔦𝔰 𝔚𝔬𝔯𝔨 𝔦𝔰 𝔍𝔫𝔰𝔠𝔯𝔦𝔟𝔢𝔡,

IN ADMIRATION OF HIS LEARNING, HIS CHARACTER, AND HIS TALENTS,

BUT MORE

IN ACKNOWLEDGMENT OF OBLIGATIONS THAT CAN NEVER BE REPAID,

AND AS A SMALL TRIBUTE OF

A GREAT AFFECTION.

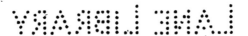
LAME LIBRARY

PHILADELPHIA:
COLLINS, PRINTER, 705 JAYNE ST.

PREFACE.

For many years past my attention has been specially directed to the subject of asthma, and from an enforced and very close observation of it I have become acquainted with many facts, both with regard to its clinical history and treatment, for any notice of which I have in vain searched the literature of the subject. To communicate these facts to others has been the principal motive that has induced me to commit the following pages to the press. This motive has been seconded by others which have not been without their influence in inducing me to lay before the profession the views, both theoretical and practical, at which I have arrived. One of these is the extreme interest of the subject in a pathological point of view, the striking illustration which the clinical history of the disease affords of the phenomena and laws of that particular form of perverted nervous action in which, I believe, it essentially consists. Another is the importance of correct pathological views in relation to the therapeutics of the disease. A third, a desire to refute the various erroneous theories that have been, and still are advanced with regard to the pathology of asthma, and to supplant by something precise and definite those loose notions about it which I find, both from conversation and from their writings, to be so common among medical men.

I earnestly hope that my book may be the means of throwing some light upon an obscure disease, and indirectly instrumental in affording some relief to the poor sufferers from it.

I can conceive no greater satisfaction and comfort to any one who has witnessed, still more who has experienced, the horrors of asthma, than the thought that he may have successfully employed, in the mitigation of its sufferings, that multiplied power which the press confers.

6, MONTAGUE STREET, RUSSEL SQUARE,
April, 1860.

CONTENTS.

CHAPTER I.

CHAPTER II.

CHAPTER III.

CHAPTER IV.

CLINICAL HISTORY OF ASTHMA (*continued*).—PHENOMENA OF THE INTERVALS.

CHAPTER V.

VARIETIES OF ASTHMA.

CHAPTER VI.

THE ÆTIOLOGY OF ASTHMA.

CHAPTER VII.

CONSEQUENCES OF ASTHMA.

CHAPTER VIII.

TREATMENT OF THE ASTHMATIC PAROXYSM.—TREATMENT BY
DEPRESSANTS.

CHAPTER IX.

TREATMENT OF THE ASTHMATIC PAROXYSM (*continued*).—TREATMENT
BY STIMULANTS.

CHAPTER X.

TREATMENT OF THE ASTHMATIC PAROXYSM (*continued*).—TREATMENT
BY SEDATIVES.

CHAPTER XI.

TREATMENT OF THE ASTHMATIC PAROXYSM (*continued*).

CHAPTER XII.

DIETETIC AND REGIMENAL TREATMENT OF ASTHMA.

CHAPTER XIII.

ON THE THERAPEUTICAL INFLUENCE OF LOCALITY.

CHAPTER XIV.

HYGIENIC TREATMENT OF ASTHMA.

CHAPTER XV.

PROGNOSIS OF ASTHMA.

APPENDIX.

ON ASTHMA.

CHAPTER I.

PRELIMINARY INQUIRY INTO THE TENABILITY OF THE THEORIES OF ASTHMA.

Theory 1. That bronchial spasm is not necessarily present in asthma; Laennec's "Asthma, with puerile breathing;" Copland's "Nervous asthma;" Walshe's Hæmic asthma." These dyspnœas not true asthma.—2. Dr. Bree's theory of a specific irritating mucus.—3. That asthma is the dyspnœa of bronchitis; the "Bronchite à râles vibrants" of M. Beau.—4. The "Humoral" theory.—5. Dr. Todd's theory of a poisoning of certain portions of the nervous centres, or nerves of respiration, by a specific materies morbi.—6. That asthma is nothing but the dyspnœa of emphysema.—7. That the phenomena of asthma are due to spasm or paralysis of the respiratory muscles.—8. That asthma is *paralysis* of the bronchial tubes.—9. That there is no such thing as asthma, as a substantive disease.

SPASMODIC asthma—paroxysmal dyspnœa of a peculiar character, generally periodic, with intervals of healthy respiration between the attacks—although not a very common disease, cannot, in this country, be said to be by any means rare, and I believe that all who direct their attention to it will find it to be much commoner than is imagined. Cases of perfectly *pure* asthma, that is, without the slightest organic complication, are, however, rare, unless they have existed a very short time, and for this reason—that asthma, if it is at all severe and its attacks frequent, cannot long exist without inflicting permanent injury on the lungs, and even on the heart. If in asthma of long standing the lungs and heart remain healthy and uninjured, we may be sure either that the attacks are very mild, so as to produce but little disturbance in the lung, or that they are very rare, so as to allow ample time for the recovery of the injury produced by one attack before the occurrence of another. But asthma is not the less asthma because it has produced certain organic changes which complicate it; and many cases are primarily and essentially asthma that ultimately become, and are called, emphysema and heart-disease.

But not only is asthma not an uncommon disease, but it is one of the direst suffering; the horrors o f the asthmatic paroxysm far exceed any acute bodily pain; the sense of impending suffocation, the agonizing struggle for the breath of life, are so terrible, that
2

they cannot even be witnessed without sharing in the sufferer's distress. With a face expressive of the intensest anxiety, unable to move, speak, or even make signs, the chest distended and fixed, the head thrown back between the elevated shoulders, the muscles of respiration rigid and tightened like cords, and tugging and straining for every breath that is drawn, the surface pallid or livid, cold and sweating—such are the signs by which this dreadful suffering manifests itself. And even in the intervals of health, the asthmatic's sufferings do not cease; he seems well, he goes about like his fellows and among them, but he knows he is altogether different; he bears about his disease within him wherever he goes; he knows he is struck—"*hæret lateri lethalis arundo;*" he is conscious that he is not sound—he cannot be warranted; he is not certain of a day's, perhaps not of an hour's health; he only knows that a certain percentage of his future life must be dedicated to suffering; he cannot make an engagement except with a proviso, and from many of the occupations of life he is cut off; the recreations, the enjoyments, the indulgences of others he dares not take; his usefulness is crippled, his life is marred; and, if he knows anything of the nature of his complaint, he knows that his sufferings may terminate in a closing scene worse only than the present.)

And not only is asthma thus comparatively common and superlatively distressing, but it is peculiarly and proverbially intractable. The asthmatic is generally looked upon as an asthmatic for life, as one who, though he should suffer many things of many physicians, would be nothing bettered, but rather grow worse, and the treatment is regarded as palliative. It must be admitted that the remedies for asthma are of very irregular and uncertain operation: that probably there is no single remedy that is not inoperative in a large number of cases; that that which is useful in one is valueless in another, while there are many cases that resist all remedies. If this intractability of asthma were doubtful, the large number of remedies that have been suggested would be a sufficient proof of it.

But besides this, asthma is a disease about whose pathology more various and discrepant ideas prevail than about any other disease that could be named, and to this day, if we appeal to the written opinions of living authors, its absolute nature must be considered as still *sub judice.*

I think, then, I shall not be undertaking a useless task if I attempt to throw some light upon the pathology, and lay down some rules for the treatment, of a disease so comparatively common, so distressing, so intractable, and so obscure.

Before attempting to enunciate or enforce any views of a disease that have, either in themselves or in the arguments adduced in their support, anything of novelty, or against which commonly received opinions are ranged, it seems to me desirable to pass in review pre-existing theories, and test their tenability by the standard of a recent physiology and pathology, that so, if any of them abide this scrutiny and prove irrefragable, they may contest the exclusive claims of the new theory, or if, on the other hand, they are found to be untenable, they may be swept away, and the ground that they occupied left clear for something more true and enduring.

And especially is such a preliminary inquiry desirable in the case of asthma, from the great number and variety of the theories that have been suggested in explanation of its phenomena, from the *primâ facie* reasonableness of many of those theories, and from the high names by which they have been endorsed.

Doubtless there are many circumstances peculiar to asthma that go far to explain why such vague and, as I think I shall show, erroneous notions should be entertained with regard to its absolute nature, such as the rarity of death in cases of uncomplicated asthma, the slightness and unconspicuous character of the *post-mortem* appearances of such cases, or the total absence of any appreciable morbid change, and the remoteness of the actual pathological condition from the manifest phenomena of the disease.

Let me, then, as the first step in the inquiry into the absolute nature of asthma, analyze in order, and see if they bear investigation, the many theories respecting it which are current, and which have either been inherited from past authority or coined in the present generation.

The first of these theories is, that contraction of the bronchial tubes is not necessary to constitute asthma—that asthma may exist without it.

Laennec abandoned the principle of the necessity of bronchial spasm as the only possible cause of asthma, inasmuch as he divided asthma into two varieties: one, asthma attended with *puerile respiration*, in which the vital expansibility of the lungs is *increased* from a temporary augmentation of the respiratory necessities of the system, occasioned by some unknown modification of the nervous influence; the other, *spasmodic asthma*, from a spasmodic contraction of the air tubes. Dr. Copland adopts the same view, and describes Laennec's "asthma, with puerile respiration," as *nervous asthma*, defining it thus—"anhelation from a feeling of want of a more complete respiration than the patient enjoys, the pulmonary expansion distinctly taking place with promptitude, completeness, and uniformity, so as to furnish a general puerile sound on auscultation." Dr. Walshe describes just the same thing under the name of "hæmic asthma," believing the difficult breathing to depend upon morbid conditions of the blood, which probably interfere with its ready oxygenation, directly or indirectly, the breathing being instinctively increased in frequency to make up for the deficient amount of oxygen supplied to the system by each separate inspiration. The dyspnœa, he correctly remarks, has much the character of the breathlessness following over-exertion in health, is not frequent in the ratio of its apparent labour, and is unaccompanied by any physical signs, cardiac or pulmonary, to explain the morbid state of the breathing.

Now that you may have a dyspnœa characterized by laborious respiratory action and an exaltation of the sense of want of breath, and, at the same time, accompanied by a free inflation of the lungs, is not to be doubted; but it is no more asthma than bronchitis is asthma; it has not one character in common with asthma that would justify such an alliance. In the circumstances under which it occurs, in the *kind* of dyspnœa, in its whole clinical history, it presents the strongest contrariety to asthma; and it would be strange indeed if two kinds of dyspnœa, so unlike in character, had anything in common in their essential pathology. There is an absence of the distress, of the characteristic wheeze, of the intolerance of the recumbent posture, of the evidence of deficient oxygenation, of the repetition of the attacks, of the periodicity, of the exciting causes, indeed of every feature characteristic of asthma. It certainly is dyspnœa, and so is asthma, and that is just what they have in common, and nothing more; but to make that the warrant for calling them both asthma would be to call all forms of dyspnœa asthma—bronchitic, emphysematous, cardiac— indeed, it would be to make asthma and dyspnœa synonymous terms.

It may be said that this is a mere dispute about names, and that it is not of any consequence whether this kind of dyspnœa is called asthma or not. But I contend that it is; because the adopting of such a nomenclature involves the confounding of things utterly dissimilar, and the surrender of the essential pathology of the disease. Besides, it is not in the interest of correct nosology, or rational treatment, that such errors in nomenclature should be allowed to stand.

I am perfectly familiar with this variety of dyspnœa, and have been accustomed to call it " subjective dyspnœa;" because I conceived there was no *objective* cause for it, nothing wrong in the condition of the lungs that could give rise to it—nothing to produce such arrears in the respiratory changes as would legitimately account for such deep and accelerated breathing—but that it arose from some perversion of the perceptive endowments of the respiratory nervous system, or of the centres, inducing a spurious kind of stimulation to respiratory effort. The cases in which I have seen the best marked specimens of it have been in narcotic poisoning, uræmia, and anæmia. The resemblance of the dyspnœa, in cases of diabetes terminating in suppression of urine, to that of chlorosis, and of both of them to common out-of-breathness from exertion, long ago struck me. I see no objection to calling this form of breathlessness " hæmic dyspnœa," instead of " subjective dyspnœa;" indeed, I think it a better name, because I think it very likely that there *is* an objective cause for it, an imperfection, namely, in the respiratory changes going on in the lungs; and that that consists in a diminished oxygenation and decarbonization of the blood, in consequence of its peculiar constitution in these respective cases. In the hypothesis which he has thrown out to this effect Dr. Walshe is probably quite correct, and it offers a rational solution of what, to my mind, was always a difficulty. I have often been puzzled at the panting dyspnœa of a chlorotic girl, not only on exertion, but when at rest, and have never before been able to give myself a satisfactory explanation of it. But, adopting Liebig's view of the part which the red globules play as the oxygen carriers, we see at once how anæmia would suspend the due oxygenation of the blood, inasmuch as it would directly diminish the agents concerned in that process; if there were half the blood globules, for example, half the oxygenation would go on; and we can easily understand how such arrears in the respiratory changes would give rise to instinctive respiratory efforts, with the object of re-establishing the balance. The dyspnœa of anæmia thus becomes at once intelligible, and furnishes, in my opinion, a most interesting confirmation of the correctness of Liebig's views as to the relation of the red globule to blood-oxygenation. The fact is, the dyspnœa, in these cases of chlorosis, is as much an integral part of the diseased condition as any other symptom—the panting shortness of breath is as characteristic as the pallor of the complexion.

If, then, this dyspnœa is no asthma at all, the free lung-expansion that characterizes it in no way invalidates the belief in the universal presence of bronchial stricture in true asthma.

Many years ago an original and ingenious view of the pathology of asthma was advanced by Dr. Bree, in a work entitled, "A Practical Inquiry into Disordered Respiration, distinguishing the Species of Convulsive Asthma." He endeavours to show that the asthmatic paroxysm, and all the excessive muscular action that attends it, is merely an extraordinary effort to get rid of some peccant and irritating matter existing in the air tubes, in the same way as tenesmus and spasmodic contraction of the bladder are extraordinary efforts to get rid of some source of irritation in the rectum and bladder respectively—feces of a particularly irritating character, or a stone; that this irritating matter exists in the lungs antecedently to the attack; and that the asthmatic paroxysm is the means and mechanism of its discharge. And this view he founds on the argument of analogy, on the fact that in continued asthma there is some permanent and immovable source of irritation in the lungs, and that in the great majority of cases of spasmodic asthma there is a copious secretion of pituita towards the end of the paroxysm, with the discharge of which the attack passes off. Dr. Bree maintains his argument with a great deal of ingenuity, and presses many facts into the service of his theory; but the most superficial reflection would suffice nowadays to show that it is utterly untenable; and had Dr. Bree enjoyed the light that now shines on us from those two important points, the stethoscope and our acquaintance with excito-motory action, he would never have broached the doctrine he did: the one would have shown him the fallacy of his views, the other would have opened to him a solution of his difficulty— the stethoscope would have shown him that the conditions of an extraordinary discharging power are not present in an asthmatic attack; indeed, that the power of getting rid of anything in the lungs is very much diminished by it; and the knowledge of reflex nervous action would, in connection with anatomy, have displayed the true nature of the disease, and made all its discrepant and scattered phenomena conspire to the production of its true and simple theory.

A word or two will suffice to show the fallacy of Dr. Bree's views, and where his error lay.

Was this peccant matter, that Dr. Bree supposed to be the exciting cause of an asthmatic paroxysm, thrown off and got rid of by expiration merely, as the carbonic acid and some of the constituents of the expired air are, or was coughing necessary for its expulsion? In either case, asthmatic breathing, so far from affording additional excretory power, would indicate a very great reduction of it—a reduction below the most moderate standard of the equable and tranquil respiration of health. For if the air simply breathed, without any assistance from coughing, be the medium of its discharge, of course, extraordinary discharging power can only be obtained by an extraordinary amount of air respired. Now, any one who listens to the chest of an asthmatic during a fit of his disease will see that the amount of air respired is very small indeed, much below the natural standard; that the vesicular murmur, even when not drowned by rhonchus and sibilus, is either inaudible or very feeble, and he will see that the amount of movement of the parietes of the chest, in spite of the violent muscular efforts and its great distension, is very slight. If a person suffering from asthma tries to blow his nose, he finds he cannot make a sufficiently full inspiration, or get enough air into his chest, to perform that act efficiently: he makes a little, short, and soundless blow that drives nothing from his nostrils; the same with coughing. A case so clearly illustrative of this once came under my observation that I cannot forbear relating it. A great sufferer from asthma had a double polypus in his nose, which so blocked up his nostrils, that he could not, in health, breathe with his mouth shut without making a loud, sniffing, snoring noise, both at expiration and inspiration, and, indeed, could not breathe at all for any length of time without opening his mouth. But when his asthma was on him, he could breathe with his mouth shut without producing any of the sniffing sound, and without increasing the embarrassment of his breathing—in fact, as well as with it open. The fact was, the amount of air respired was so small, that the narrow chinks between the polypi and the walls of the nares were sufficient for its transmission.

Supposing, on the other hand, coughing to be necessary to the expulsion of this irritating material, as some of Dr. Bree's observations indicate, a similar extraordinary respiratory power would be necessary, for an extraordinary inspiration must precede an extraordinary coughing effort. But we find asthmatic dyspnœa destroys the power of efficient cough. We find, too, that in the majority of asthmatics the greater part of the paroxysm is free from cough—it is dry; the wheezing dyspnœa is the only thing that troubles the patient. How, then, can the coughing and spitting explain the antecedent dyspnœa? or how, if the coughing is necessary for the expulsion of the offending pituita, can the preceding laboured breathing be an excretory act at all? The fact is, Dr. Bree mistook the effect for the cause. The inordinate mucous secretion, the expulsion of which gives so much relief at the termination of a paroxysm of asthma, is the result of the congestion into which the capillaries have been thrown by the long-continued imperfect respiration, and the secretion, by unloading these congested capillaries, relieves one of the most pressing causes of the dyspnœa; the expectorated matter *exists not* in the first part of the attack of which Dr. Bree considers it the exciting cause. This accumulated mucus is, no doubt, an additional source of dyspnœa, by blocking up the bronchial tubes; when the bronchial spasm ceases, this is the only source of dyspnœa that is left, and its expectoration is therefore attended with immediate and complete relief. This expectoration never takes place without a marked abatement of the dyspnœa, for the simple reason that until the dyspnœa does abate, until the bronchial spasm is passing off sufficiently to allow the chest to be freely filled with air, efficient cough, adequate to the free discharge of this accumulated mucus, cannot be effected. Expectoration cannot take place till the intensity of the dyspnœa is already subsiding. The order of events then is this: Air shut off from the lungs by bronchial stricture; consequent pulmonary congestion—in fact, a state of partial asphyxia; relief of the loaded vessels by abundant mucous exudation; inability to expectorate this material, in consequence of not being able to get sufficient air into the lungs to cough efficiently; abatement of spasm; consequent recovery of coughing power; free expectoration, and complete relief.

A great deal more might be advanced in demolition of Dr. Bree's theory, but what has been said is, I think, quite sufficient; indeed, I should not have been at such pains to notice and disprove his views as I have, were it not that the book is so well known, and caused some sensation, and made many converts, when it came out. It is so well written, however, the arguments, as far as the author's knowledge went, so well and ably supported, and, in spite of the theoretical errors, there is so much sound practical advice in it, that it really forms a valuable addition to the medical literature of this subject.

Some authors have asserted that asthma is nothing more or less than the dyspnœa of bronchitis. Of these, some have attributed the dyspnœa and wheezing to plugging of the tubes by bronchitic

mucus, while others, recognizing in the occasional entire absence
of mucus in asthma, and other facts, an insuperable objection to
this explanation, have attributed the symptoms to inflammatory
thickening of the bronchial mucous membrane. The former of
these views, analogous to Dr. Bree's in so far as it attributes the
phenomena of asthma to a mucous exudation, but differing inasmuch as it does not assign to that mucus the character of a specific
irritating humour, nor consider the muscular phenomena of asthma
convulsive efforts for its discharge, was advocated by M. Beau,
some ten or twelve years ago, in a memoir on "A Distinction of
Two Forms of Bronchitis." He considers asthma to be a phenomenon of a particular form of bronchitis which he calls "*bronchite
à râles vibrants,*" and that the wheezing and the dyspnœa alike
depend on the obstruction of the air tubes by the inflammatory
products of this bronchitis. Speaking of the spasm-theory of
asthma, he says:—

"This opinion, adopted by many conscientious physicians from
respect for medical traditions, is no longer capable of being maintained, since auscultation and percussion have given us the means of
seeing (so to speak) what occurs in the chest. It has, in fact, been
ascertained, with the assistance of these two methods of inquiry,
and in a manner the most positive, that there is no asthmatic dyspnœa without an obstruction of the bronchial tubes, which causes
vibrating *râles*, and which, producing an obstacle to the exit of
the inspired air, forces it to react on the vesicles and to dilate
them."[1]

I quote the above from an able review on this subject by Dr. W.
T. Gairdner,[2] who, in commenting on this very passage of M. Beau,
so happily exposes the untenability of the bronchitis-theory of
asthma, and so exactly expresses the objections to it that have
struck my own mind, that, although I have elsewhere shown the entire independence and distinctness of the two affections, I cannot
forbear quoting his words:—

"We had thought that the experiments of Williams, of Longet,
and of Volkmann, which are, or ought to be, well known in France,
might have saved the spasm-theory of asthma from being consigned
so very coolly, as it is in the first sentence of the above paragraph,
to the limbo of medical tradition; more especially as there never
has been any doubt, even among the most hazy and 'traditional'
of the spasm-theorists, as to the existence of an obstruction in the
bronchial tubes. The wheezing and 'vibrating râles' were too evident a portion of the asthmatic paroxysm to be overlooked, even
before auscultation and percussion were introduced. M. Beau
has entirely missed the real point of the controversy, and has not
offered the shadow of a proof on the real matter at issue—viz.,

1 Archives Générales, vol. lxxviii. p. 155.
2 Med.-Chir. Review, vol. xi. p. 476.

whether the vibrating râles, the obstruction of the tubes, and the consequent dyspnœa, are caused by mucous secretions, as he himself maintains, by sudden inflammatory engorgement of the mucous membrane, as others have supposed, or by spasmodic narrowing of the tubes generally or locally, as is the common opinion in this country.

" On the part of the mucus-theorists, it is alleged that the paroxysm of asthma is almost always terminated by expectoration of a thick, semi-transparent mucus, and that its accumulation was in all probability the cause of the paroxysm. We admit the fact to be true, but doubt very much the correctness of the inference; at least it is certain that, in ordinary bronchitis, enormously greater accumulations of mucus take place with comparatively few signs of general obstruction. We think this position must be admitted by every unbiassed observer; and it is, in our opinion, fatal to this theory. Nor can we find more probability in the theory of inflammatory or congestive thickening of the bronchial mucous membrane. That such a lesion should become the source of most serious dyspnœa in ten minutes (an incident of frequent occurrence in the violent forms of asthma); that it should subside with almost equal rapidity; that it should almost never produce a directly fatal result by asphyxia, and very rarely issue in the expectoration of pus, while, on the other hand, far more severe forms of inflammatory bronchitis often produce comparatively little evident dyspnœa—these are, in our opinion, ample reasons for rejecting the congestion theory of asthma, and maintaining the spasmodic as probable, even had the power of the bronchial fibres to produce sudden and rapid obstruction not been positively ascertained."

There is another school of pathologists who maintain that the essence of asthma is humoral, that each attack depends on the development of some specific humoral disturbance, that without that particular humoral disturbance you cannot have the asthma, that the difference between the asthmatic and one who is not so lies in the disposition or indisposition to produce this specific humoral condition. Now I do not deny that in some cases the exciting cause of the attack is humoral; but what I would deny is, that the humoral derangement has any higher place than that of an exciting cause; and what I would insist upon is, that the heart and core of the disease is nervous, that the essential peculiarity of the asthmatic is a vice in his nervous system, a peculiar morbid irritability of it, whereby a certain portion of it is thrown into a state of excitement from the application of stimuli which in another person would produce no effect at all, or a very different effect. Take an example. Two men make a hearty supper—one wakes with asthma, the other with vomiting; two men get drunk—one wakes with asthma, the other with a violent headache. These I consider to be instances of the production of different results from the application of identical sources of irritation to constitutions of different diseased tendencies. There is probably a humoral disturbance in both cases, in both the blood is contaminated with the products of deranged digestion; but there is no reason to believe that in the asthmatic the humoral disturbance is specific, or that it differs from that of the other case. A general expression, like that of a theory of a disease, should fulfil all conditions and explain all cases. But how will the humoral theory of the disease explain an attack of asthma brought on within one minute after drinking a glass of wine? What will be said of the humoral nature of an attack of asthma instantaneously brought on by a fit of laughter? What will be said of the humoral nature of an attack of asthma brought on by lying lower at head than usual by the amount of one pillow? What will be said of the humoral nature of an attack of asthma brought on in a minute or two by walking near a hayfield? No; the essential pathological condition in asthma consists, as I shall endeavour to show,[1] in the irritability of the part irritated, and not in the production of any specific irritator.

In an interesting clinical lecture, published in the *Medical Gazette* for December, 1850, Dr. Todd advances the opinion that asthma depends upon a poisoning of the nerves of respiration, or those portions of the nervous centres with which they are connected, by a particular *materies morbi*, by which their function is so perverted, that a spurious and morbid sense of want of breath is engendered; that this central or subjective breathlessness is the first step in the morbid phenomena; that it need have no real objective cause in the lungs themselves; that bronchial spasm is an accompaniment, not a cause, of the dyspnœa of asthma; and that you may have asthma without any bronchial contraction whatever.

Dr. Todd's argument is this—In many points asthma resembles gout; gout is humoral; therefore asthma is humoral. Again—you may have asthma with puerile breathing; with puerile breathing the bronchi cannot be contracted; therefore asthma may co-exist with uncontracted bronchial tubes.

But let me give in his own words the views of one whose opinions always carry with them so much weight.

"Like asthma," says Dr. Todd, "gout comes on quite suddenly; there is no warning. A man may go to bed quite or nearly well, and may wake up early in the morning with a fit of the gout in his great toe. There is another disease, epilepsy, in which we have exactly the same phenomenon. A patient, with or without warning, falls down foaming, livid, and convulsed; the paroxysm goes off and leaves him in his ordinary good health, and he may go on for years and not have another. Again—we know a fit of the gout leaves no organic lesion if it occurs once or twice, but, if it is often repeated, it leaves permanent injury in the joints it attacks. The same of asthma; the organic changes are all secondary, and a few attacks leave no traces behind them.

[1] Chapter II.

"The theory at present most in favour with regard to gout is, that it is a disease of assimilation, and that this defective or vitiated assimilation gives rise to some *materies morbi*. When this matter is eliminated from the system the attack passes off; when it accumulates the attack comes on. In asthma defective assimilative power is a frequent coincident. Gout, too, and rheumatism, and all humoral diseases, resemble asthma in being inherited.

"When the *materies morbi* of asthma has been generated, its effect is to irritate the nervous system, not generally, but certain parts of it, those parts being the nerves concerned in the function of respiration, viz., the pneumogastric, and the nerves that supply the respiratory muscles, either at their peripheral extremities or at their central termination in the medulla oblongata and spinal cord; extreme difficulty of breathing is the result, and, as a consequence of this, ultimate disease of the lungs.

"Many pathologists ascribe all the phenomena of asthma to spasm of the circular muscular fibres of the bronchi. The first link in the chain of effects of the immediate exciting cause of asthma would be, according to them, spasm of the bronchial tubes, then dyspnœa. Undoubtedly, a state of spasm of the bronchial tubes would produce a great deal of dyspnœa; but what I want to point out to you is, that this state of spasm of the bronchial tubes ought rather to be regarded as one of the accompaniments, one of the phenomena, of asthma, than as its cause. The feeling of breathlessness, or, in other words, a peculiar state of certain nerves, or of a certain nervous centre, the centre of respiration, is the first link in this chain of asthmatic phenomena. The spasm of the bronchi follows sooner or later upon this, and often it follows so quickly upon it as to appear to come simultaneously with it. Does it ever precede it? I doubt this.

"Undoubtedly you may have severe asthma without severe spasm of the bronchial tubes. I remember a well-marked instance of this in a gentleman whom I attended for a chronic disease—cancer, as I thought, of the liver. For nearly a week before his death he suffered from the most frightfully distressing asthma, which nothing could control, and which lasted without interruption till he died. I examined his chest repeatedly at all parts, and could hear nothing but the most perfect, loud, and puerile breathing, which is quite inconsistent with a state of spasm.

"Again, a section of the vagi nerves of animals produces phenomena exactly like those of asthma. Whatever be the cause of the dyspnœa in these cases, it is clear it cannot be bronchial spasm, as the muscles of the bronchi would be paralyzed after a section of their nerves."

With regard to the first part of Dr. Todd's theory, founded on the supposed analogy of asthma to gout—that you have in asthma a specific *materies morbi*—I do not think that the existence of points of analogy in the clinical history of the two diseases in any way implies identity of pathology. To how many diseases are headache, shivering, loss of appetite, thirst, an accelerated pulse, and loaded tongue common, between the pathology of which there is no affinity whatever? With regard to the second part of his theory—the co-existence of asthma with uncontracted bronchial tubes—I believe that the case that he quotes is one of that subjective dyspnœa, not asthma at all, to which I have already referred. In the anhelitus consequent upon the division of the vagi, I can see nothing resembling asthma. Altogether, I cannot but think that the arguments brought forward by Dr. Todd are inadequate to meet the mass of evidence that can be adduced in proof of the necessity of bronchial spasm and the non-necessity of humoral disturbance in asthma.

In the twenty-third volume of the *Medico-Chirurgical Transactions*, Dr. Budd, after controverting both the necessity and the existence of muscular elements in the bronchial tubes, offers the following theory of the pathology of asthma :—

"The idea of spasm was suggested by Cullen, and has been generally adopted, from inability to explain in any other way the symptoms of asthma. The necessity of such a supposition has, however, in great measure ceased, in consequence of modern discoveries in morbid anatomy. Corvisart first pointed out diseases of the heart and large vessels as an occasional cause of fits of dyspnœa, formerly regarded as nervous, and confounded under the name of asthma. Laennec, and more recently Louis, have shown that emphysema of the lungs is the most common cause of this group of symptoms ; and the physical signs of dilatation of the air-cells may be discovered during life in most persons who present the symptoms of asthma.

"Many of these persons can vary the capacity of their chests to a degree only just sufficient to supply them with the requisite quantity of oxygen in favourable circumstances. Whenever their circulation is quickened, by exciting passions or by exercise—or their power of expanding the chest is a little diminished, by the obstacle which a distended stomach offers to the descent of the diaphragm—or air is prevented from freely entering the air-cells, in consequence of secretions in the bronchial tubes—or the proportion of oxygen in a given volume of air is diminished—whether by increased temperature, as in heated apartments, or by diminished pressure, as in elevated situations, and in those states of the atmosphere which precede storms ; in fact, whenever, from any cause, their need of oxygen increases or their means of inhaling it diminishes, these persons experience difficulty of breathing, or a fit of asthma.

"There still, however, remain some cases, which at present we can only explain by supposing the dyspnœa to be nervous. It seems probable that the number of such cases will be still further diminished, and that many of those fits of asthma, which we are now forced to consider nervous, will be discovered to depend on

some organic change which has as yet escaped our observation, perhaps on some morbid condition of the blood itself.

"In fits of asthma really nervous, the difficulty of breathing
must result from spasm, or from suspension of the normal action,
of the diaphram and other muscles of inspiration."

It will be seen, then, that Dr. Budd recognizes two forms of
asthma, in neither of which does he admit bronchial spasm : in
one the asthma is nothing but the dyspnœa of emphysema ; in the
other it is a spasm or suspension of the normal action of the
muscles of inspiration.

Is either of these theories tenable? If asthma is but the dyspnœa of emphysema, or heart-disease, it can never occur without
them. Now we know that, in numberless cases of asthma, there is
not only no emphysema or heart disease, but no appreciable organic
disease whatever—that asthma may invade health without a flaw,,
and lapse again into health without a flaw. To assume organic
disease in such a case would be purely gratuitous. I know that
the dyspnœa of emphysema has been *called* asthma ; but what form
of dyspnœa is there that has *not* been called asthma? According
to Dr. Budd's second theory, the muscular phenomena of asthma
are primary. Now, all asthmatics tell us that they are preceded by
an intolerable sense of want of breath, to which they are secondary,
which enforces them, and to which they are always proportionate.
Moreover the action of the inspiratory muscles in asthma has
nothing of spasm or paralysis about it ; it is rhythmical, symmet-
rical, and forceful. Why, in spite of such effort, the inspiratory
movements are at such a dead-lock, I shall endeavour to explain in a
succeeding chapter.

Yet another theory has been suggested for asthma, a theory for
the suggestion of which it would be difficult to offer any explanation, except that pathologists were resolved that no conceivable
hypothesis should want an advocate. It is, that asthma depends
not upon spasm, but upon *paralysis* of the bronchial tubes.

Now, this theory would not be for a moment tenable except on
the supposition that the bronchial tubes were engaged as active
agents in respiration ; if they are not concerned in respiration it is
manifest that the loss of their muscular power would be immaterial,
and would leave respiratory phenomena unaffected. Supposing
they *were* a part of the active machinery of respiration, they could
be engaged in *expiration* only, and would assist by their contraction in emptying the lungs. And it must be admitted that there are
two phenomena of asthma that such a paralysis of expiratory force
would very conveniently and readily explain, and which might possibly have suggested this very theory. One is the extreme difficulty
and prolongation of expiration ; the other, the permanent state of
distension at which the chest is kept during the asthmatic paroxysm
—its girth increased, the ribs elevated, the intercostal spaces wide
—as if it could not be emptied of its air. There can be no doubt

that the difficulty of getting air out of the chest in asthma is much greater than that of getting it in, and supposing the bronchial tubes engaged in expiration, this is exactly what would result from their paralysis.[1] But I think it is now admitted on all hands that they *are* not, because they *can* not be, agents of respiration. There is one reason that, independent of many other considerations, forbids the possibility of it; it is that respiration is under the influence of the will, that it may be varied at pleasure—quick or slow, superficial or deep—while the contraction of the bronchial tubes, like that of all organic muscles, is essentially involuntary. This conclusive argument is so well urged by Dr. Budd, in his paper on Emphysema and Asthma in the *Medico-Chirurgical Transactions*, to which I just now referred, that I cannot do better than quote his words:—

"It can be shown," he says, speaking of the circular muscular fibres of the bronchi, "that these fibres are not muscles performing a part in the ordinary acts of breathing. Supposing them to be muscular, it is evident, from their arrangement and microscopic characters, that they belong to the muscles of organic life, or that they are involuntary muscles. But all the external muscles of respiration are voluntary muscles. Hence we should have engaged, to accomplish the act of breathing, a voluntary and an involuntary power. The function would be easily performed as long as these powers acted in unison—that is, as long as the involuntary muscles contracted only during expiration. But, by varying the rapidity of our breathing, we should soon have two powers opposed to each other—the involuntary muscles acting to close the bronchial tubes, while the voluntary muscles acted to expand them. We should then be able to dilate the chest only when we adjusted the inspira-

---

[1] Dr. Walshe, in his work on *Diseases of the Lungs and Heart*, p. 337, adopts this paralysis-theory as explanatory of some, though not all, cases of asthma. He says:—

"Bronchial asthma may depend on a *plus* or a *minus* state of the contractility of the muscular fibres of the bronchial tubes; in the former case it is spasmodic, in the latter paralytic.

"Laennec ascribes the peculiar air-distension of the lungs, found in persons asphyxiated by the mephitic gases of cesspools, to paralysis of the vagi nerves; Mr. Swan noticed similar distension in animals whose eighth pair had been divided in the neck. In both cases, the *contractile force of the bronchial muscles concerned in expiration* is more or less completely annulled.

"If, then, as we have seen, there be motive to believe that nervous asthma commonly depends on spasmodic action of the bronchial muscular apparatus, here are speculative reasons for presuming that paralysis of the apparatus may cause a variety of the affection. Clinically, too, we meet with examples of asthma in which the *comparative facility of inspiration, and difficulty of expiration, suggest of themselves the probability of a minus rather than a plus state of power in bronchial contractibility.*"—Walshe, *Diseases of the Lungs and Heart*, p. 337.

It is clear from the above that Dr. Walshe believes in bronchial muscular contraction as an efficient expiratory power; the first sentence that I have italicized asserts it, the last implies it—it is the inevitable third element of his syllogism.

For what I believe to be the true explanation of the distended thoracic cavity and prolonged expiration of asthma, I must refer the reader to Chapter III.

tory movements to the actions of the involuntary muscles. But we never perceive any necessity for such an adjustment. The test which this circumstance affords us is one of extreme delicacy. For, if the two powers were not exactly in unison, there would occur intervals, like the *beats* in music, when they would coincide with or be opposed to each other. The inspiratory acts would be alternately easy and difficult, according as the voluntary and involuntary muscles were in the same or opposite phases. But however rapid we make our breathing, we perceive no difference in the ease with which successive acts of inspiration are performed. This circumstance is a proof the most decisive, that the fibres of the bronchi have no independent rhythmical motions of contraction."

Discarding, then, the theory of bronchial expiration, the theory of bronchial paralysis, as a cause of asthma, falls to the ground.

Finally, I may mention, but I need hardly attempt to refute, the views of those, and they are not a few, who deny the existence of asthma altogether as a substantive disease, who hold it to be a generic and not a specific condition, and that it and dyspnœa are convertible terms.

In the above *résumé* I have not alluded to those authors who have advocated what I believe to be the only true theory of asthma—the spasm-theory—because my purpose has been simply to clear away the obstruction of erroneous notions; and if this paper *asserts* anything of the true pathology of asthma, it is strictly in a negative and exhaustive way. But there is one author, Dr. W. T. Gairdner, to whose writings[1] I feel bound to refer, not so much on account of the correctness of his views and the conclusiveness of his reasoning as to do an act of justice both to him and to myself: to him, that I may admit, which I do entirely, that in some of my writings Dr. Gairdner has anticipated me, not only in my substantial opinions, but in the arguments I have adduced and the very phraseology I have employed: to myself, that I may state that it is only within the last few months, after the principal part of this work was in type, that I became acquainted with Dr. Gairdner's admirable papers. I would fain hope that our unconscious coincidence of views depends upon our both having read nature sincerely and successfully.

[1] Edinburgh Monthly Medical Journal for 1851. Med.-Chir. Review, 1853.

CHAPTER II.

THE PATHOLOGY OF ASTHMA.—ITS ABSOLUTE NATURE.

Asthma essentially a nervous disease.—The phenomena of asthma immediately dependent upon spastic contraction of the organic muscle of the bronchial tubes. —Evidence derived from the dyspnœa and sounds of asthma.—The four ways in which the bronchiæ may be narrowed.—The phenomena of asthma mostly excitomotory or reflex.—The portion of the nervous system involved differs in different cases, being sometimes restricted to that of the lungs themselves.—Different degrees of remoteness of irritant.—Irritant sometimes humoral; a contaminate pulmonary blood.—Physiological argument: Spasm-theory confirmed by the purposes of the bronchial muscle in health.

HAVING endeavoured in the preceding chapter to give a fair summary of the various theories that are entertained with regard to the nature of asthma, and to inquire if those theories are such as are fairly borne out by the phenomena of the disease, I purpose in the present one to develop what I believe to be its true pathology.

What I shall endeavour to show is this:—

1. That asthma is essentially, and, with perhaps the exception of a single class of cases, exclusively, a nervous disease: that the nervous system is the seat of the essential pathological condition.

2. That the phenomena of asthma—the distressing sensation and the demand for extraordinary respiratory efforts—immediately depend upon a spastic contraction of the fibre-cells of organic or unstriped muscle, which minute anatomy has demonstrated to exist in the bronchial tubes.

3. That these phenomena are those of excito-motory or reflex action.

4. That the extent to which the nervous system is involved differs very much in different cases, being in some cases restricted to the nervous system of the air-passages themselves.

5. That in a large number of cases the pneumogastric nerve, both in its gastric and pulmonary portions, is the seat of the disease.

6. That there is a large class of cases in which the nervous circuit between the source of irritation and the seat of the resulting muscular phenomena involves other portions of the nervous system besides the pneumogastric.

7. That there are other cases in which the source of irritation, giving rise to the asthmatic paroxysm, appears to be central—in the brain; consequently, in which the action, though excito-motory, is not reflex.

8. That there is yet a class of cases in which the exciting cause of the paroxysms appears to be essentially humoral.

Let us now examine these propositions in the order in which I have stated them, and see what proofs can be brought in their support.

1. The reasons that force upon one's mind the conviction that asthma is essentially a *nervous* disease are very numerous, and not less forcible and convincing; but I shall here be able only briefly to indicate them, as their fuller consideration would involve too great space. They are principally derived from the following considerations:—*a*. The *causes* of asthma; *b*. its *remedies*; *c*. its *associated and precursory symptoms*; *d*. its *periodicity*; *e*. the *absence of organic change*; *f*. the circumstance that the phenomena of the disease are *muscular*.

a. We see, in the first place, that the *causes* of asthma are such as affect the nervous system, and such as give rise to other diseases acknowledged on all hands to be nervous. Thus, fatigue and physical exhaustion, and sudden or violent mental emotion, will bring on an attack. I was informed, some short time since, by my friend, Dr. Theophilus Thompson, of a case in which, on two occasions, severe asthma was brought on in a gentleman by sudden fear, from his having, as he imagined, administered accidentally an over-dose of belladonna to his wife. I knew the case of an asthmatic boy, some years ago, who used constantly to be warned by his parents not to over-excite himself, as if he did he would be sure to have the asthma the next day; and lately I met with another case, in which I was told that when the asthmatic was a little boy, he found in his disease a convenient immunity from correction; "Don't scold me," he would say, if he had incurred his father's displeasure, " or I shall have the asthma;" and so he would; his fears were as correct as they were convenient. Venereal excitement will bring on asthma; a gentleman once told me that one of the severest attacks he ever had in his life was brought on in this way. Moreover, many well-known and recognized causes of asthma can only act on the lungs through the intervention of certain parts of the nervous system; thus, gastric irritation can produce spasm of the bronchial tubes only through the intervention of the pneumogastric nerve—it is the only connecting link between the two organs, either physiologically or anatomically.

b. Again, the *remedies* of asthma are such as appeal to the nervous system—as antispasmodics, sedatives, direct nervous depressants, &c.; tobacco, for example, stramonium, antimony, chloroform. Perhaps the effect of chloroform is, of all remedies, the most striking, and at the same time the most illustrative of the purely nervous nature of the affection—a few whiffs, and the asthma is gone; a dyspnœa that a few seconds before seemed to threaten life is replaced by a breathing calm and tranquil. Now, remembering the action of the drug, that it is the nervous system to which it appeals,

3

it is impossible to help seeing in this the most conclusive proof that the symptoms are due to a nervous cause. And besides these ordinary remedies, there are other circumstances that will put a stop to the paroxysm, that eminently prove its nervous nature; one of these is mental emotion—any strong or sudden passion, such as fear, fright, or surprise. It is a curious thing that mental emotion should have the effect both of inducing and relieving asthma, but so it is; and there are not wanting facts analogous to this—*e.g.*, shock will bring on chorea, and shock will cure it. I think the *immediate* effect of emotion is always to cut short asthmatic spasm, if it exists, by a sort of nervous revulsion; whereas its tendency to induce it is *remote*, and only shown after some time, as the next day; and it acts, I think, by producing an exaltation of nervous impressibility —and thus facilitating the induction of excito-motory action. Nothing, indeed, in the whole range of pathological phenomena is to my mind more remarkable than the effect of emotion upon asthma. Dr. Todd has told me that he has had patients come to him who have lost their asthma the moment they have entered his house; suddenly, and without any apparent cause, except the mental perturbation at being within the precincts of the physician, the difficulty of breathing has vanished. We see just the same thing in toothache—the sight of the dentist's house is enough to cure it. I witnessed once myself so striking an example of this sudden disappearance of asthma under the influence of alarm that I cannot forbear relating it.

A gentleman, a confirmed asthmatic, was suffering an unusually bad attack of his complaint, so bad that he was unable to move from his chair, or speak even, except in catchy monosyllables. He had been suffering all day, and in the evening his sister was going to give him an emetic of ipecacuanha, when she suddenly fell down in an hysterical fit, to the occurrence of which she was subject. The suddenness of her attack and the severity of her sufferings so alarmed him, that he sprang from his chair and ran to her relief, and as soon as he had placed her in a position of safety ran down two flights of stairs to procure the restoratives that were usually administered; having run up stairs again with the same speed, and applied the remedies, he found to his surprise that his asthma was gone, and indeed it was its sudden departure under the influence of alarm that. had alone enabled him to perform such a feat; a man who, two minutes before was unable to speak or move, had, under the influence of an absorbing alarm, ran down two flights of stairs and up again, and found himself after his exertion breathing with perfect freedom. The asthma gradually returned, and within an hour he was as bad as ever. I do not think it possible to adduce a stronger proof than this of the purely nervous nature of asthma. I might cite many such cases.[1]

[1] A remarkable exception to this curative power of excitement once came under my

c. Again, the *periodicity* of asthma implies its nervous nature—that is, such a periodicity as characterizes asthma. There are three kinds of periodicity in disease. One, in which it is produced by the periodical return of its cause, as in the recurrence of hay-fever every summer, the morning expectoration after a night's rest, indigestion every day at a certain time after dinner. Another, in which the periodicity seems to depend upon that rhythmical impress which is stamped on the functions, that sort of diurnal oscillation in which the body is swung by the constant recurrence, at one unvarying daily interval, of the habitual actions and passions of the body; I think that hectic and ague acquire their periodicity from this diurnal heat into which the body falls. But there are other diseases whose rhythmical recurrence cannot be explained on either of these suppositions, whose periodicity has no relation either to the diurnal interval or to the renewal of the cause, but which must be intrinsically periodic; such are epilepsy and asthma. In these the interval is long and of no certain standard—that is, though tolerably constant in the same individual, it differs very widely in different cases—the period is peculiar to each case, is an integral part of the pathological condition. This last kind of periodicity, and this alone, it is that points at all to the nervous nature of a disease.

d. Furthermore, the associated and precursory symptoms of an asthmatic attack are such as point to its nervous character. The quantity of limpid water passed in the early part of the paroxysm, white as pump-water, like the nervous water passed in the students' "funking-room," or like the urine of hysteria, or that of nervous headache; the neuralgia, which I have often noticed; the frontal headache; the drowsiness and languor of the previous day, by which the approach of the attack is foreknown; or, on the other hand, a peculiar and unwonted hilarity and animation and sense of health —all these are just such symptoms as we meet with in various diseases of the nervous system, such, for example, as hysteria and epilepsy.

e. Another circumstance in favour of the view that asthma is essentially nervous, in fact consistent with no other, is the possible absence of appreciable organic change, as shown by *post-mortem* examination, in cases where the disease has not been of long standing. A man may have been known during his life to have had attacks of asthma, he may have seemed over and over again almost *in articulo mortis* from want of breath; and yet if death from some other cause[1] gives an opportunity of examining his lungs, they may be found apparently in every way healthy—no trace of inflammation or its products, the vesicular structure perfectly normal, the passages leading to it lined by a healthy and unchanged membrane, the cavi-

observation, in the case of a woman who suffered from a violent attack of asthma the whole of the time she was in labour.

[1] I say *from some other cause*, because if asthma kills, it always does so by producing organic change in the heart or lungs, or both.

ties of the pleura free from all abnormal contents, their surfaces smooth and apposed, the heart sound. The disease shows no cause, and has left no trace, either in the respiratory or circulatory systems—in fact, no trace anywhere. Where, then, shall we locate it? What is its starting-point? We may, I think, lay it down as a rule that all those diseases that leave no organic trace of their existence produce their symptoms through the nervous system.

f. Lastly, the phenomena of the disease are muscular, the proximate diseased condition is situated in the muscular system, and whenever the proximate derangement is muscular, we may always, with one or two exceptions, safely affirm that the primary disease is nervous. In epilepsy, tetanus, chorea, paralysis agitans, hemiplegia, child-crowing—in all these the obvious departure from health is in the muscular system; but the essence of the disease is nervous. The only exceptions that I know of are the cases in which the muscles are either poisoned by some material present in them, as, for example, in the paralysis of lead-palsy, the cramps of cholera, or disorganized by fatty degeneration, as we see in the heart, the muscles of disused limbs, &c. In these cases, the disease is radically and primarily muscular. In all other cases, muscular disturbance is but the index of nervous disease. Hence the very fact that the phenomena of asthma are muscular is all but proof positive that the nervous system is the seat of the primary derangement.

2. *That the phenomena of asthma—the distressing sensation and the demand for extraordinary respiratory efforts—immediately depend upon a spastic contraction of the fibre-cells of organic muscle, which minute anatomy has demonstrated to exist in the bronchial tubes.*

Although this is a proposition that many perhaps might think it hardly worth while to set about proving, yet I think it will be well not to assume it, partly for the reasons I have already mentioned (the general absence, namely, of precise pathological views on the subject), partly because it is a necessary stepping-stone to the succeeding propositions, and partly because I think its proof will be the best way of expressing my notions of the ultimate pathology of the disease and my reasons for them. It will certainly be an advantage if it can be shown beyond cavil that spasmodic stricture of the bronchial tubes is the only possible cause of asthma, that it is adequate to the production of all the phenomena, that it is a form of perverted physiology that may exist pure and uncomplicated with any organic disease, and that the view that would assign it as the sole essential condition in asthma is—what all pathological views should be—physiological and rational. I think perhaps the eliminative or exhaustive method of proof will be as good as any.

I will suppose a case of severe uncomplicated asthma, such as we sometimes see. Now, what have we here? We have, as the sole constituent symptom, *dyspnœa*—dyspnœa of a peculiar kind—sudden in its access, intense, and agonizing, following a state of perfect apparent health and ease, and relapsing as suddenly, perhaps speedily, and, it may be, without any expectoration, into ease and tranquillity again. What, then, can give rise to such phenomena as these? We know that the only way in which such an arrear in the respiratory changes as produces a sense of dyspnœa can be brought about, is by a derangement of the supply of one or both of the two fluids, the air or the blood, or by a disorganization of the functioning portion of the lung. On what recognized diseases, then, can we fall back, as supplying in such an instance the necessary conditions? On heart-disease possibly, bronchitis, and emphysema. But if we examine the heart we find it, in the case supposed (that is, in a case of uncomplicated asthma), perfectly healthy—it cannot then be that. The mucous membrane of the air passages could not assume and relinquish a condition of inflammation so suddenly; and moreover, to produce such dyspnœa the inflammation must be intense, and could not fail to give rise to the results of inflammation, yet none such are thrown out. There is not necessarily any mucous exudation; crepitation or expectoration may both be absent. Besides, it would be impossible for bronchitis to exist to such an extent as to give rise to the amount of dyspnœa, without producing the constitutional signs of inflammation; but none such are present—the patient is not ill, he is wheezing and labouring—he passes from a state of health to a state, not of illness, but of dyspnœa, and back again from dyspnœa to health; there are no sequelæ, there is no convalescence. It cannot therefore be bronchitis. Emphysema we know it is not, for the dyspnœa of emphysema is constant and unvarying, and moreover, we listen to the breathing before and after the attack, and find evidence that the spongy structure of the lung is perfectly healthy. We see, then, that in none of the three ways in which dyspnœa is ordinarily produced—on the side of blood-supply, on that of airsupply, or on that of injured functioning structure, by heart-disease, emphysema, or bronchitis respectively—can the symptoms of asthma be explained. Moreover, the character of the dyspnœa is altogether peculiar; it is utterly unlike either of the three dyspnœas that have been mentioned. Heart-dyspnœa is intolerant of the slightest exertion, or of the recumbent position, and sitting up, or stillness, may cure in two minutes the most violent paroxysm. The breathing, too, has rather a panting and gasping than the wheezing, labouring character of asthma. Bronchitic dyspnœa is short, crepitous, and accompanied with cough; asthma, often long-drawn, dry, and without cough. In pure emphysema, the dyspnœa is abiding, varies but little, and has no wheeze.

But the dyspnœa of asthma tells a plainer tale than this; it tells us not only what it is not, but what it is. It gives the most positive evidence of narrowing of the air-passages. The asthmatic's breathing is what our forefathers called "strait," what we call "tight;" he feels as if a weight were on his sternum, as if his chest were compressed, as if a cord bound him, as if it would be the greatest relief to him if some one would cut his breast open and allow it to

expand; he rushes to the window to get air, he cannot tolerate
people or curtains about him, his clothes are loosened, and all the
muscles of respiration tug and strain their utmost to fill his chest.
But he can neither get air in nor out, he can neither inspire nor
expire—his respiration is almost at a dead lock; he cannot blow his
nose, can hardly cough or sneeze, cannot smoke a pipe, and if his
fire is failing, cannot blow it up; he has hardly air enough to produce the laryngeal vibrations of speech.   The chest is distended,
indeed, to its greatest possible limit, the cavity of the thorax is
enlarged, both in the costal and diaphragmatic directions; the costal
distension is shown by the fact that the clothes that ordinarily fit
will not meet over the chest by from one to two inches, while the
descent of the diaphragm is shown by the increased girth of the
abdomen, and by the heart being drawn down to the scrobiculus
where it is seen beating plainly; such are the violent instinctive
efforts of the respiratory muscles to overcome the obstruction to the
access of air.   But they are unavailing; the air that is without
cannot get in, and that which is within is locked up.   In spite of
the violent muscular effort there is hardly any respiratory movement,
the parietes of the chest cannot follow the action of the muscles;
on listening to the chest the respiratory murmur is inaudible, even
when not drowned by the wheezing; respiration is almost *nil.*
Where, then, can this obstruction to the introduction and exit of air
be?   It must be in some part of the air-passages—the larynx,
trachea, or bronchial tubes.   In the larynx and trachea we know,
from the symptoms, it is not.   The fact of bronchial stricture, then,
is certain.

The very intensity of the dyspnœa, too, its agonizing and laborious character, implies that the seat of the mischief is in the air-
passages.   Dyspnœa is essentially remedial, and tends directly, both
by its sensory and muscular phenomena, to diminish and relieve its
cause.   As soon as respiration is not going on satisfactorily, the
sense of dyspnœa, or want of breath, at once prompts to more violent respiratory efforts, which tend to relieve it.   The distressful
sensation is an essential link in the chain; it gives warning of the
condition to be remedied, and is the irresistible stimulus to the
remedial efforts.   But this sense of dyspnœa, being in its nature
remedial, would be likely to be felt only in those cases in which the
condition giving rise to it could be remedied by those extraordinary
respiratory efforts to which it irresistibly prompts.   Now, consistently with this view, I think I have noticed a very curious law with
regard to dyspnœa; it is this, that it is proportionate not to the
amount of injury done to the organ, but to the amount of relief that
the condition admits of by extraordinary respiratory efforts.   If the
parenchyma of the lung, its functioning structure, is injured, no
amount of respiratory effort will better the condition, and accordingly violent dyspnœa is not induced.   Thus, half the lung may be
destroyed by phthisis or solidified by pneumonia, and the tranquillity

of the respiration be hardly interfered with : a little hurried, per- haps, but with no distress or violent effort. But if, while the lung- substance is healthy, the free access of air is prevented, violent and distressing dyspnœa is immediately induced, as in croup, laryngitis, the sudden infarction of a large bronchus. For here, if the air could only be got in sufficient quantity to the healthy functioning structure, the balance of the function would be completely restored ; hence it is that such cases are always characterized by those violent respiratory efforts which have for their object the freer introduction of air, and that urgent sense of want of breath which is the consti- tuted stimulus to these efforts. We recognize, therefore, in the very urgency of asthmatic dyspnœa evidence that the mischief is in the air-passages, and that it is of such a nature as to shut off the air-supply.

But the *sounds* of asthma give us perhaps still more certain and circumstantial evidence as to the condition of the bronchial tubes. We know in health that respiration is noiseless, but that when the breathing becomes asthmatic, it is accompanied with a shrill sibilant whistle. We know, too, that hollow tubes give no musical sound, when air rushes through them, if they are of even calibre, but if they are narrowed at certain points, if their calibre is varied, the air in them is thrown into vibrations and they become musical instru- ments. The wheezing of asthma, then, is as positive evidence of bronchial contraction as if we could see the points of stricture—it is physical demonstration.

Now, in what ways may the bronchial tubes be narrowed? In

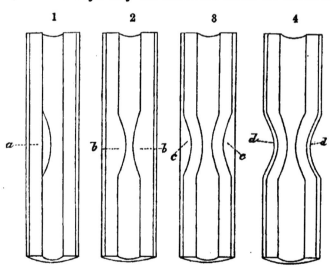

Diagram showing the four ways in which the bronchial tubes may be narrowed.
1. Bronchial catarrh. 2. Recent bronchitis. 3. Old bronchitis 4. Asthma.

four, I think, as shown in the accompanying diagram. By a plug of tenacious mucus partly closing the passage, Fig. 1, *a;* by congestive or inflammatory thickening of the mucous membrane, Fig. 2, *b*; by plastic exudation thrown out in the submucous areolar tissue in severe bronchitis, and undergoing subsequent slow contraction (in the same way as we see in œsophageal and urethral stricture), Fig. 8, *c*; and by contraction of the circularly-disposed organic muscle which exists in the bronchial wall, Fig. 4, *d*. This last is spasmodic stricture, the other three are not; the first is no stricture of the tube at all; and the second and third are inflammatory stricture; the second recent, vascular, and mucous; the third old, fibrous, and sub-mucous. In all these ways the column of air in a bronchial tube may be constricted, and the tube converted into a musical instrument, the seat of a sound that will be sonorous or sibilant rhonchus, of high or low pitch, according as the tube is large or small. Now, which is the cause of the sound in the case before us—the sibilus of asthma? The sibilus depending on a plug of tenacious mucus sticking to the side of the tube is generally (always *ultimately*) relieved by coughing; the sibilus of asthma is never affected by coughing. Inflammatory tumidity of the mucous membrane can never be dissociated from the symptoms of existing bronchitis, and the sibilus arising from it is not of transient appearance and disappearance; the sibilus of asthma, however, may come one minute, and the next be gone, and is ever changing; moreover, the signs of bronchitis are absent. The sibilus arising from the contraction of plastic exudation thrown around the tube is unvarying and irremediable, a permanent condition, and must have been preceded by some recognized attack of severe bronchitis; the wheeze of asthma, on the other hand, ceases with the paroxysm, and there need not have been bronchitis in any part of the previous history of the case. We have thus got rid of three of the possible causes of sibilus; we have seen that in the case before us (asthmatic wheezing) it cannot be produced by mucous plugging, by vascular tumidity of the mucous membrane, or by the slow contraction of old plastic exudations thrown around the tube. Muscular spasm alone remains. And should we have in this a condition consistent with all the phenomena, and sufficient for their production? Perfectly. The supposition of spasmodic stricture of the air-tubes would explain the sudden access and departure of the dyspnœa, for it is a state that may be instantaneously induced, and may instantaneously vanish; it is consistent with perfect health in all other respects, with the absence of all organic disease or vascular disturbance in the lungs (except that which results from it), with the kind and characters of the sounds generated, with the particular type of the dyspnœa, with the effects of remedies, and with all those circumstances that point to the nervous nature of the disease, such as its causes, the effect of emotion, its periodicity, &c.; for only by the production of muscular contraction of their walls can nervous stimuli affect the condition of the bronchial tubes; everything, therefore, that points to the nervous nature of the disease points to spasmodic bronchial stricture as its proximate pathological condition.

Thus we see, by evidence as certain as sight, that in asthma bronchial spasm must and does exist, and that no other conceivable supposition will explain the phenomena. And we see this independently of that anatomical and physiological support that dissection and experiment supply, and that has hitherto been the chief evidence adduced.

But we find in the muscular furniture of the bronchial walls and the nervous furniture of the whole bronchial system a valuable confirmation of the correctness of these views, both negatively and positively, for while their absence would be a sad stumbling-block in the way of our inferences from other evidence, their presence supplies exactly the required machinery. Nay, more, it is the most positive proof that could possibly be that muscular contraction of the bronchial tubes does take place. For, what is the purpose of circularly-disposed muscle, if not to vary the calibre of the tube it invests? The muscular coat of the bronchiæ consists of circularly-disposed bands of fibre-cells, forming a continuous layer immediately beneath the mucous surface; these fibre-cells may be seen in tubes of great minuteness, as small as one-tenth or one-twelfth of a line in diameter. The nervous system of the lungs is derived from the vagus, the cervical portion of the sympathetic and the anterior and posterior pulmonary plexus, and is from these origins furnished with wide-spread and varied connections. It is these wide-spread nervous connections that can alone explain some of the phenomena of asthma to which I shall have presently to refer. The nervous system of the lungs, thus derived, consists of ramifying plexuses, supported by the bronchial tubes as upon a scaffolding, and conducted by them to every part of the lungs. These plexuses form a sort of network, investing the bronchial tubes, even to their finest ramifications, and are furnished with microscopical ganglia.

But, besides this anatomical evidence, we have the positive proof of direct experiment; for Volkman, C. J. B. Williams, and others, to whose accounts I must refer the reader, have clearly shown that the bronchial tubes undergo contraction, in some cases even to complete occlusion, from the application of various stimuli, both to the tubes themselves and to the trunks of the pneumogastric nerves. This completes the chain of evidence that the essential condition in asthma is bronchial spasm.

3. *That the phenomena of asthma are those of excito-motory or reflex action.*

Whenever the peripheral application of a stimulus results in muscular motion, we say that the phenomena are reflex. And so they are, universally. As far as our present knowledge goes, we believe that a stimulus applied to a sentient surface or organ must first be transmitted to a nervous centre by incident, and thence reflected by motor filaments, before it can affect the muscular tissue, and stimulate it to contraction. The nervous centre may be a ganglion of microscopical minuteness, and the filaments emanating from it to their peripheral distribution may be of extreme shortness; but still, however near the seat of movement may be to the seat of stimulation (and they may be completely coincident), such a centripetal and centrifugal course, and such an intervention of a centre, are essential. We see a very good example of this kind of reflex nervous action in the peristaltic movement of the intestines. In this case the stimulus travels along a perceptive filament to one of the ganglia of the abdominal portion of the sympathetic; there it comes into relation with a motor filament, and is by it transmitted to the muscular wall of the intestine. Of just such a nature is the contraction of the bronchial tubes in obedience to sources of irritation applied to their internal surface; the filaments distributed to the mucous surface receive the impression, along them it travels to some of the scattered ganglia of the pulmonary plexuses, and thence returns by motor filaments to the bronchial muscle to which these are distributed. This is the normal function of the bronchial nervous system; it is for the production of bronchial contraction, in obedience to stimulus thus applied, that it is especially organized. It is by this reflected path that surface-stimulation arrives at and contracts the muscular wall. It is in this way that the bronchi know when and where to contract: that a plug of mucus produces a circumscribed strait through which cough drives it with greater force; that exudation occupying the capillary bronchial tubes is expelled by their peristaltic contraction; that offending material that has found ingress through the glottis is shut off by bronchial stricture from reaching the ultimate lung-structure—supposing, that is, such actions really to take place.[1] In asthma from the effluvium of hay, and of certain animals, as cats and rabbits; asthma from inhaling the emanations from ipecacuan powder; asthma from breathing ammoniacal or carburetted fumes; asthma produced by certain airs; asthma complicating bronchitis—in all these the bronchial spasm is of this natural, physiological character; the seat of the application of the stimulus and its reflected path being the same as that by which ordinary stimuli arrive at, and produce contraction of the bronchial muscle.

But one of the peculiarities of asthma is, that it may be induced by stimuli applied to remote parts; in these cases the nervous circuit is much longer, and the phenomena of reflexion clearer and more conspicuous. Take, for example, that most common of all the varieties of asthma, what we may call *peptic asthma*, in which the induction or prevention of attacks is entirely controlled by the state of the digestive organs; in which an error in diet—the eating some particular thing, eating too largely or late in the day—is sure to bring on an attack; while a certain dietetic abstention is as certain to be attended with immunity from the disease. Here the reflex character of the phenomena is clear, and the nervous circuit by which the reflexion is completed conspicuous and evident. I think there

[1] This point will be further discussed in the concluding paragraphs of this chapter.

are three degrees of remoteness of the application of stimulus producing asthma, and thus three groups into which we may divide these clearly reflex cases.

1st. Those that I have just.mentioned, in which the source of irritation is alimentary, and generally gastric. Here the nerve irritated is the gastric portion of the pneumogastric by which the stimulus is conducted to the medulla oblongata; this is probably the seat of the central reflexion, and transmits the stimulus immediately to the lungs by the pulmonary filaments of the same nerve, the bronchial muscles contracting in obedience to this reflected stimulation, just as they would have done if it had been primarily pulmonary. Here we have only one nerve concerned—the pneumogastric, but two portions of it, one of which plays an afferent and the other an efferent part, while the portion of the centre involved is confined to the origin of the nerve—to the seat of implantation of these respective gastric and pulmonary filaments.

2d. Those cases in which the irritation is more remote, but is still confined to the organic system of nerves; e.g., asthma produced by a loaded rectum.

3d. Where the cerebro-spinal system is the recipient of the irritation which is the provocative of the attack; for example, a remarkable case related to me by Dr. Chowne, in which the application of cold to the instep immediately produced the asthmatic condition.

Of these two last groups of cases I know of very few examples, and I may dismiss them with a few words. A case came under my observation some years ago in which the patient could regulate his asthma entirely by the condition of his bowels. They were, as a rule, relieved every evening: if the customary relief took place, and he retired to bed with an empty rectum, he awoke the next morning well; but if he neglected to relieve his bowels, or his efforts to do so were abortive, he was quite sure to be awoke towards morning by his asthma. Strange as this may appear, it is strictly true. Dr. Copland remarks that the attack is often preceded by costiveness and inefficient calls to stool—an observation quite in accordance with the case I have just related; and I should be disposed to think, myself, that these were not only precursory and premonitory symptoms, but that they had something to do with the causation of the asthma that followed them—that the attack had a *propter* as well as a *post* relation to them. Of a strictly analogous nature are those cases of hysterical asthma in which the attacks are preceded by recognized symptoms of uterine irritation. The remarkable case communicated to me by Dr. Chowne to which I have already referred, was as follows: J. G., a man of about fifty years of age, made application to an insurance office for the assurance of his life. In reply to the questions of the physician of the office, he stated that he was liable to spasmodic asthma. He stated that he was subject to these attacks if by any accident cold water fell upon his instep, or his instep in any other way became cold. The impression on the mind of my informant, who was the medical man who examined him, was that this was the commonest, but he is not sure it was the only, cause of the attacks. The asthma came on suddenly and *immediately*, and the attacks were very severe. The circumstances were considered so curious that great pains were taken thoroughly to sift the case, and the result was that the facts were clearly established, and the man's life refused in consequence.

But while cases illustrating in this remarkable way the excito-motory nature of asthma, and the distance from which stimuli may reach and influence the innervation of the lungs, are rare, cases of peptic asthma, in which the attacks are caused by pneumogastric irritation, are so common, that I think few cases could be found of true spasmodic asthma in which the disease is uninfluenced by the state of the digestive organs, while in a very large number it is entirely under their control. This fact is so patent and so generally recognized, that it has by many writers been made the basis of their classification of asthma; thus Dr. Bree and Dr. Young erect into a distinct species those cases that are dependent on gastric irritation. Therapeutically, the full appreciation of this fact is most important; more is to be done for our patients on the side of the stomach than in any other direction. An observant and thoughtful physician once said to me that he considered dietetic treatment *the only* treatment of asthma.

But there is yet again another class of cases that have suggested to my mind the belief that asthma is sometimes *central*, not reflex, in its origin; that it may originate in irritation of the brain itself, or the spinal cord. The two following cases appear to me to be examples of this kind of "*central*" asthma. The first was communicated to me by my brother, Mr. James Salter, and occurred under his own observation. The patient was a boy of about ten years old, and the disease acute hydrocephalus, which ran a fatal course in about a fortnight. Five days before his death he was suddenly seized with an attack of dyspnœa of the asthmatic kind; it was very severe, lasted about half an hour, and then entirely vanished. The following day he was seized with a precisely similar attack; but this was the last; the symptoms never reappeared, and the patient sank in the ordinary way, from the brain disease, about four days afterwards. He had never before suffered from asthma; there were no chest symptoms either before or after the attacks, no cough, no expectoration. My brother is very precise as to the nature of the dyspnœa; he says there was nothing cardiac about it, no panting, no orthopnœa, but that it had the labouring, "difficult" character of asthma. I conceive that in this case the bronchial spasm was a phenomenon of deranged innervation from central irritation, analogous to the jactitations, rigidity, and convulsions characteristic of hydrocephalus.

The other case was that of a man of about fifty years of age, subject to epilepsy. His fits had certain well-known premonitory symptoms, and occurred with tolerable regularity, I think, about once a fortnight. On one occasion his medical attendant was sent for in haste, and found him suffering from violent asthma; the account given by his friends was, that at the usual time at which he had expected the fit he had experienced the accustomed premonitory symptoms, but instead of their being followed, as usual, by the convulsions, this violent dyspnœa had come on. Within a few hours the dyspnœa went off, and left him as well as usual. At the expiration of the accustomed interval after this attack the ordinary premonitory symptoms and the usual epileptic fit occurred. On several occasions (I do not know how many) this was repeated, the epileptic seizure being, as it were, supplanted by the asthmatic. Of these four points my informant, who was the medical attendant, seemed certain: that there was nothing amiss with the lungs either before or after the attacks, that the character of the dyspnœa was asthmatic, that each attack of asthma occurred at the usual epileptic period, and that they were preceded by the premonitory symptoms that ordinarily ushered in the epilepsy. I think that such a case admits of only one interpretation—that the particular state of the nervous centres that ordinarily threw the patient at certain periods into the epileptic condition, on certain other occasions, from some unknown cause, gave rise to bronchial spasm; that the essential diseased condition was one and the same, but that its manifestations were altered, temporary exaltation and perversion of the innervation of the lungs supplanting unconsciousness and clonic convulsion. Bearing in mind the many points in their clinical history that asthma and epilepsy have in common, this case is one of peculiar interest.

To this same category of *central* asthma we must, in strictness, assign those cases in which the paroxysm is brought on by violent emotion, as in that remarkable instance I have related of the gentleman who had, on two distinct occasions, violent spasmodic asthma suddenly induced by alarm, from the fear that he had poisoned his wife. In such a case, the seat to which the stimulus is primarily applied is the brain itself.

Lastly, there is a class of cases in which the exciting cause of the paroxysms appears to be essentially *humoral*. I have stated that the most frequent of the exciting causes of asthmatic attacks are alimentary, and that an error in diet, or the mere introduction of food into the stomach, produces bronchial spasm by reflex stimulation, through the intervention of the pneumogastric nerve. But is this the only way in which the lungs can be affected by what is put into the stomach? No. Although the pneumogastric nerve is the only single structure that has a distribution common to both organs, yet the venous system affords a very close and intimate bond of connection between the stomach and the lungs; for any rapidly absorbable material introduced into the stomach is at once taken up by the venous radicles of the gastric mucous membrane, and within a few seconds, having passed through the liver and the right side of the heart, finds itself in the pulmonary circulation. In this way the blood in the lungs is liable to constant change in its composition from admixture with it of the different materials thus taken up by the gastric veins; and from the absence of secernent or elective power on the part of these veins, is ever at the mercy of the food. The chief parts of the normal results of healthy digestion, or the morbid results of depraved digestion, and that numerous class of bodies which are at once taken up without any change, are thus thrown directly upon the lungs. In the intestines we have an additional and still more direct channel for the introduction of the contents of the alimentary canal into the pulmonary circulation, namely, the lacteal absorbents. It is I believe, in this way, by the actual presence in the vessels of the lungs of the materials taken up from the stomach and intestines, that the introduction of food into the alimentary canal frequently gives rise to bronchial spasm. A contaminate blood is the irritant, and excites the bronchial tubes to contract through the intervention of the pulmonary nervous system, just as the effluvium of hay or an irritating gas would. In one case the irritant affects the surface to which the nerves are distributed, in the other the capillaries among which they lie. When I say a " contaminate" blood, I do not mean that the material present in it is necessarily peccant. I believe it may be perfectly normal, and yet produce asthma. I believe that digestion may be everything that it should be, and its results in no way different from that of a perfectly healthy person, and yet they shall, in an asthmatic, produce asthma the moment they arrive at the lungs. I believe this because some of the materials that give rise to asthma are such as undergo no change, but are at once absorbed, and must therefore necessarily be identical in the lungs of the sound man and in the lungs of the asthmatic, and also because many persons who are rendered asthmatic by taking food exhibit no symptoms of deranged stomach-action whatever. With one such case in particular I am very familiar; it is that of a lady who every day within a few minutes after commencing her dinner experiences that dry constricted straitness of breathing characteristic of asthma; even if she has her asthma at no other time, she will have it then; after lasting a quarter of an hour, or half an hour, it passes completely off. Now this lady's digestion is remarkably good, unusually powerful and rapid; she is free from the ordinary restrictions of diet that most people are obliged to acquiesce in—radishes, cucumbers, and other unwholesomes, agree with her perfectly well: and the production of the asthma does not depend upon the quality of the food; such things as I have mentioned do not seem to induce it, while she will often become asthmatic during the plainest meal. I believe in this, as in hay, ipecacuan, and other asthma, that the irritant differs not in the asthmatic and the healthy person, but that the essential difference is in the irritability of the pulmonary nervous system—that it resents that which it should not resent—that its morbid sensitiveness exalts that into a stimulant which should not be a stimulant, and that thus the pulmonary nervous system registers (as it were) on the bronchial tubes those changes in the constitution of the pulmonary blood of which it should be unconscious.

There are, however, certain, articles of diet which, either from their being peculiarly offensive when materially present in the lungs, or apt to give rise to dyspepsia and its vitiated results, or specially irritating to the gastric portion of the vagus, are very apt to induce asthma. Such asthmatic articles of food are, cheese, nuts, almonds and raisins, and sweet things in general, salted meats, condiments, potted, and preserved, and highly seasoned things, fermented drinks, especially malt liquors and sweet wines. I think malt liquor, especially the stronger sort, with a good deal of carbonic acid gas in it, is perhaps the most asthmatic thing of any ; next to that I should place raisins and nuts. I know the case of an asthmatic gentleman who cannot eat a dozen raisins without feeling his breath tight and difficult. But there is great caprice about asthma in this respect, strongly marked idiosyncrasies in individual cases. Thus, in one case, a single glass of hock would invariably bring on an attack, though any other wine might be drunk with impunity ; in another, Rhine and Bordeaux wines—hock and claret—were the only ones that could be drunk ; a dinner at which they alone were partaken of was sure never to be followed by asthma ; but if port or sherry were drunk, the asthma would infallibly come on within an hour or two. In another case, the whole mischief of a dinner, its sting, lay in its tail, in the usual post-prandial coffee; if that vicious drink was declined, no harm came of the dinner, but if it was partaken of, on came the asthma.

But why, it may be asked, do I choose to adopt the opinion that these different alimentary materials produce asthma by their material presence in the blood of the lungs, consequent on their gastric absorption ? Why is not the supposition that they act as irritants to the gastric portion of the vagus sufficient for the explanation of all cases ? I do not say positively that it is *not* sufficient; I do not say it is the sole way in which all these articles of diet excite asthma. But there is in particular one circumstance that makes me think that some of these materials at least, and in some cases, act by their presence in the lungs themselves, and it is this—that they induce the asthma in just such time as they would take to reach the lungs subsequent to their absorption ; that the interval between the taking the material and the supervention of the asthma will be long or short according as the absorption of that particular material is immediate or deferred. Thus, in a case which once came under my notice, in which the taking of wine or any alcoholic drink was always followed by asthma, the asthma was immediate, within a minute or two;

while in another case, in which the food producing the asthma was such as would furnish material for lacteal absorption, the asthma did not come on till about two hours after taking the food; that is, when the chyle would be beginning to reach the blood which was being poured into the lungs.

But we must not forget that asthmatics are very commonly dyspeptics, and often exhibit symptoms of perverted and capricious stomach action that suggests to one's mind the belief that the innervation of the whole of the vagus is vitiated, its gastric as well as pulmonary portion, and that the dyspeptic and asthmatic symptoms are but parts of a whole.[1]

What I would wish, then, to express on this subject is—that I believe it possible that asthma is sometimes produced by particular materials admixed with the blood in the lungs, and that therefore it is so far *humoral;* but that these particular materials—whether absorbed unchanged, as alcohol, ethers, and saline solutions, or the results of healthy digestion, or of perverted digestion—have nothing particular in them, but are the same as they would be in any nonasthmatic person, and that the essence of the disease in these cases, as well as in all others, consists in a morbid sensitiveness and irritability of the pulmonary nervous system.

Great and valuable light is often thrown on pathological questions by considering the laws of the physiology of the part concerned, for pathology is often but deranged physiology, and pathological aberrations in strict subservience to physiological laws. Let us then see if we can detect in the probable purpose of the muscular endowment of the air-tubes, an explanation of any of the phenomena of asthma. What *is* the purpose of the muscular contractility of the air-passages?

This is a question that has been variously answered, and whose certain solution is beset with considerable difficulties. In one light we may look upon the bronchial system as the ramifying efferent duct of the great conglomerate gland the lungs, of whose excretion, carbonic acid, it affords the means of outdraught. Now, the ducts of all large glands are furnished with organic muscle—liver, pancreas, salivary glands, kidneys, ovaries—so that the existence of muscular elements in the walls of the bronchial tubes is in strict conformity with anatomical analogy. But when we pass on from anatomy to function, all analogy ceases. The purpose of the muscular endowment of the ducts of glands in general is the expulsion of the secretion; little waves of vermicular contraction pass along them, always in a direction *from* the gland, and thus their contents are driven along towards the orifice. Such cannot be the purpose of the muscularity of bronchial tubes, for they are permanently and necessarily patulous; indeed, throughout their greater length a

[1] For a fuller discussion of this point the reader is referred to Chapter XII., where some of these cases of asthmatic dyspepsia are narrated.

special arrangement is adopted by which their closure shall be effectually prevented, by means of the rings and flakes of cartilage scattered throughout their walls. In the larger tubes these are such and so placed that only a slight amount of contraction is possible; they are continued down, in increasing tenuity and scantiness, to tubes of a smallness of half a line in diameter, and wherever they exist perfect closure is impossible; so that in none except tubes of extreme minuteness can absolute occlusion take place. But beyond the point of the cessation of cartilage flakes muscle still exists: it has been demonstrated in tubes $\frac{1}{120}$th of an inch in diameter, and probably exists even in the ultimate lobular bronchiæ. Here, of course, perfect closure can be effected.

What are the acts, then, of which the bronchial tubes, thus constituted, are the seat? Respiration and Cough. For we must consider cough a normal act. It is the constituted mechanism of expulsion of any particles of foreign matter which may at any time be introduced with the respired air, and against whose ingress the stricture function of the glottis so imperfectly provides. Indeed, the respiratory organs have no power of selection, no means of filtering the material on which they are every moment dependent for the exercise of their function; they are ever at the mercy of the air, and of any materials that may contaminate it. The power, therefore, of expelling any foreign or offending particle that may have found entrance becomes a necessary appendage to respiration. Cough is, no doubt, often a phenomenon of disease, but it becomes pathological from the material on which it is exercised and not from the essential nature of the act. If exercised on blood, pus, or excessive mucus, it is a symptom of disease; if on some foreign particle that has found accidental ingress, it is strictly normal. It is no more pathological than sneezing is pathological, which a particle of dust or a sunbeam may cause at any time. What purpose, then, if any, has the muscular endowment of the air-passages in relation to these two acts—respiration and cough?

It has been maintained by many that the bronchial tubes contract at each expiration, and so assist in the expulsion of the air. But the character of the fluid expelled—gaseous, and the method of its expulsion—quick, transient, and iterated, are neither such as the ordinary slow vermicular contraction of organic muscle would be appropriate for; it is impossible that the bronchial tubes can expel the expired air in the same way as the ducts of glands do their secretion, it is impossible that a wave of contraction can pass from extremities to trunk of the bronchial tree at each expiration; it would be a rapidity of transit entirely at variance with all that we know of the law of organic muscle contraction. Moreover, we know that uninterrupted patulence from glottis to air-cell, both in inspiration and expiration, is an essential condition of normal breathing. If there is any bronchial contraction coincident with expiration, it must be a slight narrowing of all the tubes, in propor-

4

tion to the contraction of the entire lung, which would act, not as a special expiratory force, but would merely diminish the amount of residual air locked up in the air-passages at the end of expiration.

This slight contraction of the whole bronchial system at each expiration I am, for the following reasons, inclined to believe. I have long observed that rhonchous and sibilant râles are often only audible during expiration; that in inspiration they cease; that they are frequently confined to the end of an expiration, not becoming audible till the expiration is half performed; that the longer and deeper the expiration the louder they are; and that the inaudible respiration of persons in apparent good health, particularly the old, may be rendered wheezing by making them effect a prolonged expiration. I have remarked this, not only with the dry sounds of asthma, but the moist râles of bronchitis; the crepitous wheeze of senile bronchitis is often confined to the termination of the expirations. If you tell a person with unsound lungs to wheeze, he immediately effects a prolonged expiration, as if he knew that that was the way to produce a wheeze. Now, the source of sound—the plug of mucus, or the inflamed tumid membrane—exists as much during inspiration as expiration: why, then, should the sound be present in the one and absent in the other? On what does it depend? Manifestly on the alternate contraction and dilatation of the air-passages. The plug of mucus, or the tumid membrane, which does not narrow the tube sufficiently to give rise to a musical sound in inspiration, in expiration does. I do not know how we can explain these phenomena except by supposing that all the bronchial tubes undergo contraction during expiration, and thus magnify the effects of any sources of inequality in their calibre; for a plug of mucus, for example, that would form hardly any impediment to the passage of air in a wide and patulous tube, would form a considerable barrier, and throw the air into strong vibrations, if that tube were in a state of contraction. Moreover, I have noticed (and this is a very curious fact) that when the breathing is inclined to be asthmatical, the dyspnœa may be aggravated, and the asthmatic feeling very much increased, by a prolonged expiration,[1] while, on the other hand, the spasm may be broken through, and the respiration for the time rendered perfectly

---

[1] I am aware that this is in direct contravention of the statement of Laennec, Williams, and other authorities on thoracic diseases, who affirm that after a prolonged and deep expiration the chest may be freely distended; the respiratory murmur being audible and loud, and the spasm apparently temporarily suspended. I should be rather inclined to guess that in this case the re-establishment of the respiratory murmur and the suspension of the spasm were the result not of the *expiration*, but of the full *inspiration* that has succeeded it. At any rate, I can only say that I have never observed what Laennec and Williams affirm, and have frequently seen what I have above described; and respect for authority, however high, should never be pushed to the concession of anything positively observed.

free and easy, by taking a long, deep, full inspiration. In severe asthmatic breathing this cannot be done ; but in the slight bronchial spasm that characterizes hay-asthma I have frequently witnessed it. It seems as if the deep inspiration overcame and broke through the contracted state of the air-tubes, which was not immediately re-established.

Now all this looks as if expiration favoured, and inspiration opposed, contraction of the air-passages; in fact, I think it amounts to positive proof of it. But this does not at all imply that the bronchial tubes undergo *distinct muscular contractions* at each expiration. I think it possible to explain the phenomena otherwise. I think it possible that the diminution of their calibre at expiration may be due to the constant and unvarying tendency of their muscular and elastic walls to contract. This tendency is antagonized and overcome during inspiration, by which the tubes, like the other contents of the chest, are forcibly distended ; in expiration this tendency is no longer opposed, and, like the other contents of the chest, the tubes collapse. Still, the assumed active contraction of the bronchi is quite consistent with the phenomena, especially those which I have mentioned with regard to asthma, that a long expiration, namely, deepens the spasm, while a full inspiration may temporarily annihilate it. This looks as if bronchial contraction and inspiration were incompatible, and could not co-exist. Still, it would be possible to explain both these circumstances by supposing that prolonged expiration merely *suffered* the tube more completely to yield to the pre-existing asthmatic spasm, while the distension of expiration was too strong for it and overcame it.

In relation to cough, the opinion has been advanced that the muscularity of the bronchial tubes may, by diminishing their calibre, increase the rapidity of the rush of air driven through them by the act of coughing, and thus increase its expulsive power. If this contraction were general, and extended to the smaller tubes, the reverse would be the case, for a smaller stream of air would be brought to bear upon the obstructing material. If, however, it is a circumscribed contraction, confined to the situation of the matter to be expelled, then it would be a veritable adjuvant, and the air would rush through the point of narrowing with increased rapidity, and therefore increased expulsive power, just as narrowing an outlet of water clears and deepens the channel. But the contraction being at the seat of the matter to be expelled, and there alone, is an essential condition to this increase of expulsive power. A little glottis is, as it were, formed there, and the material inevitably driven through it.

But there is a third purpose, I think, arising from this very danger of the access of deleterious matter to the lungs, more important than either of the other two to which I have referred, and which I believe to be *the* purpose, *par excellence*, of the muscularity of the air-tubes. It is the guarding the delicate ultimate lung-structure, the shutting off from the air-cells, and preventing reaching them, any deleterious material that may have gained entrance through the glottis. After having passed the glottis there is no other means by which the further progress of any foreign matter may be arrested; and its arrest ere it reaches the pulmonary structure seems as essential to the well-being of the lung as its subsequent expulsion by cough. We know, in fact, that very little of the foreign particles contaminating the air reaches the air-cells; that it is almost entirely arrested and expectorated; and we know, too, that the respiration of air charged with any irritating or noxious material, such as the smoke of burning pitch, pungent vapours, dust, &c., will immediately produce in many people the symptoms of bronchial stricture.

Another office that has been claimed for the muscularity of the bronchial tubes is the regulation of the supply of air to those portions of the lung in which they terminate, in the same way as the muscularity of the arteries regulates the blood-supply to the capillaries. We can easily understand how, when one lung or one portion of a lung is injured, a relaxation of the bronchial tubes of the other portion would enable them to deliver to it a freer supply of air, and thus capacitate it better for doing double duty. On the other hand, we can imagine how, in certain violent inspiratory efforts a narrowing of the bronchial tubes would limit the supply of air, and exercise a conservative and protective influence by preventing too great and sudden a distension.

But if we would form a correct idea of the purposes which are stored up in an organ, our attention must not be restricted to its working in health, but must embrace also those exceptional processes that arise in the course of disease, those latent, and, during health, inoperative powers kept in store, as it were, against the emergencies they are to meet, by the possession of which in its different organs the body becomes not only a self-maintaining and self-regulating, but a self-correcting machine. Have the bronchial tubes any such exceptional office, adapting them to a pathological exigency? Such a one has been assigned them. It has been maintained that when the smaller bronchial tubes become filled with secretion, as they so commonly do in disease—with mucus, for instance, as in capillary bronchitis, or with muco-plastic matter, as in pneumonia—they empty themselves of it, and pass it on into the larger tubes, by a peristaltic contraction. This would be the acquisition in disease of the same kind of action as the ducts of most glands have in health. There are two strong negative reasons in favour of this view. One is that there is in these minute bronchial tubes an absence of that anatomical peculiarity that would prevent anything like a peristaltic contraction of the larger ones—namely the flakes of cartilage. The other is that these ultimate tubes are wanting in the ordinary mechanism of discharge by which the bronchial system keeps itself empty—the *vis à tergo*, namely, of cough; for, having behind them only so small a volume of air—that contained in the lobule or group of lobules in which they terminate—sufficient explosive force cannot be brought to bear upon the mucus obstructing them—there is no air behind it to drive it forth. The larger the tubes, the more effectual cough becomes, because the greater the portion of lung with which they correspond, and the larger the volume of air on which the parietes of the chest exercise their pressure in the explosive expiration of cough. The ultimate bronchiæ, then, being deficient in this power of clearing themselves, we should naturally expect that some succedaneum would be provided, and this we recognize in the peristaltic contraction of which they are probably the seat. Were it not for this, one can hardly conceive by what mechanism they would empty themselves of the materials by which, as shown by the sounds of respiration during life and *post-mortem* examination, they are so apt to become infarcted.[1]

Now can we see in these real or probable purposes of the muscular contractility of the bronchial tubes any explanation of the phenomena of asthma, and any clue to the ultimate pathology of the disease? Yes, I think we can, most clearly. We see that the purpose of this muscular furniture of the bronchial tubes is that they should contract under certain circumstances, and on the application of certain stimuli; and seen by this light we recognize in asthma merely a morbid activity—an excess—of this natural endowment; the tubes fall into a state of contraction with a proneness, a readiness, that is morbid; the slightest thing will throw them into a state of spasm, the irritability of the muscle is exalted, the contraction violent and protracted, that becomes a stimulus to contraction which should not be, and the nervous and muscular system of the lungs is brought within the range of sources of irritation applied to such distant parts as ordinarily in no way affect them. Any healthy man may have his bronchial tubes temporarily thrown into a state of asthmatic spasm by the inhalation of ammoniacal or carburetted or other irritating gases; but only by such materials, whose exclusion is necessary for the safety of the lung, will this natural asthma be brought about. A greater degree of bronchial sensibility is shown in those cases, by no means uncommon, of what is called "hay-asthma," in which the stimulus to bronchial spasm is the effluvium of hay; a still greater, in those cases, much rarer, in which the emanations from ipecacuan powder will at once give rise to asthma; a still greater in that numerous class of cases of asthma in which the disease is called into activity by certain atmospheric peculiarities which are altogether inappre-

---

[1] I wrote this early in 1858. About a year after, I had my attention directed to a mine of interesting and valuable matter, comprised in some papers by Dr. Gairdner, of Edinburgh, on "The Pathological Anatomy of Bronchitis," published in the *Monthly Journal of Medical Science* and the *British and Foreign Medico-Chirurgical Review* in 1851 and 1853. Those who are familiar with these important essays will recognize the close resemblance that exists between Dr. Gairdner's views and my own, and the process of reasoning by which they are arrived at.

ciable, as where an attack of asthma is inevitably brought on by
going to a certain place, living in a certain house, sleeping in a certain room.   All these cases fall strictly under what we may call
the formula of health; they are physiological; they are instances
of the contraction of a muscular tube in obedience to stimulus
applied to the mucous membrane that lines that tube; the nervous
system engaged is the *intrinsic* nervous system of the tubes, its
own ganglia and perceptive and motor filaments, in the same way
as in œsophageal deglutition or intestinal peristalsis; the error is
merely a morbid exaltation of a normal irritability.   But there
are other cases in which the error is more than this, in which the
nervous apparatus involved in the phenomena is abnormally extended; in which certain outlying and distant parts of the nervous
system are the recipients of the stimuli that give rise to the bronchial spasm, as in those cases, to which I have referred, where an
attack is induced by an error in diet, a loaded rectum, the application of cold to the instep, mental emotion; in which the gastric
filaments of the pneumogastric nerves, the sympathetic, the cutaneous nerves of the foot, and the brain, are respectively the recipients of the stimulus that gives rise to the bronchial contraction.
In the former class of cases the bronchial spasm takes place in
obedience to the wrong stimulus applied to the right place; in the
latter, place and stimulus are alike wrong; the relation of the
asthma to its cause is in the one case immediate or primary, in
the other, remote or secondary—mediate, through the intervention
of some part of the nervous system extrinsic to the lungs.

In what, then, does the peculiarity of the asthmatic essentially
consist?   Manifestly, in a morbid proclivity of the musculo-nervous
system of his bronchial tubes to be thrown into a state of activity;
the stimulus may be either immediately or remotely applied, but in
either case would not normally be attended by any such result.
There is no peculiarity in the stimulus, the air breathed is the same
to the asthmatic and the non-asthmatic, the ipecacuan powder, the
hay effluvium, is the same in both; nor, probably, is their any peculiarity in the irritability of the bronchial muscle; the peculiarity is
confined to the link that connects these two—the nervous system,
and consists in its perverted sensibility, in its receiving and trans-
mitting on to the muscle, as a stimulus to contraction, that of which
it should take no cognizance.   In those cases where the spasm is
produced by some irritant applied to the air-passages themselves, this
perverted irritability is confined to the bronchial nervous system.
The exact seat of the perverted nervous action in those other cases
where the stimulus is remote, is more doubtful.   Take, for instance,
that case in which cold water thrown on the instep immediately
produced asthmatic dyspnœa.   Was the cerebro-spinal nervous system in fault here?   Did it transmit to the nerves of the lungs a
morbid stimulation, or was the fault, as in the other cases, confined
to the pulmonary nervous system—to its being morbidly affected by

a nervous impression perfectly normal? These are questions that in the present state of our knowledge it would be difficult or impossible to answer. At any rate, it is clear that the vice in asthma consists, not in the production of any special irritant, but in the irritability of the part irritated.

These considerations, I think, tend to rationalize our notions of asthma, and to impart at once an interest and an order to its phenomena.

CHAPTER III.

CLINICAL HISTORY OF ASTHMA.—PHENOMENA OF THE PAROXYSM.

Premonitory and initiatory symptoms.—Drowsiness, dyspeptic symptoms, headache, excitability, profuse diuresis, neuralgic pains.—Time of attack, the early morning. Why?—Description of access of paroxysm—Appearance of the asthmatic in the height of the paroxysm.—Pulse.—Itching under the chin.—Muscular phenomena.— Enlargement of capacity of chest.—Modification of respiratory rhythm.—Auscultatory signs.—Conclusions.—Length of paroxysm.—Necessity of starving during the attack.—Expectoration.—Its physical and microscopical characters.—Hæmoptysis.

IN considering the phenomena of asthma, I shall take first the phenomena of a paroxysm, and then the phenomena of the disease generally; and I shall adopt this order because the phenomena of the paroxysm are so much more pronounced and marked, and constitute so much the body of the malady, while those of the disease generally, in opposition to those of the paroxysm, are rather the phenomena of the intervals, and consist of certain permanent conditions influencing the paroxysms, or produced by them.

As in epilepsy, we have premonitory symptoms in the form of the *aura epileptica*, spectra, and other subjective phenomena; then the establishment of the paroxysm; then those conditions of the nervous and muscular systems which constitute its climax; and then its abatement and the post-epileptic sleep; so in asthma we have certain precursory symptoms, and then the attack in its accession, perfect establishment, and departure.

The precursory symptoms of a fit of asthma are liable to a great variety in different individuals; some persons never experience any, but having been guilty of some imprudence, or the regular period of an attack having recurred, the seizure of the dyspnœa upon them is the first indication of its approach. But I think that the majority of asthmatics *do* know that an attack is coming on them by certain feelings in themselves, or certain conditions of which they are aware. These symptoms generally show themselves on the night previous to the attack; but in some cases for a longer time. The patient will feel himself very drowsy and sleepy, will be unable to hold his head up or keep his eyes open, and that without having undergone any particular fatigue or done anything that could account for it.[1]   I remember one case in which this was very strikingly marked; the asthmatic always knew when he was going to be ill the next day by the extreme drowsiness that overpowered him at night; he would go sound asleep over his reading or writing, or whatever he might be engaged in, and that at an early hour of the evening. It was in vain for him to rouse himself; in spite of all his efforts, and in spite of the prophecies of those about him that he was going to be ill, and his convictions of what awaited him, to bed he must go. And probably any resistance of these feelings would have been of no avail, and would neither have postponed nor modified the attack; the asthma was not the *result* of the heaviness, but the heaviness merely indicated the approach of the asthma; it was the commencement of that particular nervous condition of which the succeeding respiratory phenomena were but the more complete development; in fact, it must be looked upon as an integral part of the paroxysm. I find this precursory drowsiness to be the commonest of all the premonitory symptoms of asthma.

Others, again, know by extreme wakefulness and unusual mental activity and buoyancy of spirits that an attack awaits them; and I knew one case in which an attack of ophthalmia always ushered in the asthma: the man was liable to inflammation of his conjunctiva, it was always worse before his attacks than at any other time, and he invariably knew by the state of his eyes when he was going to suffer a paroxysm. It might be thought that this was a case of mere catarrh, that the asthma was caused by the inflammation of the eyes creeping down through the nasal mucous membrane into the air-passages; but this was clearly not the case—there was no coryza, no bronchitis; the ophthalmia was strumous, and I believe that an exacerbation of the strumous cachexia, a more debilitated, and therefore a more irritable condition of system, was the cause alike of the inflammation of the conjunctiva and the spasm of the air-tubes. At other times the precursory symptoms are connected with the stomach, and consist of loss of appetite, flatulence, costiveness, and certain peculiar uneasy sensations in the epigastrium; but here I think we have something more than mere premonitory signs; I think the relation of these symptoms to the spasm which follows is often that of cause and effect.

Of all the circumstances attending the commencement of an asthmatic paroxysm, none is more constant than the time at which it occurs. This is almost invariably in the early morning, from three to six o'clock. There are some cases in which the usual time is the evening, some just after getting into bed, before going to sleep, and some in which there is no particular time, but the attack

---

[1] Floyer, who wrote in the sixteenth century, was perfectly aware of this premonitory sign, having noticed it in his own person. "There appears," he says, "a great dulness and fulness of the head, with a slight headache and great sleepiness on the evening before the fit."

may come on at any hour of the day or night, on the occurrence of some exciting cause, such as a fit of laughter, a full stomach, change of wind, &c. In nineteen cases out of twenty, however, the dyspnœa first declares itself on the patient's waking in the morning, or rather wakes him from his sleep when he has had but half a night's rest.

Now, I think there are two reasons for the attack coming on at this time: one is the horizontal position of the body, the other the greater facility with which sources of irritation, and, indeed, any causes of reflex action, operate during sleep than during the hours of wakefulness. The first cause acts thus: When a person lies down and goes to sleep, the recumbent position favours the afflux of blood to the right side of the heart, and therefore to the lungs; in addition to this, the position of the body places the muscles of respiration at a disadvantage, especially the diaphragm, against the under surface of which the recumbent position brings the contents of the abdomen to bear; to this may be added the diminished rate at which the vital changes go on during sleep; and lastly, the lowered sensibility of sleep, which prevents the arrears into which the respiration may be getting from being at once appreciated. Here, I think, we have a sufficient explanation both of the time at which the attack generally comes on and of the amount of dyspnœa that may accumulate before the asthmatic is roused from his slumbers. He goes to bed perhaps quite well; the position of his body and the torpor of sleep soon throw his lungs into arrears, and they become congested. This goes on for some time, gradually increasing, without producing any particular effect; but, by and by, this pulmonary congestion reaches such a pitch that it becomes itself a source of great local irritation, and gives rise to asthmatic spasm; this, in its turn, cuts off the supply of air, and increases the congestion, and thus the asthma and the congestion, the cause and the effect, mutually augment one another, till they produce such an amount of dyspnœa as is incompatible with sleep, and the patient suddenly wakes with all the distress of an asthmatic paroxysm full upon him. Now, in this case, all the causes I have mentioned act together, but we know that each individually has its separate agency in producing the effect, because by removing any one of the causes you may prevent the result; we know that the position of the body tends to induce the attack, because an extra pillow may prevent it; we know that the disadvantage at which the muscles of respiration are placed during sleep conduces to it, because the attack may in some cases be prevented by laying the head on the arm, so as to make the shoulder a fixed point, from which the accessory muscles of respiration can act;[1] lastly, we know that the greater proneness to excito-

[1] An asthmatic friend, with whose case I am familiar, tells me that he always sleeps much better on a sofa than on a bed; no amount of bolstering can impart to a bed the comfort and ease of a sofa. This he attributes to the fixed support that the side of the sofa affords on which to rest his arm, and the leverage thereby furnished for the accessory muscles of respiration.

motory action during sleep has to do with it, because some asthmatics. do not dare to go to sleep after the commission of any imprudence, whereas they may be guilty of any irregularity with impunity, if they only keep awake for some time afterwards. I know one asthmatic who often sits up half the night after taking a supper (breathing perfectly freely), because he knows that if he goes to sleep, his asthma will come on immediately; but by thus sitting up till his supper is fairly digested, his stomach empty, and the source of irritation thus removed, he may go to sleep fearlessly, and have a good night's rest.

One cannot help seeing the striking resemblance that exists between this and the orthopnœa of cardiac disease; only, in the one case, the extreme dyspnœa is brought about by the obstruction which the heart-disease opposes to the circulation through the lungs; in the other by the sparing amount of air admitted through the obstructed bronchi; in both the congestion of the lungs is first induced by the position of the body, and the sense of arrears—the *besoin de réspirer*—blunted, and the respiratory efforts postponed by the insensibility of sleep. But in the orthopnœa the violent and extraordinary respiration that succeeds the starting from sleep soon re-establishes the balance; whereas in the asthma the constriction of the bronchi which persists after waking precludes the admission of the necessary amount of air, and the dyspnœa remains.

One curious circumstance with regard to time is that it may be varied according to the intensity of the cause; the more intense the source of irritation the shorter will the sleep be before the asthma puts a stop to it. I once knew an asthmatic who was always awoke by his disease with an earliness proportionate to the size of the supper he had taken; certain airs disagreed with him as well as food before sleeping, and if the two causes acted conjointly, he would wake with asthma much earlier than if they acted singly; thus, if he went to a place that did not agree with him, he might awake about five o'clock with his asthma; the same if he ate his supper in a place that *did* agree with him; but if he ate a supper when staying at a place that did *not* agree with him, he would get no sleep after two or three o'clock. This may seem singular and an over refinement, but it is strictly true; I have watched it over and over again.

How essentially characteristic of the disease this occurrence of the attack in the early morning is—how inherently a part of it—is shown by the fact that, in the great majority of cases, at this time and at this time alone will the attack come on, at whatever time in the twenty-four hours the exciting cause may be applied. For instance, in some cases over-exercise will bring on an attack; in many cases that have come under my care this has been so; but although the asthma was in these pretty sure to follow such over-exertion, it never came on immediately, never till the next morning; the exertion might be followed at the time by a little shortness of breath, not much exceeding that of a healthy person, which would speedily and entirely disappear, and the patient would pass the rest of the day, and go to bed, in perfect health; but as surely as possible he would be awoke the next morning at the usual time with his asthma. And it would make no difference at what time of day the over-exertion had been taken, morning or evening: at the stated time, and at that only, neither earlier nor later, would its results declare themselves. Now, here we have an exciting cause actually and inevitably bringing on an attack, but powerless to do so, its effect suspended, as it were, and laid dormant until the characteristic time had come round. Nothing could show, as I think, more clearly than this both the tenacity with which the disease sticks to its favourite time of occurrence and its essentially nervous nature. For through what but through the nervous system could such exciting causes maintain their influence suspended, and finally produce their effects after so long an interval, during which the respiratory and circulatory systems had been in a normal and tranquil condition?

I have always believed that this morning occurrence of asthma is the result of the causes I have mentioned, the horizontal position and sleep, and the conditions of circulation and respiration that they induce, and I cannot but believe that this is its true explanation. But about six months ago a case came under my observation which seemed to imply that this feature of asthma was an essential part of its natural history, and not dependent on external circumstances. The case was that of a night porter, whose duties compelled him to turn day into night and night into day. He went to bed at seven o'clock in the morning, and slept through the early part of the day. But though the ordinary times of sleeping and waking were thus transposed, the asthma came on at the usual time, from five to six in the morning, towards the end of his vigil, when he was up and awake, and when none of the determining causes that I have mentioned could have been in operation. If the asthma had come on in this case at a time having the same relation to sleep and recumbency as in ordinary cases, it would have made its appearance about eleven or twelve o'clock in the day. This case certainly looks as if the particular period that the paroxysm affects depended on some inherent and inveterate habit of the disease. But the teaching of a single case like this is not to be taken in contravention of reason or unsupported by further evidence. It is, however, I think, worth putting on record, and worth bearing in mind.

One of the symptoms frequently attendant on the first stage of an attack of asthma is *profuse diuresis;* the patient will half fill a chamber-pot with pale, limpid water, exactly like the urine of hysteria. This abundant secretion generally comes on soon after the asthma commences, but I have known it to come on so early that the patient was awakened from his sleep by the distension of his bladder, when the difficulty of his breathing was only just commencing. It generally lasts for the first three or four hours, and then ceases altogether. I believe the secretion of this abundant white urine to be of the same nature as the hysterical urine that it resembles—that it is nervous; and I regard it, as I have shown elsewhere,[1] as one of the many evidences of the nervous nature of asthma.

Another early symptom which I have often observed is *neuralgic pains*, a deep-seated aching in the limbs and joints; the testicles, too, are very apt to be affected with it, and I knew one case in which the testicle, and the tibia, from the knee to the ankle, were always affected on the same side, sometimes the right testicle and tibia only, sometimes the left, sometimes both; but always the tibia and testicle on the same side. The pain is constant, deep-seated, and wearying.

Let us now consider the phenomena by which an attack of asthma is generally ushered in. The patient goes to bed in his usual health, with or without premonitory symptoms; he goes to sleep, and sleeps for two or three hours; he then becomes distressed in his breathing, and dreams, perhaps, that he is under some circumstances that make his respiration difficult; while yet asleep, the characteristic wheezing commences, sometimes without disturbing the patient himself, to such a degree as to wake those in the same or an adjoining room, as if a whole orchestra of fiddles were tuning in his chest; perhaps he half wakes up and changes his position, by which he gets a little ease, and then falls asleep again, but only to have his distress and dreams renewed, and again partially to wake and turn. Shortly the increasing difficulty quite wakes him, but only perhaps for a minute or two: he sits up in bed in a distressing half-consciousness of his condition, gets a temporary abatement, sleep overpowers him, and he falls back to be again awoke and again sit up; and so this miserable fight between asthma and sleep may go on for an hour or more, the dyspnœa arousing the sufferer as soon as sleep is fairly established, and sleep again overpowering him as soon as the wakefulness and change of position have a little abated the extremity of his suffering. By and by the struggle ceases, sleep is no longer possible, the increasing dyspnœa does not allow the patient to forget himself for a moment, he becomes wide awake, sits up in bed to lie back no more, throws himself forward, plants his elbows on his knees, and with fixed head and elevated shoulders, labours for his breath like a dying man.

When once the paroxysm is established, the asthmatic offers a very striking and very distressing spectacle. If he moves at all, it is with great difficulty, creeping by stages from one piece of furniture to another. But most commonly he sits fixed in a chair, immovable, unable to speak, or even, perhaps, to move his head in answer to questions that may be put to him. His back is rounded and his gait stooping; indeed, his whole figure is deformed. His chest, back, shoulders, and head are fixed; he cannot even turn his head from side to side, but when he looks from object to object merely turns his eyes, like a person with a stiff neck; his shoulders are

---

[1] Chapter II. p. 85.

raised to his ears, and his head thrown back and buried between
them. In order the better to raise his shoulders, and at the same
time spare muscular effort in doing so, his elbows are fixed on the
arms of his chair, or his hands planted on his knees, or he leans
forward on a table, or sits across a chair and leans over the back
of it, or he stands grasping the back of a chair and throwing his
weight upon it,[1] or leaning against a chest of drawers or some piece
of furniture sufficiently high to rest his elbows on in a standing
position. At every breath his head is thrown back, his shoulders
still more raised, and his mouth a little open, with a gasping movement; his expression is anxious and distressed; the eyes are wide
open, sometimes strained, turgid, and suffused; his face is pallid,
and, if the dyspnœa is extreme and long, slightly cyanotic; the
labour of breathing is such that beads of perspiration stand on his
forehead, or even run in drops down his face, which his attendant
has constantly to wipe. He is so engrossed with his sufferings and
the labour of breathing that he seems unconscious of what is going
on around him; or else he is impatient and intolerant of the assi-
duities of those who are in vain trying to give him some relief.

If the bronchial spasm is protracted and intense, the heat of the
body falls; the oxygenation of the blood is so imperfectly performed,
from the sparing supply of air, that it is inadequate to the maintenance of the normal temperature. The extremities especially get
cold, and blue, and shrunk; I have known the whole body deathly
cold, and resist all efforts to warm it, for four hours. But while the
temperature is thus depressed, the perspiration produced by the
violent respiratory efforts may be profuse, so that the sufferer is at
the same time cold and sweating. It is this union of coldness and
sweat, combined with the duskiness and pallor of the skin, that gives
to the asthmatic so much the appearance of a dying man, and that
even sometimes makes the initiated fear that death is impending.

The pulse during severe asthma is always small, and small in
proportion to the intensity of the dyspnœa; it is so feeble sometimes
that it can hardly be felt. The explanation of this is very simple.
The imperfect supply of air produces capillary arrest—partial stasis
—of the pulmonary circulation; but a small quantity of blood is
therefore allowed to pass on to the left side of the heart, so that the
volume on which the left ventricle contracts, and which it impels
into the arterial system at each pulsation, is extremely small, and
barely sufficient to register itself at the wrist. That the small pulse
is due to pulmonary capillary arrest, itself due to the shutting off of
air from the lungs, is proved by the fact that immediately the paroxysm yields the pulse resumes its normal volume. I have never known
the small pulse absent in severe asthma; its very explanation proves
that it could not be.

[1] I have known a patient stand in this position for two days and nights, unable to
move.

One curious symptom of asthma, which I have found present in a large number of cases (I am not sure it is not universally present), but which I have never seen noticed in any treatise on the subject, is *itching under the chin*. I have often known that the breathing of asthmatics was tight, and told them so, from seeing them scratching and rubbing their chins. The itching is incessant, and of an indefinite, creeping character; but although it is impossible to help scratching it, the scratching does not relieve it. It is often accompanied with the same itching sensation over the sternum and between the shoulders, especially between the shoulders. It appears the moment the first tightness of breathing is felt, and goes off when the paroxysm has become confirmed—indeed, I think it is more pronounced in those slight and transitory tightenings of the breathing to which asthmatics are so liable (as, for example, after laughing) than in regular attacks. But I think it is the most strongly marked of all in the asthma that accompanies hay-fever. The sternal and interscapular portion of this itching is, I think, of easy explanation; its distribution to the chin is less easy to understand. According to the law that the pain arising from the irritation of a viscus shall be referred to the superficies, front and back, in the middle line and at a level with the viscus (a law illustrated by the seat of the pain in stomach, bowel, and uterine disease), the seat to which the sensation from bronchial irritation is referred is the sternum and between the blade bones. Thus, in bronchitis, the raw, scraping feeling that accompanies cough is sternal and interscapular; so that in relation to this asthmatic itching the fact would appear to be simply this—that while the impression on the bronchial nervous system produced by inflammation of its mucous membrane gives rise to sternal and interscapular *pain*, that produced by spasm of these tubes gives rise to sternal and interscapular *itching*. The itching of the chin must, I think, be of the same reflex character, and admit of the same explanation, but the reason of its locality is less apparent.

On stripping an asthmatic in the height of a paroxysm, an admirable example is seen of the immense array of muscles that become, on an emergency, accessory to respiration, and some idea is formed of the toil of the asthmatic, and the extremity of those sufferings that necessitate for their relief such extreme labour. All the muscles passing from the head to the shoulders, clavicles, and ribs are rigid, and the head is rendered a fixed point from which they can act on their respiratory attachments. Ordinarily these muscles, such as the splenii and scaleni, have their inferior attachments fixed, and move the head and neck; but now their upper attachment is fixed, and from it they act as mediate or immediate elevators of the ribs and distenders of the thoracic cavity; and this is how it is that the asthmatic is incapable of moving his head. By the contraction of the *trapezius* and *levator anguli scapulæ* the shoulders are raised to the ears, in order that the muscles proceeding from the shoulders to the ribs may act at advantage as elevators of these latter. The muscles of the back are so engaged in respiration that they cease to support the trunk, and the gait becomes stooping. At every inspiration the *sterno-mastoids* start out like cords, and produce by their sudden prominence a deep pit between their sternal attachments. I have already referred to the gaping descent of the lower jaw at each inspiration. Now, what is the explanation of this? What is its mechanism? I think the *rationale* of it is this: By its endeavours to raise the scapula the homo-hyoid muscle is strongly contracted at each inspiration; but its hyoid attachment being by far its most movable extremity, the contraction of the muscle tends rather to draw the hyoid bone down than to elevate the shoulder; and as the elevators of the hyoid bone—the mylo-hyoid, genio-hyoid, and digastric—are firmly contracted with a view of fixing it, the drawing down of the hyoid bone also draws down the jaw, and thus is produced the descent of the jaw at each inspiration, so that this gasping movement really depends on one of the depressors of the hyoid bone being, by virtue of its scapular attachment, also an accessory muscle of respiration, and being at the same time, from the loose and floating character of its superior attachment, unable to effect that interchange of its fixed and moving points that takes place with regard to the other extraordinary muscles of respiration. In the case of other accessory muscles of respiration, either extremity can be made the fixed one, and thus render the action of the muscle respiratory or non-respiratory, according to circumstances; if the lower extremity is fixed, as is ordinarily the case, the head or neck is moved, and the muscle is non-respiratory; if the upper extremity is fixed, the shoulders or ribs are raised, and the muscle is respiratory. But the upper attachment of the homo-hyoid not being firmly fixable, the muscle cannot transfer its contractions to its respiratory extremity, and thus, though theoretically, it is not actually a respiratory muscle. This explanation, if correct, is not uninteresting, as it offers an example of the maintenance of a type of action in spite of disturbing circumstances that necessarily make the action inoperative; it is an instance, if I may so express it, of morphological physiology, bearing the same relation to function as the retention, in obedience to type, of superfluous or modified appendages does to structure. I am not sure that the other depressors of the hyoid bone do not share in the action.

Meantime, all the muscles that increase the capacity of the chest are straining their utmost and starting into prominence at each inspiration; as each breath is drawn, every muscle is thrown out into bold relief, and since there are hardly any muscles of the trunk that are not mediately or immediately respiratory, the whole muscular system of the trunk may be mapped out in every part of its detail. The straining muscles are rendered all the more conspicuous from asthmatics being generally so thin.

But violent and laborious as are these respiratory efforts, they are abortive; although the muscles that should move the parietes of the chest are contracting to their utmost, no corresponding movements take place—the chest is almost motionless, its walls are fixed as in a vice, as if they could not follow the traction of their muscles, and this is really the case. This immobility, in spite of the violent action of the moving agent, is one of the most singular and striking appearances of asthmatic breathing. How different from the wide range of movement that follows even less considerable respiratory effort in one to and from whose lungs the ingress and egress of air is free!

One result of these straining efforts to fill the chest is a permanent distension of it; its walls are kept fixed in a condition of extreme inspiration. So great is this enlargement of the chest during the paroxysm that any article of dress that would ordinarily fit the waist cannot be brought together by two inches. But the chest is enlarged in every way; the diaphragm therefore descends, the abdomen therefore seems fuller, and its girth increased. This, I believe, is the principal cause of that abdominal distension of which asthmatics complain, and which is generally assigned to flatulence. As soon as the paroxysm goes off the chest and abdomen resume their original size. I do not see that anything is gained by this distension of the thoracic cavity; the only difference is that the volume of air locked up in the chest is rather larger, but no more is changed at each respiration, and it is the amount so changed, and not the quantity contained in the lungs, that relieves the demand of respiration. But air is the thing that is wanted, and inspiration is the act that ordinarily relieves that want; this keeping the chest, therefore, at a condition of extreme inspiration must be looked upon as an instinctive but blind and abortive effort to remedy that which is irremediable.

But let us take a nearer view, let us scrutinize more closely the breathing of the asthmatic in the height of his paroxysm.

It will be observed, in the first place, that the breathing, though intensely difficult, is not short; on the contrary, it is even sometimes longer than natural, so that not more than nine or ten respirations are taken in a minute. And this simple fact of the lengthening of the respiratory interval would of itself be sufficient to my mind to show what the condition of the air-tubes must be: that with such a demand for a rapid and often-renewed supply of air its supply and renovation should be so tardy cannot but be due to some difficulty of ingress and egress.

The coincidence of respiratory distress with prolonged respiratory interval always implies, I believe, stricture of some part of the air-passages; it implies a capacity for the full volume of air, with such a tenuity and penury of supply that the required quantity can only be got in and out by long and tedious effort. In a case of chronic laryngitis, in which the patient was literally dying from want of breath, I once counted the respirations, and found them seven in a minute, so slender was the stream of air and so long did it take before the required quantity could be drawn or driven through the narrowed glottis.

It will be further observed that the relative length of the inspiration and expiration is reversed—that instead of the inspiration being longer than the expiration, as is normally the case, the expiration is longer than the inspiration; that while the inspiration is very little longer than usual, sometimes even shorter, the expiration, instead of being the short and gentle collapse of natural breathing, is a difficult and prolonged effort by which the air is slowly and painfully driven out of the lungs; and so great sometimes is this lengthening out of the expiratory act that I have known it four or five times as long as the inspiration, occupying nearly the whole respiratory interval, instead of being half the length of it, or less, as in health. I know nothing like this modification of the respiratory rhythm in any other disease; I believe it is peculiar to asthma. In phthisis and emphysema there is a certain amount of prolongation of expiration, but nothing like this. In the most intense asthmatic breathing the difficulty of getting the air out of the chest is so great, the expiratory movement (with all its effort) so slight, and the quantity of air expelled so small, that, as if aware that the chest would never be emptied at that rate in time for the next inspiration, a violent involuntary effort comes to the assistance of the expiration, and pumps out the remainder of the air with a sudden jerk. This termination of a prolonged, ineffectual, and almost motionless expiration by a sudden expiratory jerk is characteristic of the intensest asthma, and occurs in no other form of dyspnœa whatever; whenever we see it we may be sure that the bronchial spasm is extreme. It is at expiration, too, that the asthmatic experiences the greatest distress.

Now, why should the impediment to respiration in asthma tell more on expiration than inspiration? Either there must be a greater obstacle to the egress than to the ingress of air, or, the obstacle being the same, the expiratory force is feebler than the inspiratory. The former of these suppositions I do not believe; I do not believe, for the reasons I have mentioned elsewhere, that there is increased bronchial contraction synchronous with each expiration: the latter of these suppositions physiological experiment contradicts;—it has been demonstrated that the expiratory force is *greater* than the inspiratory. Still, I believe the impediment affecting inspiration less than expiration does depend on an excess of inspiratory over expiratory power. I believe expiration in asthma to be actually, though not potentially, weaker than inspiration—that it has the power in reserve, but does not make use of it. Inspiration is normally muscular; expiration is not; and it seems that the muscular apparatus of expiration is less easily set in motion than that of inspiration. That there is the expiratory power in reserve, and that it is adequate to the instantaneous completion of the expiratory act, is

5

proved by the sudden jerk that expels the remainder of the inspired air.

As in all other dyspnœas, so in asthma, the moment the expiration is completed the inspiration begins—there is no pause, the
normal post-expiratory rest is lost.

Thus it will be seen that the breathing in asthma differs from
that of health in these particulars: 1st. Its frequency is modified,
sometimes being more, sometimes less frequent than natural; 2d.
Its rhythm is altered, expiration being greatly prolonged, and sometimes wound up by an involuntary effort peculiar, I believe, to
asthma; 3d. Expiration, instead of being a case of simple elastic
recoil, as in health, is a violent muscular effort; 4th. There is no
post-expiratory rest.

Such being the external phenomena of the breathing of asthmatics, what are the auscultatory sounds that accompany them?
They are exactly such as we should expect—exactly such as are
consistent with these external phenomena, and such as imply, if
the spasm is severe, an almost impassable bar to the ingress and
egress of air. On applying the ear to the chest we hear—respiratory murmur *none*; and that is not because it is drowned by other
sounds; if no other sounds are present it is equally inaudible; it is
because the conditions of its production do not exist, because sufficient air is not admitted to generate it; just as there is no respiratory murmur in the long-drawn inspiration of whooping-cough, or
beneath thoracic parietes fixed by pleurisy or intercostal rheumatism. And this suppression of the ordinary breathing sound is a
proof of the depressed standard at which respiration is being carried on, and of the completeness with which air is locked out of and
into the chest. The sounds that *are* heard are dry tube-sounds,
large and small—sonorous and sibilant rhonchi of every variety, of
every note and pitch, and in all parts of the chest, converting it
into a very orchestra; but the sounds are mostly sibilant, high and
shrill, resembling the chirping of a bird, the squeaking of a mouse,
or the mewing of a kitten. And this smallness of sound makes me
think that it is almost exclusively the smaller tubes that are the
seat of the constriction, whilst the diffusion of the sounds all over
the chest shows that constricted tubes exist everywhere.

There is one other fact, in relation to the sounds of asthma, that
I think is instructive, and that seems to me to imply that the points
of stricture are constantly changing their place, that spasm is constantly disappearing in one part and making its appearance in
another; and that fact is, that the sounds are continually changing
their character and site. On listening over a part of the chest
where a few minutes before you heard a loud shrill sibilus you find
it gone, while a part that just before was silent is the seat of a cho-
rus of piping. Now, if the sounds were of a moist character, if
they where caused by mucus, I grant that such an inference could
not be drawn, for sounds so caused may be, and constantly are,

suddenly removed by cough, or other dislodgment of the accumulated secretion; but in the early part of an attack of uncomplicated
spasmodic asthma there is no accumulation of mucus in the air-tubes
—they are dry; the narrowing of the tube, therefore, that gives
rise to the musical sound, being solely dependent on bronchial
spasm, solely admits of removal by the relaxation of that spasm;
and the frequent cessation and change of place of the pipings shows
that the spasm that causes them is transient and wandering.

The auscultation, then, of the asthmatic shows us these things:—
a. The almost perfect stagnation of air in the chest, in spite of
   the violent respiratory efforts.
β. That the tubes affected are generally very small.
γ. That tubes in all parts of the chest are simultaneously affected.
δ. That the points of constriction are constantly changing place.

Such, very feebly described, and with too much detail to make a
telling picture, is a fit of asthma. To be fairly imagined it should
be witnessed—to be fully appreciated it should be experienced.

The length of time required for the attack to attain its maximum
intensity differs very much in different cases. In some within a
quarter of an hour of the first seizure the patient seems at the point
of death, in others the dyspnœa creeps slowly on, getting deeper
and deeper for hours. The time that it lasts, too, differs greatly—
from a few minutes to many days. It is very rarely that it remains
long at its state of greatest intensity, in an hour or two the severity
of the paroxysm gives way, and, even if it does not completely
disappear, the patient experiences a sense of inexpressible relief.
In others the attacks come quickly on and as quickly and completely subside, so that in half an hour the whole thing may be over
and the patient as well as ever. This, however, is very rarely the
case, except as the result of the immediate adoption of remedial
measures, as when the patient on finding the asthma on him at once
gets out of bed and sits or stands, leaning against some piece of furniture, keeping himself thoroughly awake, or smokes *ad nauseam*, or
takes an emetic. Under these circumstances the attack will speedily and quickly pass off. In many cases it subsides soon after
breakfast, or towards noon, but the patient is *non compos* for the
rest of the day. In others it lasts the entire day, gradually abating
towards evening; the patient has a good night, and wakes well the
next morning. In others it gets gradually worse as night comes on,
and the second night is worse than the first. In some cases the
access and departure of the spasm are alike sudden, in others they
are both gradual. There is generally a marked time at which the
spasm yields and the patient passes from a state of agony to one of
very endurable suffering; he generally knows when this has taken
place and feels that the crisis of the fit is over, and often knows
exactly when to expect it, for the attacks are commonly very uniform
in this respect. In some cases the spasm remains at an unvarying
standard, and the sufferer grinds on all day without respite: much

more commonly, however, he experiences aggravations and abate-
ments, for half an hour breathing perhaps as if each breath would
be his last, then getting an hour or two's *comparative* ease, then
another paroxysm, then another exacerbation, and so on throughout
the day. These aggravations are frequently due to some exciting
cause—the taking of food, laughing, bodily exertion, yielding to
sleep—against which, therefore, as long as his attack lasts, the asthmatic is obliged most scrupulously to guard himself. Nothing is so
certain as food to induce these exacerbations, and since asthma in
no degree interferes with appetite the enforced starvation to which
the patient is reduced becomes an additional source of suffering;
fainting with hunger, he dares not let a particle of food pass his lips,
and as long as his paroxysm continues so long must he starve. I
have known several cases in which each attack involved from thirty-
six to forty-eight hours of total abstinence from food. In one, for
example, the patient habitually ate nothing after an early dinner;
on his asthmatic days he took nothing whatever, went to bed exhausted but with his asthma gone, and awoke the next morning very
weak but perfectly well. If he yielded to the temptation of taking
any food his asthma got worse instead of better towards evening,
the night was sleepless, and the second day as bad as the first: so
that on the occasion of each attack he took nothing from dinner on
one day to the breakfast of the next day but one, an interval of
forty-two hours; in this way alone could he limit the duration of his
attacks to a single day. The more inane and exhausted the asthmatic is, the more disposed is his paroxysm to give way—it seems
starved out, as it were.

When the spasm finally subsides it generally does so coincidently
with the first appearance of expectoration. Up to that time the
wheezing has been dry, and there has been no cough, or, if any, a
short, single, dry one; the first appearance of moist sounds and
loose cough is the harbinger of relief. It was this circumstance
that induced Dr. Bree to believe that the exciting cause of asthma
was some offending humour in the bronchial tubes which the expectoration discharged and which the previous asthma was the abortive
attempt to get rid of. For the reasons of my rejection of Dr. Bree's
theory, and for what I believe to be the true explanation of the relation of this mucous expectoration to the spasm and its final relief,
I must refer the reader to the Introductory Analysis of the Theories
of Asthma. The amount of this expectoration and the length of time
that it lasts depend on the length, and probably also in some degree
on the intensity, of the previous attack. If the attack is very short
—an hour or so—the expectoration of a pellet or two of mucus is all
that takes place; if it lasts the entire day, in addition to the expectoration in the evening which winds up the attack, it will appear
again the next morning and even for two or three mornings after;
if, however, the attack is protracted over several days, the expectoration may continue for a week or two. It is curious after how

slight and transient a tightening of breathing, this mucous exudation will invariably appear. Many asthmatics are liable, after laughing, or after taking food, or inhaling dust or smoke, to little paroxysms of the true asthmatic dyspnœa, lasting perhaps five or ten minutes, and then over; each of these little attacks is sure to be followed in a few minutes by the expectoration of one or two little portions of this mucus, sometimes so immediately that its discharge appears to be the occasion of the relief of the breathing.

In character this mucus is very curious; it is in distinct little pellets, about the size of a pea, that are coughed up and expectorated with the greatest facility, unattached to anything else: they are of the consistency of jelly or thick arrowroot, of a pale gray colour, of an opalescent transparency, and a saltish taste.

On examining a portion of this material with the microscope it is seen to consist of a nearly homogeneous viscid matter, containing innumerable corpuscles of a peculiar appearance, and of whose nature I am at the present time not at all certain. I am not aware that I have seen any exactly similar bodies in any other material. Most of them are spherical, but not round, being many of them polyhedra with the angles rounded off. They are pale, homogeneous, or so slightly granular as to be nebulous, and look darker or lighter according as they are in or out of focus. (Fig. 2, a a.) They remind one, the roundest of them, of pus cells more than anything else, and in looking at some specimens you might almost imagine you are looking at pus; but they differ from pus in being rather larger, in not being perfectly spherical, and in containing no nuclei. It is impossible to make out a cell-wall in them. They are in diameter about $\frac{1}{1800}$ of an inch. The above description applies to the most spherical of them, but there are others mixed with these of very different forms—oval, oblong (b), fusiform (c), caudate (d), some almost linear—but evidently identical in nature, of the same refracting power, and passing into them by inseparable gradations of form. Though these structures look cellular, I cannot make out in them the elements of a true cell—nucleus, nucleolus, and cell-wall; and there are certain appearances about them that make me think they are rather spheroids of a firm but softish material not contained in any envelope. One of these

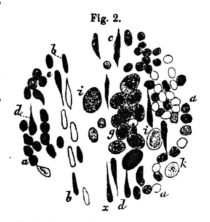

Fig. 2.

Cellular elements in sputum of asthma × 200

appearances is that many of the elongated particles are linearly and parallelly arranged (b b), as if they were drawn out, and as if their shape had been altered from that of the sphere by the traction of the viscid material in which they were suspended: this change of form from the drawing out of the mucus in which they are imbedded would imply considerable softness.   Another appearance is that some of them are drawn out into thin processes, making them caudate, or fusiform.   Some of these processes end indefinitely—melt away gradually, and become invisible, and are evidently not bounded by cell-wall (x).   Some of the fusiform and caudate forms are distinctly granular, and have a granular and indefinite outline, and yet, through connecting links of form and appearance, we can see they are the same as the clear homogeneous spheroids.

What are these bodies?   Are they pus cells?   Clearly not, as I have already intimated; their size, shape, diversities, reaction of acetic acid, and the absence of nuclei, all forbid.   Are they modifications of epithelium cells?   This, in spite of what Kölliker says as to the rarity with which the epithelium of the respiratory mucous membrane is detached, I was at first inclined to believe; especially did some of the caudate or conical forms look like columnar epithelium (e); but to this view, too, the absence of nuclei, the softness and homogeneity of the cells, if cells they can be called, and the forms of many of them, seem an insuperable objection.   Are they nuclei of epithelium?   They seem to be more like this than anything else—large, rapidly-generated cytoblasts.   If so, it would appear that the congested mucous membrane in asthma is the seat of an exuberant development of cell-germs, excessive in size as in number, and so soft that the slightest pressure or traction alters their form.

Besides these, there are numerous large spherical or oval cells (g) from $\frac{1}{500}$ to $\frac{1}{800}$ of an inch in diameter, mostly occurring in groups, which are coarsely granular and opaque from being filled with particles of black carbonaceous matter.   These cells are always numerous in those gray patches so abundant in the sputum of those who breathe a smoky atmosphere.   In some sputa, as those of forgemen and smiths, these patches are almost black, and here these cells are very abundant.   I have never seen them in the white expectoration of those who breathe a pure country air.   There can be no doubt that the particles with which they are filled are the carbonaceous contamination of the respired air.   How do these particles get into the cells?   Are there certain cells generated by the respiratory mucous surface, whose special *rôle* it is to attract within themselves, and thus isolate and throw off, atmospheric impurities?   Are they cells at all, or are they mere aggregations of carbon particles with a mucous investment, assuming a spherical form in obedience to mere physical laws?   I think the appearance of a cell-wall round them is too decided for this supposition; but I am at a loss to understand how particles of such a size as some of the granules are can get inside of the homogeneous membrane of the cell-wall.

There are, lastly, a few cells exactly like these carboniferous cells in size and form—large, oval, delicate—but instead of being filled with carbonaceous matter, they are pale and finely granular (*i i*); some of them have the slightest trace of opaque black particles in their centre (*k*), and they are all evidently, to my mind, identical with the others, minus the carbon granules.

Sometimes, however, the pulmonary congestion is so great that the vessels relieve themselves in another way. We all know that it is not at all an uncommon event in the clinical history of some cases of heart-disease (especially obstructive mitral) for hæmoptysis to occur —the obstruction of the pulmonary circulation arrives at such a pitch that the congested vessels are unable any longer to resist their contents, they give way and blood is poured out. (I have seen this hemorrhage from congestion prove fatal in a few hours.) Just the same thing happens in asthma. If the shutting off of air by the constricted tubes is very complete the decarbonization of the blood is arrested to such a degree, and the consequent capillary *stasis* becomes so considerable, that, as in the other case, the vessels give way under the pressure of their contents, and relieve themselves by rupture. The intensity of the asthma, however, is not a measure of the probability or the amount of hemorrhage, for in some of the most severe cases it never occurs. There must be, I think, some concurrent condition—heart-disease, or a hemorrhagic tendency—for it to happen. But severe the asthma *must* be; it never comes on in slight attacks. Its access is sudden, its cessation or subsidence gradual, and it lasts sometimes for hours, or even days, after the attack has gone off. I have known it last a month before it has entirely ceased. Where it has once occurred it is very apt to occur again; the fact being, I suppose, that where the pulmonary circulation has once been subjected to such tension, and had to bear the stress of so considerable an obstruction, it never quite recovers its original tone, and is ever afterwards more disposed to yield when again subjected to the obstructing force.

In quantity the blood is generally not more than streaks and patches mixed with the mucus. Sometimes, however, perfectly pure blood is coughed up and although the quantity is generally small—a teaspoonful or so—I have known it amount to profuse hemorrhage, from half a pint to a pint.

CHAPTER IV.

CLINICAL HISTORY OF ASTHMA (*continued.*)—PHENOMENA OF THE INTERVALS.

Periodicity. A characteristic but not constant symptom.—Diurnal periodicity that of organic asthma; weekly; monthly; annual, as in winter, hay, and æstival asthma. —Intrinsic and extrinsic periodicity.—Tendency to habitude. Cases.—Change of type.—Capriciousness.—Caprice of the disease in general; caprice of individual cases. Physiognomy.—Time of life of first access. Influence of sex: its implication.—Is asthma hereditary?

HAVING in the previous chapter described the phenomena of the asthmatic paroxysm, I purpose in the present one to direct attention to those general features of asthma that characterize it as a whole —those different events that develop themselves in the course of the disease, and whose variations and combinations impart the distinctive features and individuality to each case. Such general features of the disease arise from the relations of the paroxysms to each other, their relations to the subject of them in respect to age, sex, &c., the modifications they undergo, and certain of the effects they produce, and may be called, in opposition to the phenomena of the *paroxysm*, the phenomena of the *intervals*, or, perhaps more correctly, the phenomena of the *disease*.

Of these events in the clinical history of asthma, the principal are the following:—

1. Periodicity; 2. Habitude; 3. Change of Type; 4. Tendency; 5. Capriciousness; 6. Physiognomy; 7. Time of life of first access; 8. Influence of Sex; 9. Hereditariness.

I. *Periodicity.*—Asthma is one of the few diseases that can be strictly pronounced periodic. It is not merely paroxysmal, it is periodic; the paroxysms occur at regular and definite periods. And this periodicity may be said to be typically characteristic of the disease; it is the most pronounced in those cases that are in other respects the most uncomplicated and best marked specimens of it. But although the absence of periodicity in a given case deprives the disease of one of its best marked features, it is by no means constant; in some cases it is but slightly marked—the periods vary a good deal; and in some it is entirely lost. In others, however, the regularity is most curious; as the period characteristic of the particular case recurs, the attack is predicted with the greatest certainty and never fails to appear at the right time—never misses, never anticipates, never postpones. In the length of the intervals, although in each

case it is constant and characteristic, there is the greatest variety
—from a day to a year. Many of these intervals appear to be
arbitrary, and one cannot make out at all why they should be, as it
were, chosen: many of them, however, are natural—the measures of
certain cycles, the period of recurrence of certain conditions, either
in the external world or within the body, so that their agency in
determining the frequency of the paroxysms is easily intelligible,
inasmuch as they measure the interval from one occurrence of the
exciting cause, or the condition of susceptibility, to another. Such
periods are a day, a week, a month, a year; and these are all of them
very common measures of the asthmatic interval. For example,
diurnal asthma is very common. A patient comes to you and tells
you that every morning precisely at the same hour, say four o'clock,
a dry wheezing difficulty of breathing wakes him, and obliges him
to sit up in bed, or leave his bed altogether, and go through, in short,
all the sufferings of a regular asthmatic attack. Such a case is at
the present time under my observation. A poor woman, aged 52
(Mary Baker, Case 33, Appendix), who had never had asthma before, came to me at the hospital, and told me that for the last five
months she has been awoke every morning between four and five
o'clock with severe dry wheezing dyspnœa, obliging her to sit up
for about an hour, or get out of bed, labouring for her breath with
great distress. After that time the urgency of the dyspnœa abates,
the wheezing gets moister, a slight expectoration comes to her relief, and she is able to lie back and get a little imperfect sleep: it is
not, however, till she has been up about an hour—that is, about
eight o'clock—that the difficulty of breathing entirely leaves her.
When I saw her, in the middle of the day, she was breathing as well
as I was; and so she continues all day. She goes to bed quite well,
lies down as well as ever, and sleeps undisturbed till four or five the
next morning when she is awoke as before.

Now this diurnal period is very common where asthma is associated with chronic bronchitis, heart-disease, &c. Indeed it is *the*
period of impure asthma, of asthma grafted on organic disease of the
heart or lungs; and wherever I meet this invariable morning recurrence I always suspect it is not simple asthma, and look out for some
permanent heart or lung mischief. And one can easily understand
why this should be so. The condition of sleep, and the recumbent
posture, bring a diurnal aggravation of the permanently existing
conditions giving rise to the bronchial spasm; and the time of the
night at which the asthma comes on and the patient is awaked depends upon the length of time required for this diurnal aggravation
to produce such an amount of asthmatic contraction of the bronchial
tubes as to render the continuance of sleep impossible. If the organic cause of the asthma exists to any considerable extent the
patient will be sure to have the asthma every night; for the organic
condition is *constant*, and it will be impossible for the patient to assume the horizontal position and the condition of sleep long without

this aggravation of conditions giving rise to asthma. The impeded circulation through the lungs in heart-disease, or the inflamed and irritable state of the bronchial mucous membrane in chronic bronchitis, is not adequate, while the patient is awake and erect, to the production of bronchial spasm; but recumbency and sleep soon render them so, partly by aggravating them, partly by exalting reflex susceptibility in the way I have more fully explained in the second chapter.

Once in the twenty-four hours the patient lies down and sleeps, and, therefore, once in the twenty-four hours he has an attack of asthma. But were it not for the organic disease (say heart-disease), the mere sleep and horizontal position would not produce that embarrassment and arrears of the respiratory function which induce the asthmatic spasm.

I would say then, wherever the asthmatic period is diurnal look out for organic disease. But this rule does not always hold good. The nightly recurrence of asthma does not necessarily imply that it has an organic basis. In the woman I mentioned just now there was not a trace of organic disease. The respiratory sounds were perfectly natural; there was no prolongation of expiration; the breathing was very deliberate with plenty of surplus time; the post-expiratory rest was long; the heart was quite normal. I have at the present time under my care another case precisely similar in this respect (Mary Anne Frost, Case 25, Appendix).

Where the asthma is dependent upon the state of the digestion the diurnal period is very common. The patient will have an attack every afternoon after dinner, lasting for two or three hours till digestion is over. This is so very common that I shall not cite cases of it. As a rule we may say that where the period is diurnal the attack depends on some daily-recurring exciting cause. But even this is not universally true; for I have known cases where the attack recurred daily under such varying circumstances, and at times so free from any discoverable exciting cause, that the reason of its daily rhythm appeared to be unaccountable. In these cases we must seek another explanation of the diurnal period, to which I shall refer presently.

Once a week is a very common interval—at the same hour of the same day, as the week comes round, and at no other time. I remember one very remarkable instance of this in an asthmatic boy, who for years had an attack every Monday morning. On every other morning in the week he awoke well; but as surely as Monday morning returned so surely did his asthma appear. A suspicion arose on the part of his parents that he was malingering. His lessons on Monday morning were different from those on other days, and they thought he might be shamming, or at any rate making the most of his complaint, in order to escape school. It was not till this had been going on for a long time that the real cause became evident:—on Sunday evening he took supper, on other evenings not, and the Monday morning's asthma was caused by the Sunday evening's supper. On taking supper on other occasions it was found that asthma invariably followed, and this cleared up the Monday morning's mystery. He left the suppers off, and the regular Monday morning's asthma vanished. It is probable that in most asthmas with the weekly period the interval is due to the recurrence of the same exciting cause in some part of that seven days' circle in which life, in all Christian countries, moves.

The fortnightly interval, which is by no means a rare one, is probably due to the same cause; the weekly rhythm determining the period, but the interval proper to the case being longer than once a week. I have such a case under my care at the present time, in a young asthmatic who for some years past has had an attack regularly once a fortnight, and, as in the preceding case, always on the Monday morning. He cannot however attribute it to eating supper on Sunday night, for he never does so; but he can and does assign it to something peculiarly characterizing Sunday, and believes that it is caused by the unusual amount of exercise that he takes on that day.

The monthly interval, as far as I have observed, is due to the menstrual period. I have never seen nor heard of any case of it, well and regularly marked, except in women, and in cases of what appeared to be clearly hysterical asthma. But of hysterical asthma it is, as might be expected, the characteristic interval; and I should always in a monthly asthma in a woman look out for a uterine cause.

Asthma occurring once a year is almost always winter asthma, and almost always a complication of asthma with bronchitis—muscular spasm engrafted on inflammation of the mucous membrane of the air-passages. These cases, as I shall show elsewhere, are not really cases of asthma at all; that is, not primary and idiopathic asthma. Asthma they must be; wherever there is paroxysmal constriction of the air-passages there is asthma; but the asthma is not the substantive disease, it is a mere appendage to the bronchitis. Such cases are always well from spring to autumn, and their winter asthma is not one attack but an irregular succession of attacks, varying as the bronchitis. There is, however, one kind of annual asthma that is not a winter asthma but a summer asthma; and that is, that curious disease called *hay-fever* or *hay-asthma*. This begins and ends with the hay season, and varies in the time of year according as the hay season is early or late. As long as the grass is in flower it persists, with that it ceases. Its visits are therefore restricted to about a month or six weeks in the early summer. It is not constant throughout this time as one attack, but comes and goes with those other symptoms of irritation of the respiratory mucous membrane of which it is a part. The neighbourhood of hay, bright, hot, dusty sunshine, a full meal, laughter, &c., suffice at any time during the hay season, to bring it on. It often affects a sort of diurnal rhythm, being generally worse at night. While this condition lasts the asthma is often so severe as to deprive the sufferer of sleep for nights together, and he leaves his bed in the morning pallid, blear-eyed, and worn out. When the hay season is over every symptom vanishes, and for ten or eleven months the patient may calculate on a perfect immunity from even the slightest asthmatic sensation.

I find there is a third form of annually-recurring asthma besides these two, the winter and the hay asthma, it is asthma whose severe attacks are confined to the hot weather of the late summer and early autumn. It is not at all uncommon for asthma to be so much worse at this time of the year—about August, and a little before or after—that it may be almost said to be confined to this period; the manifestations of the asthmatic tendency at other times of the year being so slight as hardly to attract any attention. I possess the notes of several cases in which this autumnal recurrence of the disease was well marked. Why asthma should be worse in hot weather I think would be difficult to explain; of the fact there is no question. Even in cases that exist all the year round it will frequently be found to be worse in sultry July weather than at any other time, and more especially if the weather is thundery as well as hot. I have the notes of as many, I should think, as six cases in which the connection between thunder and asthma was well marked.

The intervals, however, which many cases of regular periodic asthma choose, are, though constant, quite arbitrary, as, for instance, ten days, a fortnight, three months.

There is one curious circumstance about asthma that clearly shows that its periodicity is inherent—part of the disease. It is, that each attack seems to impart, for a time, an immunity from a repetition of it. For some time after an attack, the time varying according to the interval characteristic of that particular case, the patient may expose himself to the ordinary exciting causes of the paroxysms without the slightest fear of inducing one. As this period draws to a close, exposure to the provocatives of the attacks is attended with more and more risk; and when it has transpired the slightest imprudence is certain to bring on a fit. Indeed, so great does the asthmatic tendency after a while become, that no amount of care will succeed in warding it off.

For example, suppose that the exciting cause of the attacks is food, unwholesome in character, or taken late in the day, and suppose that the interval is monthly. For a week or two after the attack the patient may take supper with impunity; towards the end of the month he does so at great risk; when the month is up he does so with the certainty of bringing on his disease; but he may keep it at bay for some days by extraordinary care in his diet. Beyond that time, however, the most scrupulous care will not avail to postpone the paroxysm. This curious feature, in which asthma so much resembles epilepsy, suggests to one's mind the idea that each attack is a sort of clearing shower; that in the intervals between the attacks an unknown something—that particular condition of nervous system in which the peculiarity of the asthmatic consists—accumulates, and that each paroxysm is the discharge of this accumulated condition. At any rate, this is the sort of idea that the phenomena suggest to one's mind, and I am not sure, a mere analogy as it appears, that it does not come nearer to the true expression of the pathology of the truly periodic non-organic cases than any other illustration or explanation that could be offered.

But we must not run away with the idea that an exact periodicity is by any means a constant feature of asthma. In the *majority* of cases, if asthmatics are asked how often their attacks occur, they will mention some definite period, although their specification may not be precise, or may be accompanied with the qualification that it varies a little—*about* every ten days or a fortnight, or *about* every two months. In those cases in which the occurrence of an attack depends on the occurrence of some known exciting cause the degree of regularity will, of course, depend upon the regularity of the recurrence of that cause, which is often a mere approximative regularity; and it so happens that many of the provocatives of asthma are quite arbitrary in the period of their recurrence, as, for instance, a debauch, a late dinner, a fog, and may, some of them, be varied at will. In these cases of course all exact periodicity would be lost; the cause being irregular, so will be the attacks; and in those cases where the cause is entirely under the control of the individual, as, for instance, where it depends on the kind of food or time of taking it, the attack may be brought on at any time and as often as the asthmatic wills; or, by rigid abstention from the exciting cause, the period may be indefinitely prolonged. I have known, for example, the same asthmatic bring on an attack twice a week because he dined late and unwholesomely twice in that time, and keep off an attack for many months by simply abstaining from this one exciting cause. Of course if he had dined late and largely once a week, or once a month, his asthma would have been periodic, with those respective intervals.

There are, however, a large number of cases of pure, uncomplicated spasmodic asthma, in which, without any recognized exciting cause of irregular recurrence, all trace of periodicity is lost. The patient does not know when to expect his attack. He may have one in a twelvemonth, he may have one to-morrow, he may have four in a month, he may go years without one; it may never occur at two intervals alike, and when it does occur he is perfectly at a loss to say why it should choose that particular period. The time of its recurrence and its frequency are alike inexplicable. He may be living in perfect health and daily dread.

To express summarily, then, what appear to be the facts with regard to the perioditity of asthma, we may say—

1. That asthma is typically periodic.

2. That, though there is a period for each case, there is no particular period for the disease in general.

3. That the periodicity of asthma is of two kinds, *intrinsic* and *extrinsic*, the latter a spurious periodicity, dependent on the periodic recurrence of the exciting cause; the former, the true essential periodicity, independent of all external circumstances.

4. That periodicity, though a common, is not a universal feature of asthma.

II. *Tendency to Habitude.*—All those who are familiar with asthma, must have observed in it a disposition to habitude—a disposition to maintain and constantly repeat any peculiarity it may have acquired. And this is probably due to the very same tendency of the affection that makes it periodic, to the tendency to repetition, to its being essentially a repetitive disease—the attacks are repeated not only in respect to the interval at which they occur, but in all other circumstances and particulars—the time of day or night at which the paroxysms come on, the length of time they last, their provocatives, *lœdentia* and *juvantia*, and peculiarities in every respect. And that this maintenance of all the circumstances, both in the intervals and the attacks, *does* depend upon this disposition to habit, this disposition to repeat again what once has been, and that it is not due to the phenomena of each case being an essential and inherent part of the disease, is proved by the fact, that if the spell of this repetition is in any particular once broken, the feature that has thus lapsed will stay away; that its absence (although, perhaps, in the first place due to some temporary cause) will be, like its presence, repeated; and, on the other hand, that any peculiarity that has once been acquired (although, perhaps, from some transient and accidental circumstance), will, as the time comes round, recur, and thus be finally adopted among the symptoms, and become a constituent part of the clinical phenomena. There are hardly any circumstances of the disease that may not thus be lost and acquired, and therefore hardly any whose exact maintenance is not due to this tendency to repetition, rather than to their being an essential part of the disease. And thus it happens, that though there are no two cases of asthma that do not strikingly differ, and although in a course of years the features of any one case may be entirely changed, yet there is no disease of a paroxysmal nature in which the consecutive attacks are more exactly the counterpart of each other, or in which an uniform type of phenomena is more rigidly adhered to.

One of the results of this is, that the asthmatic becomes thoroughly "up" in his own case; every symptom is an old acquaintance to him; he recognizes the slightest indications, and can predict every event of his disease exactly as it will happen; he knows when an attack is coming on long before others can see any sign of it; he knows when it will go off; he soon comes to learn, too, by this exactly repeated experience, what he may do, and what he may not; what will do him harm, and what good; and thus often becomes his own best physician. I know of no disease in which the medical attendant gets more valuable hints from his patients, and none in which the opinion of the latter is more to be relied on.

A clearer idea of this peculiarity of asthma will perhaps be obtained by the narration of a few illustrative cases, than by any attempt at a general statement or description of it.

A gentleman, who had long suffered from violent spasmodic asthma, went in the summer of 1843 to Ryde. He awoke, the morning after his arrival, miserably bad, and had to rise from his bed about five, and sit leaning forwards on pillows placed on a table; in this position, in an hour or two, he got ease, and remained well for the rest of the day; and, as he had been to Ryde before and been as well there as elsewhere, he hoped his attack had passed away. The next morning, however, he awoke at four o 'clock, still worse; the next, at three, worse; the next night he hardly lay down at all, and left his bed at two. He then thought it was time to be off, and left by the steamer that morning. He was, however, too bad to proceed farther than Southampton that day. The next morning, after a good night, he awoke perfectly well, and stayed at Southampton a week. He then thought he would go back to Ryde, and try the experiment again. He returned, and the next morning, to his delight, found himself well. He then felt he was safe, and stayed at Ryde a month, with a degree of immunity from his disease quite unusual for him at his ordinary residence—indeed, without any asthmatic sensation the whole time; and I have no doubt he might have stayed there six months with an equally unbroken immunity. His second visit began well, and therefore continued well; but if he had persisted in his first attempt his visit would probably have been one of uninterrupted asthma. His return to Southampton broke the habit, and enabled him to start afresh.

An asthmatic patient, living in a county town in the South of England, informed me that there was a village about two miles from the town, to which his family went in the summer, but to which he never dare go, because his breathing was so bad there. One summer he went there, expecting to be obliged to leave the next day as usual; but, to his surprise, awoke the following morning well. He took the hint, and stayed there three months in unbroken health, free even from the mild form of asthma to which he was accustomed in the town. On his return to the town his usual asthma reappeared. All subsequent attempts to repeat the experiment have failed; he has never been able to make another "good start."

A gentleman, who lost his asthma some years ago on going to London, has found since that whenever he goes into the country it returns. It frequently begins the very evening of his arrival; and even if he goes to bed well it is sure to wake him about three o'clock in the morning, Then, for the rest of his visit, he has no peace; he has to sit up half the night, and gets no more than two or three hours' sleep before he is obliged to get up again. Nothing will do but his return to London. On some rare occasions, however, for some unknown reason, the asthma has not appeared on the night of his arrival in the country, and then he is sure to be well for the whole of the rest of his visit, however long it may be. As the first night is, so will be all. But when a visit to the country has once lit up his asthma, so inveterate is the tendency of the disease to keep up what has once been set going, that, although he returns to London, and to the same conditions and habits as before in every respect, it may be weeks before the asthmatic tendency which has been excited subsides. I have known him pass nine and even twelve months in Town without a symptom of asthma, as free from it as a person who has never suffered from it, so that he has said he had almost forgotten what the feeling of asthma was—could lie low at head, eat a supper, and take any liberties he liked with himself. But after a visit to the country has thrown his disease into a state of activity, although returning to London to the same house, the same room, the same occupations and habits, he has experienced for weeks his old morning asthmatic sensations, has been obliged to sleep higher at head, to eschew suppers or even late dinners, and to take the same precautions as he would in the country. After a time these symptoms have gradually died out, and he has shaken down into his old condition; so that he looks with great dread upon going into the country, not so much on account of the asthma during the few days he is there, as because, when it has once been set going, he does not know how long it may continue after his return to Town.

One patient informs me that whenever he is well at the commencement of a frost he is sure to be well as long as the frost lasts. Another states that although his dyspnœa was usually confined to the morning, he would often for a month together experience a slight attack every day after dinner, lasting for two or three hours, so that he has sometimes gone without his dinners to avoid the attack. Then for three or six months, perhaps, he would be free from these after-dinner fits, and then they would come on again. Sometimes they would habitually come on after supper; sometimes for weeks together his breath would be very bad of an afternoon, and then clear up in the evening, and he would have a good night; at others he would be quite well throughout the day, and bad at night; *but always the same for many days and weeks together*—the habitude, the diurnal rhythm, always strongly marked.

I might go on multiplying examples to almost any length, but I think I have cited enough to prove and illustrate this curious feature of the disease.

The rule, then, appears to be, that if asthma is subjected to unchanging external influences its cycle of phenomena will go on repeating themselves with a marvellous exactness, but that the maintenance of this unvarying repetition is strictly dependent on the maintenance of identical external conditions, and that any change, however trifling, is capable of breaking the existing habit and of introducing fresh phenomena. Hence we get a practical rule of considerable importance.—If the asthmatic is going on well, leave well alone; keep him as he is; do not try any experiments with him; for an unfavourable change, once acquired, may persist with unmanageable pertinacity. If, on the other hand, he is going on ill, if his case has got into a rut, give it a shake, make some change, *any* change, no matter whether the object is very definite or the therapeutics very rational, in the hope that by breaking the existing habit the patient's condition may be improved. It is a hazardous thing to make any change in the "surroundings" of an asthmatic, if his symptoms are quiescent; for while the caprice and uncertainty of the disease deprive us of the power of saying what the result of that change will be, its tendency to repetition deprives us of the power of saying when it will end. On the other hand, the most blind and purposeless treatment may be attended with the happiest results, merely by acting as a disturbing force and breaking the chain of repetition.

III. *Change of Type.*—Having directed attention to two characteristics of asthma—its periodicity and habitude—in which it shows a tenacity of type and an aversion to change, I must now say a few words *per contra*, and show that in certain ways it affects change and is a peculiarly mutable disease. This may at first sight appear somewhat inconsistent and contradictory, but, if true, it *cannot* be so; and a closer examination will show that it *is not* so. The changefulness of asthma is quite consistent with its periodicity and its tendency to habitude. Its sameness is an iterated sameness, a constant and frequent repetition of like phenomena; its changes, on the other hand, are slow, gradually brought about by slight and almost imperceptible variations in these recurrent phenomena. This applies to one form of its changefulness—its tendency to change of type: the other, its capriciousness, must be admitted as qualifying, and rendering less marked and perfect, both its periodicity and habitude.

It is very rare to meet a case of asthma over which considerable changes do not pass in the course of years. In the severity of the attacks, in their character, in their duration, in the length of their intervals, in the time of day at which they occur, in their provocatives, in the remedies that control them, in the condition of the patient in the intervals, in the simplicity or complicity of the disease —in all these points asthma is prone to change. Independently of the changes that necessarily take place in the progress of a case, either towards a more severe or confirmed state or towards recovery, there are others that can neither be considered progressive nor regressive, but which are so considerable, and which so completely alter the features of the case, that in a few years it would not be recognized as the same. From being irregular the symptoms have perhaps become confirmed; from being occasional they have become stated; attacks that were formerly confined to the morning now extend throughout the day; remedies that were formerly infallible

6

have now become worthless; a more scrupulous care is necessary in avoiding possible excitants, whose number is greatly increased; the time in the twenty-four hours in which the paroxysm occurs is changed from morning to evening, or from evening to morning; and so on.

One very common change in the type of asthma—so common that it may be said to be its normal history—is as follows: At first the paroxysms are of great intensity, and occur at distant intervals, and between them the breathing is perfectly free and clear. As the case progresses the attacks become milder but more frequent. At last they become so mitigated that there can hardly be said to be any exacerbations of the dyspnœa at all. But in the meantime there has gradually grown up a constant dyspnœa, which never goes off in the intervals between the paroxysms, and which, from being at first very slight, almost inappreciable (indeed, in the first part of the case not existing at all), becomes very considerable, and an abiding source of distress to the patient, embarrassing his conversation and impeding his movements, but often, strange to say, less observed by the sufferer himself than by those about him. Thus, by the mitigation of attacks and the gradual development of dyspnœa in the intervals, a paroxysmal has been changed for an abiding condition. This is in part a change for the better, in part a change for the worse; for while the asthmatic no longer suffers from the agony of his paroxysms, and may be said rather to experience inconvenience than suffering, yet he now never feels the lightness and freedom of untrammelled breathing. Moreover, an abiding dyspnœa, however slight, affects more the general health than any intensity of paroxysm, implies a worse state of things for the present, and is more ominous for the future.

This gradual change in the phasis of asthma, which is the history of the majority of chronic cases, arises from the operation of three coexisting causes: a gradual diminution of nervous irritability as life advances, diminishing the tendency to spasm, and mitigating the paroxysm; a gradual loss of reparative power, so that the temporary mischief to the lung left by each attack is less recovered from in the intervals; and thirdly, the accumulated disorganization of the lung from the continued operation of its cause. The process goes on for years; and the change is so gradual that it is only by comparing himself with what he was some time before, that the patient recognizes it. The experience of many asthmatics will, I am sure, bear me out in this description.

IV. *Capriciousness.*—One of the most singular features of asthma, and one which it possesses to a degree perhaps not possessed by any other disease except by hysteria, is its unaccountable *caprice*. It is always puzzling its victim and his friends by the exhibition of some unexpected vagary, giving him pleasant and unpleasant surprises, raising his hopes and then disappointing them, and altogether confounding his calculations. One may say of asthma as Horace did of Tigellius—"Nil fuit unquam sic impar sibi."

Asthma is doubly capricious: the disease in general is capricious, and each case is capricious in itself.

The caprice of the disease in general is shown in the extreme un-likeness of different cases to one another. Not only are they unlike, but they exhibit the strongest contrarieties and oppositeness—in their behaviour to remedies, in their causation, in their paroxysms, in every point, in fact, of their clinical history. One case is better in dense crowded cities, another in the open country; one likes a low damp situation, another a high and dry one; one a relaxing air suits, another a bracing one; one flies from the place which another seeks; one is confined to a spot in which another would die in a year; one is better in winter, another in summer, a third is equally bad all the year round; in one the attacks are entirely under the influence of the stomach, in another food makes no difference; one knows as well as possible when he is going to have an attack, another has no warning; in one the attacks occur with the regularity of clock-work, in another there is not a trace of periodicity; in one ipecacuan is the cause, in another it is the cure; in one nitre-paper acts like a charm, in another it is worthless; one patient says he would as soon be without life as without stramonium, another might as well smoke so much dried cabbage-leaves.

There are three questions in relation to the clinical history of asthma on which, in concluding this part of my subject, I would make a few observations.

At what age is asthma most disposed to come on?

What appears to be the influence of sex as affecting liability to asthma?

Is asthma hereditary?

V. *Time of Life of First Access.*—There appears to be no time of life at which asthma may not make its appearance—from the earliest infancy to old age. The extremes of life, and any part of life between those extremes, are obnoxious to it. A few days after birth the infant may give unmistakable evidence of it; or the old man, after spending a long life without an asthmatic symptom, may suddenly become the victim of it. There are some periods of life, however, at which it is more apt to declare itself than at others; and, as one age is obnoxious to one cause of asthma, and another to another, cases of asthma differ in kind very much according to the age at which they commence. Thus the cases that come on in early life are usually due to the bronchial disorders of childhood—infantile bronchitis, measles, whooping-cough—acting on a constitution pos-sessing a congenital proclivity to the disease. There is commonly, in these cases, a sensitive bronchial mucous membrane, and often some pulmonary collapse and emphysema. The cases that come on in youth and early manhood are generally specimens of the pure spasmodic form, without any organic complication. Those that come on late in life are commonly cases of organic asthma—either asthma complicating chronic bronchitis, or cardiac asthma.

I find that in thirty-eight cases, in which I have noted the time of first access, in seven it occurred during the first year of life. In one of these, distinct symptoms of asthma were recognized at fourteen days old, in another at twenty-eight days, in another at three months, in another at one year, and in three "during the first year," but the exact time is not remembered. I have long known that early infancy is accessible to asthma, and that many of the best-marked and purest spasmodic cases start from this early date; but until I examined my cases I was not aware so large a proportion, nearly one in five, occurred within the first year of life. In some of these the disease appeared so early that it would be difficult to say that it was not truly congenital. Within a few days of birth the breathing had the true asthmatic character. The constitutional tendency must be strongly marked indeed that would develop itself so early. And it is worthy of remark that in all those cases in which the disease made such an early appearance there was a history of inheritance; and this is quite consistent with what one would expect: its inheritance would imply its constitutional character; its being constitutional would make it probable that it would early declare itself.

The following is a table showing, in the forty-seven cases in which I have noted this point, the relative frequency in which asthma develops itself in the successive decades of life:—

During the first year	9 } 19
From one to ten	10
From ten to twenty	8
From twenty to thirty	7
From thirty to forty	6
From forty to fifty	3
From fifty to sixty	4
	——
	47

It would appear from this that the first appearance of asthma is less and less likely to occur as life advances up to old age, when there is an increase. And this is exactly what one might expect from the constitutional nature of the disease. All constitutional diseases are, *ipso facto*, disposed to declare themselves early; the stronger the constitutional tendency the earlier; and the longer they pass without appearing the less likely are they to appear. This table, it must be remembered, is not a table of the number of asthmatics at different ages, but of those who have *become* asthmatic at those respective ages. It is strictly a table of the relative frequency at the different periods of life of the *first access* of the disease.

Almost all the cases of which I have taken notes are uncomplicated cases. Of a large number of cases of senile bronchitic asthma that have come under my observation I have preserved no record;

if I had, the number of cases commencing between fifty and sixty, and upwards, would have been much larger. The number four in the table by no means indicates the proportionate frequency of the commencement of organic asthma in old age.

VI. *Influence of Sex.*—In fifty-four cases in which I have noted the circumstance of sex, thirty-six have been in males, and eighteen in females, or exactly twice as many in the former as in the latter. To what does this fact point? It unmistakably asserts that the causes of asthma are circumstances to which men are more exposed than women, such as the inclemencies of the weather, the wear and tear and hardship of life, the stress of violent and sustained respiratory efforts as in heavy labour, and intemperance. Unless these are the causes of the difference we must suppose it to depend upon some greater proclivity to asthma on the part of the male nervous system than the female. Now this I do not believe. Indeed, I believe the reverse. An asthmatic nervous system is a mobile, sensitive nervous system, and certainly the female nervous system is more mobile and sensitive than the male.

Consistently with this, I believe it will be found that idiopathic asthma—the pure neurosis—is as common in women as in men, and that the cases by which so large a preponderance is given to men are cases starting from bronchitis. Senile asthma (chronic-bronchitic and cardiac) is, I should say, ten times commoner in men than in women.

VII. *Is Asthma Hereditary?*—I think there can be no doubt that it is. Not that I would take this fact for granted, or on the common assertion that it is so; for I think this a point on which error might be apt to arise. In all diseases a certain number of cases will be found in which on the mere doctrine of chances, the parents, or other members of the family, have been similarly affected. But I think the number of cases in which there is a family history of asthma is greater than will admit of this explanation. Out of thirty-five cases in which I have noted this circumstance I find distinct traces of inheritance in fourteen; in twenty-one not. It appears, therefore, to be inherited (and my numbers are sufficient to give some evidence) in two cases out of every five; that is, in the proportion of two to three. The kind of inheritance differs very much; sometimes it is direct, sometimes lateral; sometimes immediate, sometimes remote; as will be seen in the following specification of the inheritance in these fourteen cases:—

1. Inherited from the father.
2. Father a confirmed asthmatic.
3. Inherited from the father.
4. Father a confirmed asthmatic, brother suffers from hay asthma.
5. Grandfather a confirmed asthmatic.
6. Brother and paternal grandmother asthmatic.
7. Father, two paternal uncles, and paternal grandfather.
8. Inherited from father, paternal sister died of it.

9. Father died asthmatic at forty-seven.

10. Several indirect branches of the family asthmatic but neither parent.

11. Mother slightly asthmatic, maternal grandmother severely.

12. Grandfather now suffers from asthma.

13. Grandfather and uncle both asthmatic.

14. Sister and paternal grandmother asthmatic, brother with hay asthma.

With regard to the inheritance of asthma, I have observed one curious fact, which suggests an interesting general pathological question. It is, that several brothers and sisters in a family may be asthmatic without the parents having been so. This would seem to suggest, in respect to disease, a principle with which breeders of cattle are familiar—that certain *combinations* produce certain results, and lead to the *creation* of certain peculiarities, and that the qualities of the progeny are not the mere resultant of the combined qualities of the parents—just as we sometimes see a family of red-haired children, both the parents of which have black hair.

<hr />

CHAPTER V.

VARIETIES OF ASTHMA.

Idiopathic or uncomplicated asthma ("spasmodic"), and symptomatic or complicated asthma ("organic").—Intrinsic asthma; ipecacuan, hay, toxhæmic asthma, &c.—Excito-motory; peptic, organic nervous, cerebro-spinal nervous.—Central asthma. Asthma depending on bronchitis and heart-disease.

ADOPTING the views that I have endeavoured to enforce, as to the absolute nature of asthma, we must conclude that wherever that peculiar paroxysmal tightness of breathing, so unlike anything else, that we call asthma, is present, there is present bronchial stricture; and, conversely, that wherever the bronchial tubes are the seat of spasm, there, whatever else may be present or absent, the symptoms of asthma must manifest themselves. Regarded in this light we may say that asthma is one and indivisible—that there is but one species of asthma; and as far as its essential pathology goes, there *is* but one asthma—one in its morbid anatomy, one in its characteristic phenomena. But the circumstances under which asthma may occur are so various, and the features of different cases so peculiar, and impart to those cases such an individuality that all writers have attempted, with more or less success, to make some classification of its different varieties.

I say, with more or less success; I might almost have said, with uniform want of success. Two mistakes of an opposite nature have been made by systematic writers on this disease: one, calling that asthma which is not asthma, as Lænnec's "asthma with puerile respiration," Walshe's "hæmic asthma," and what is commonly known as "cardiac asthma;" the other, denying the name of asthma altogether to those cases where, although bronchial spasm is undoubtedly present, the pathological condition is complex—saying it is not asthma, because it is not *pure* asthma. These two principal faults, together with a rejection of the simplicity of nature (as simple in disease as in health), and an absence of any one single basis of classification, have rendered the attempts to systematize the varieties of asthma singularly unhappy.[1]

Seeing that asthma may occur in individuals in all other discoverable respects perfectly healthy—in whose lungs, heart, stomach, nervous system, not the slightest lesion can be traced, and, on the other hand, may be a mere appendage, or complication, of abiding and grave organic disease, a natural division at once suggests itself into two principal species—idiopathic or uncomplicated, and symptomatic or complicated asthma: it is to the former that the name "spasmodic" has, *par excellence*, been applied; the latter is sometimes called "organic" asthma. With the first form we are familiar in the ordinary typical specimens of the disease; the second we see most commonly as asthma complicating bronchitis. Some authorities would restrict the name asthma entirely to the first form, and deny that the second is asthma at all—it is nothing more than bronchitis, they say, with paroxysmal dyspnœa. But asthma is not necessarily absent because bronchitis is present; and if the paroxysmal portion of the dyspnœa depends in these cases, as it undoubtedly does, upon spasmodic narrowing of the air-tubes superadded to inflammation of their lining membrane, then it is, to all intents and purposes, asthma, and the case, as far as this symptom and this condition go, is one of asthma. We cannot, if we adopt any strictness of definition, deny the presence of asthma in any case where there is muscular spasm of the bronchial tubes and its attendant characteristic dyspnœa.

Now, what is the essential difference in these two cases?—what is the difference between the man who, in all other respects perfectly healthy, wakes up once a fortnight in an agony of dyspnœa, which in a few hours subsides and leaves no trace behind it, and the man who, in addition to the abiding rattling wheeze of chronic bronchitis, suffers, perhaps many times a day, from paroxysms of a more intense and drier dyspnœa, bearing evidently no relation to the inflammation of the mucous surface or the amount of the secretion? What is the

---

[1] I must be pardoned for not taking up the reader's time in enumerating the different classifications of asthma adopted by different writers. The chief cause of their failure has been, I believe, a want of a simple reading of nature, its place being supplied by an unquestioning inheritance and adoption of received notions. It seems to me to be a subject in which authors have done more in the way of reading each other's books than scrutinizing their own patients.

difference, I say, in these two cases? In fifty points of their physiognomy and clinical history they differ, but these are non-essential differences; their only essential difference is that of *cause*. In the first case, an impression is made on a morbidly irritable pulmonary nervous system by some occult cause that eludes our search. In the second case, the cause is the inflamed condition of the bronchial mucous membrane acting as a local and immediate irritant, the bronchitis having just the same relation to the asthma as the inflammation of the urethra in gonorrhœa has to the spasmodic urethral stricture that so frequently accompanies it, or as the ulcerated rectum has to the tenesmus of dysentery.

Adopting these differences of causation as the basis of my classification, and I find it to be the best and the most natural that can be selected, I have arranged the varieties of asthma according to the following scheme :—

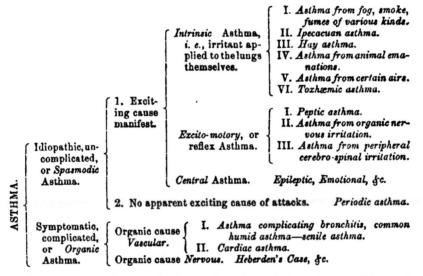

Let me say a few words in explanation of the above table, and then describe more fully, as far as they deserve separate description, the different varieties of asthma included in it.

1. It will be seen that I divide those cases of idiopathic or spasmodic asthma in which the provocatives of the attack are manifest, into three groups, according to the seat of the exciting cause.

First, cases of what I call "intrinsic" asthma, in which the irritant is applied to the lungs themselves.

Secondly, cases in which the source of irritation has a distant seat, as stomach, bowels, uterus; and which I call "reflex."

Thirdly, in which the irritation appears to be central in the brain itself.

I call the first class of cases "intrinsic," because the lungs are alone concerned; the source of irritation is applied to the very part that is the seat of the diseased phenomena. These cases are divisible, according to the nature of the irritant, into six varieties. In five out of the six the irritant is some material respired, and provokes the bronchial tubes to contract by direct contact with their mucous surface. I have placed them in order according to their tenuity or subtleness.

The first variety, produced by fog, smoke, or fumes of various kinds, is a very common one; many people suffer from slight asthmatic dyspnœa under such circumstances who never do under any other;—a foggy November morning, the smoke of burning pitch, or of a candle that has been blown out, or lighting a lucifer match, will make some people quite asthmatic who are never so at other times. This tendency, unless it is excessive and exhibited towards many things, cannot be considered morbid, as it results from the natural and salutary function with which the bronchial tubes are endowed, of guarding by their contraction against the intrusion of offending and injurious materials.

The second variety is very rare, and extremely curious; the subjects of it are always attacked with violent asthmatic dyspnœa and wheezing if *ipecacuanha powder* is used, or a bottle containing it merely opened, in the room where they are. I have only met with three cases of this variety, and, what is very curious, in none of them does asthma occur under any other circumstances—no other irritant will produce it. The subjects of the affection were each of them first seized with the sensation when using ipecacuanha in dispensing a prescription; it was quite new to them, and they were at a loss to account for it; but subsequent experience showed them what it was, and they were never able to touch ipecacuanha without a repetition of their symptoms, and were always obliged to leave the room when it was employed. They were all medical students, a circumstance which may appear remarkable, but which may be easily explained by the fact that only those engaged in using drugs would be exposed to the emanations of ipecacuan: if more people were exposed to the peculiar exciting cause the number of instances of this kind of asthma would probably be much greater.

The third variety, by no means uncommon, refers to the asthmatic portion of that curious affection known as *hay-fever*. Most people who suffer from this disease experience, in addition to the intolerance of light, lachrymation, sneezing, irritation of the conjunctiva, nasal passages and fauces, that characterize it, distinct asthmatic dyspnœa. The asthma and the other symptoms are generally proportionate, and undoubtedly arise from the same cause; in fact, the asthma is merely due to an extension into the air-passages of the same irritation that affects the conjunctival, nasal, and faucial mucous membranes. As I shall have somewhat more to say of this curious affection, I shall defer the further consideration of it to the end of this chapter.

The fourth variety very closely resembles this last, the symptoms are almost indentical—inflamed conjunctiva, watering of the eyes, an itching burning tumidity of the lachrymal ducts, nasal passages and throat, and asthma—but due, not to hay, but to nursing a cat or kitten, or rubbing the eyes after having stroked their fur. The only animals that I have known capable of producing this kind of asthma are cats and rabbits. I believe this affection is undescribed; I have never been able to meet any description of it or reference to it.

The fifth variety includes a large number of cases of asthma—all those cases, in fact, in which the asthma is induced by the air of certain localities, as, for example, asthma that is invariably brought on by going into the country in an individual who never has it in London. This is one of the commonest events in the clinical history of asthma—nothing is commoner than to find that an asthmatic can breathe perfectly well in one place, and in another can hardly live. I have collected notes of a large number of such cases, and must refer the reader for the narrative of some of them to Chapter XIII.

The sixth variety—toxhæmic asthma, or asthma produced by blood-poisoning—differs from all the preceding, inasmuch as, although the source of irritation is present in the lungs themselves, it is not applied to the surface of the air-passages, but circulates in the blood of the pulmonary capillaries. We see examples of it in those cases in which certain materials, taken into the blood by absorption (as, for instance, certain aliments—beer, wine, sweets), produce asthma as soon as they arrive at the pulmonary circulation. Some cases in which asthma comes on during each meal appear to be undoubtedly of this kind.

The second class of cases I have called excito-motory or reflex, because the source of irritation has a distant seat, far removed from the lung, and reaches and affects the air-tubes by a reflex circuit. There are three varieties of this class. *First*, Those in which the asthma follows an error in diet, or always supervenes on a full meal, which I call peptic asthma, and which I believe to depend upon irritation of the gastric filaments of the pneumogastric nerve, propagated reflexly to the pulmonary filaments, and producing through them motor phenomena, *i.e.*, bronchial contractions. *Secondly*, Those in which the source of irritation is still more distant, and the nervous circuit that transmits it longer, involving probably the sympathetic, as in asthma from a loaded rectum or uterine irritation. *Thirdly*, Those in which the cerebro-spinal system is that which receives the first irritation, as, for example, where the exciting cause is some particular condition into which the external surface is thrown.[1]

In all the preceding varieties, whether the source of irritation exists in the lungs themselves, or is applied to some part far removed (that is, whether it is what I call "intrinsic" or "reflex" asthma), the

[1] See a remarkable case, which I have related in the second chapter, in which the paroxysms of asthma were brought on by the sudden application of cold to the instep.

exciting cause has a peripheral seat. But there are many cases in which we are warranted in believing that the perverted innervation starts from the brain or spinal cord itself, that it is primarily central. Those cases in which asthma is brought on by any sudden emotion are of this "central" kind.

2. But cases of asthma are not uncommon in which *no* exciting cause of the attacks can be detected. The best-marked specimens of *periodic asthma* are of this kind. As the time for the attack comes round the asthmatic knows that it will make its appearance, and that any care he may exercise will be of no avail in warding it off. He knows perhaps to a day, when it will appear; goes to bed at night with the certainty of being awoke in the morning with his disease upon him; and yet in no respect shall his condition that night differ from what it was on any previous night. And as, on the one hand, no care will prevent its occurrence when the time has arrived, so, on the other (in some cases), no provocative will induce it before the expiration of the required interval. Soon after an attack the asthmatic may do what he likes with impunity—take cold, eat a heavy supper, anything. But as the time for an attack comes round, woe be to him unless he exercises the most scrupulous care; any indiscretion, any irregularity, and the asthma is on him. It seems as if the disease was seeking, with increasing impatience, some loophole—some excuse for making its appearance; and if that loophole is not furnished it comes without any pretence of cause whatever. In such cases the only cause of the attack is that a certain interval has transpired since the last. This is closely analogous to what we see in epilepsy—after the attack the epileptic is a free man; but when the time for the fit draws nigh it is necessary to guard him from many sources of disturbance, and the most scrupulous care will not suffice to delay the fit many days. In both cases there appears to be either an accumulation of some occult cause, which at the fit discharges itself, or, the cause being abiding, an accumulation of susceptibility to that cause, which at the fit is temporarily lost.

So far, then, for asthma that has no abiding, no organic cause, but is compatible, as far as our means of scrutiny go, with perfect anatomical integrity of every viscus of the body, and perfect health between the paroxysms.

But muscular contraction of the bronchial tubes, giving rise to dyspnœa of the asthmatic type, is very common as a direct result of organic disease. In these cases the organic lesion itself is the exciting cause of the spasm, and the cause being in its nature abiding, the resulting asthma is, in a great degree, the same. As contrasted with idiopathic asthma the paroxysms are more frequent, of easy induction at any time, the remissions between the attacks imperfect, and the health in the intervals permanently marked by the signs of the organic disease. In the vast majority of cases the organic disease that gives rise to bronchial spasm is such as immediately affects the vascular condition of the bronchial mucous membrane—the inflammation or congestion of the mucous surface appears to be the stimulus that, through the nerves of the air tubes, excites the muscular wall to contrast.

There are two ways in which the vascular condition of the bronchial tubes may be deranged—actively, by inflammation, passively, by congestion; and either seems adequate to the induction of bronchial spasm;—the former we see in bronchitis, chronic and acute; the latter in any condition suspending or interfering with respiration, or impeding the transit of blood through or from the lungs, as aneurism, heart-disease, &c. I have therefore divided organic asthma, depending on bronchial hyperæmia, into two varieties—asthma complicating bronchitis, and cardiac asthma. The only difference between the two is, that in the one case the hyperæmia causing the asthma is active, in the other passive.

I do not mean to say that heart-disease and aneurism can only produce asthma by producing an impediment to circulation through the lungs. Remembering the intimate nervous connection between the lungs and heart we cannot but see that a diseased heart may produce spasm of the air-tubes by reflex nervous irritation; and remembering the anatomical contiguity of the heart and great vessels to the pulmonary plexuses and the nerves thence proceeding we cannot but see that any enlargement or displacement of any of these structures might, by pressure upon or tension of the pulmonary ganglia and nerves, produce, as a direct irritant, bronchial stricture. Nothing that anatomically affects the roots of the great vessels can leave the pneumogastric nerves unimplicated.

I myself have no doubt that in ordinary *acute* bronchitis a good deal of the dyspnœa that ushers in the attack and accompanies the dry sore stage, when there is such a sensation of rawness beneath the sternum and between the shoulders, and coughing is so painful, is due not only to the mucous membrane being tumid from inflammation and so narrowing the calibre of the tubes, but to active contraction from the irritation and exalted sensibility that the inflammation gives rise to.

But it is in *chronic* bronchitis that the best-marked cases of organic asthma are seen, the asthmatic element being often sufficient to constitute a very important and conspicuous part of the symptoms, so that, in some instances, it is difficult to know whether to call it asthma with bronchitis or bronchitis with asthma. My own belief is, that severe chronic bronchitis never exists without asthmatic complication, more or less. I believe that in all such cases a good deal of the dyspnœa cannot be explained on any other supposition; and this opinion is based upon the close scrutiny of the hundreds of cases of chronic bronchitis with which the out-patient practice of a hospital has furnished me :—the character of the dyspnœa, the circumstances under which it occurs, its *juvantia* and *lœdentia*, the impossibility of explaining its paroxysms by any changes in the condition of the mucous membrane or the amount of the secretion, all point to asthmatic spasm engrafted on the bronchial inflammation.

This kind of organic asthma is analogous, as far as *cause* goes, to those varieties of spasmodic asthma in which the bronchial stricture is caused by irritants introduced into the air-tubes, with this exception—that in the one case the irritant is something *applied* to the membrane, in the other, it is the condition of the membrane itself.

Of *cardiac asthma* I will merely say, that a good deal of the dyspnœa in heart-disease that is called cardiac asthma is not asthma at all; it is dyspnœa of the true cardiac type, and in no way dependent on contraction of the bronchial tubes. The paroxysms of gasping breathlessness which characterize orthopnœa (which is the most characteristically cardiac of all dyspnœas) are in no way dependent on bronchial contraction. But, beyond this, there often is in heart-disease a considerable amount of genuine asthma, which has just the same relation to the bronchial turgidity and congestion which exists in heart-disease as it has in bronchitis to the bronchial inflammation. Any considerable impediment to the transit of blood through the heart cannot long exist without producing bronchial congestion (from communication of the bronchial vessels with those of the pulmonary parenchyma?); and it seems to be a fundamental law of bronchial organization that no vascular or other derangement of the lining membrane of the air-tubes can occur without a corresponding disturbance of their muscular endowment. This springs immediately and inevitably from the relation between bronchial surface and bronchial muscle (which I have endeavoured elsewhere to explain)— from the fact that the one is the recipient of impressions giving warning of the necessity of the contraction of the other. It seems to make no difference whether the bronchial hyperæmia is active or passive, except this much—that when it is active, that is inflammatory, the bronchial spasm is much more intense and protracted; the asthma that complicates bronchitis is much more considerable than that which we ever see in heart-disease.

But are the pulmonary and great thoracic vessels and the heart the only seat of organic disease engendering asthma? By no means. Many cases are on record in which the asthma was due to organic disease of the pulmonary nervous system itself, as, for instance, a tumour or exostosis pressing upon one of the pneumogastric nerves. A case recorded by Heberden, in which asthma was due to exostosis of the upper dorsal vertebræ, was probably of this kind. Dr. Gairdner, of Edinburgh, mentions a case characterized during life by " frequent difficulty of respiration," which I cannot doubt was asthmatic, and in which after death, a neuromatous tumour of the vagus was found.[1] It is very probable that many cases of asthma in which the cause is occult are of this nature; but the nervous lesion is such as to elude detection, or perhaps is never sought for.

[1] Edinburgh Medical and Surgical Journal, 1850.

94 VARIETIES OF ASTHMA.

This, I think, exhausts all the genuine varieties of asthma. I am not aware of any variety, truly individual and distinctive, that I have not referred to.

But why, it may be asked, should I make no mention of that very common class of cases in which asthma is complicated with emphysema? Is not that an organic asthma, and do not such cases constitute a distinct variety? I think not. I think that, in the great majority of the cases in which emphysema and asthma are combined, the emphysema is, as I shall endeavour to show in a future chapter, either the consequence of the asthma, or of some common cause both of the asthma and of itself. Certainly the history of such cases warrants such a conclusion; for generally the asthma exists uncomplicated for some months or years, with perfect freedom from dyspnœa between the paroxysms, before the permanent dyspnœa, and the configuration of the chest, and other signs of emphysema, develop themselves. I think the emphysema has, in this case, just the same relation to bronchial tubes occluded by spasm as it has in bronchitis (the whooping-cough bronchitis of children, for example) to bronchial tubes occluded by mucous infarction; that it is compensatory dilatation of those portions of the lung that air *can* reach, in consequence of the inability of other portions of the lung (that air cannot reach) to follow the expansion of the chest; and that it is from the completeness of the bronchial stricture that the lung is unable to dilate in spite of the violent inspiratory efforts that are brought to bear upon it. Since, therefore, I consider the emphysema that so often complicates asthma to be a consequence and not a cause of the asthma—something appended to it, and not a part of it—its presence cannot constitute a distinct variety. For, pure uncomplicated asthma, of any of the varieties that I have mentioned, may, after a time, if the paroxysms are long and severe, have emphysema engrafted upon it.

The relation between asthma and emphysema has, I know, been differently interpreted. Some authers[1] maintain that the emphysema is the cause of the asthma. But to my mind, independent of the positive proof we have that asthma really depends on bronchial spasm, the sequence of events in the clinical history of these cases, the inadequacy of such a lesion as emphysema for the production of the phenomena of asthma, and the presence of asthma in numerous cases without emphysema, all forbid our entertaining such a theory. But I must refer the reader, for a fuller consideration of this question, to a future chapter on the *Consequences of Asthma.*

[1] Dr. Budd, "On Emphysema and Asthma." Medico-Chirurgical Transactions, 1840, pp. 53 *et seq.* See Chapter I.

CHAPTER VI.

THE ÆTIOLOGY OF ASTHMA.

Two kinds of causes of asthma.—I. Causes of the paroxysms; respiratory causes; alimentary causes; nervous causes; psychical causes.—II. Causes of the disease; *a.* Organic and acquired; *β.* Constitutional and inherited.—Organic disease not necessarily at the root of the asthmatic tendency.—Is asthma in its essence a systemic or local affection?—Conclusion.

THE ætiology of asthma is undoubtedly the most obscure and difficult part of the whole subject.

The causes of asthma are of two kinds; the causes of the paroxysms, and the causes of the disease: the one the immediate provocative of the attack, the other the original and essential cause of the asthmatic tendency. And this division is strictly natural, the two kinds of cause being entirely diverse: the cause of the paroxysm not producing the disease, and the cause of the disease not producing the paroxysm.

As for the causes of the paroxysm—the immediate excitants of the asthmatic spasm—they are plain enough. The experience of every asthmatic gives him very certain information on this point. It is of the essential cause of the disease—that which has originally rendered the individual an asthmatic, that obscure something that disposes him from time to time to fall into the asthmatic state on the occurrence of the exciting cause of the attacks, the *fons et origo mali* —that I speak, when I assert the difficulty of the subject.

I.—THE IMMEDIATE OR EXCITING CAUSES OF ASTHMA: THE PROVOCATIVES OF THE ATTACKS.

Though not in logical order, I shall consider these first because they are so manifest and well known, and because they throw some light on the nature of the essential cause of the disease.

They differ entirely in different cases. There are probably no two cases alike in the list of things that will bring on an attack; what will be certain to do so in one case will be innocuous in another, and what will be fatal in the other will be innocent in the one; so that no one thing can be declared an inevitable provocative of asthma; but each case is constant, and the excitants of the spasm constitute a part of the individuality, and form an unchanging portion of the clinical history, of each case. In nothing, I think, does asthma show its caprice more than in the choice of its exciting causes; almost every case furnishes something new and curious in this respect. The mere enumeration of the whole list would be portentously long. I shall merely notice the most common and characteristic, and shall group them, for order's sake, under the four following heads:—

1. Irritants admitted into the air-passages in respiration.
2. Alimentary irritants (errors in diet).
3. Sources of remote nervous irritation.
4. Psychical irritants.

1. *Respired Irritants.*—These constitute the most numerous class of all the excitants of asthma. Some of them are such as naturally offend the air-passages, and, if admitted, produce such an irritation of the bronchial mucous membrane as secures their immediate expulsion by cough; some even, such as pungent and stifling gases will occasionally produce temporary bronchial spasm (the true asthmatic dyspnœa and wheeze) in persons that have no asthmatic tendency; ordinarily, however, explosive cough, soon over, is the only result of breathing them. But in asthmatics the case is very different; the respiration of them immediately inducing a regular fit of asthma. Dust, smoke, pungent fumes, mephitic vapours, cold air, are irritants of this kind. And in respect to them the peculiarity of the asthmatic consists, not in their irritating his air-passages, for that they do in every one, but in their producing, as a result of that irritation, not a mere cough, or a slight, transient bronchial stricture, but intense and persistent asthmatic spasm. Of these, I think the worst—the most apt to produce asthma—are dust and certain smokes, such as the smoke of pitch, or of an extinguished candle. I have known some asthmatics who could not tolerate the least dust. One in particular I remember, a clergyman, with otherwise but a slight tendency to asthma, who never dared be present at the annual assortment and distribution of blankets to the poor of his parish, as the dust and fluff disengaged always brought on a violent fit of asthma. In another case the small amount of smoke generated by the imperfect combustion of a night light was always sufficient to bring on an attack.

But there is another class of respired irritants, that ordinarily are no irritants at all, but that in certain asthmatics infallibly produce their disease; such are the emanations from hay, from ipecacuan, from certain animals. One asthmatic is obliged to expatriate himself in the hay season and take a sea voyage; another cannot stay in a room in which a bottle of ipecacuanha is opened; a third cannot stroke or nurse a cat; another cannot go near a rabbit hutch; another is immediately rendered asthmatic by the neighbourhood of a privet hedge; another cannot sleep upon a pillow stuffed with feathers; another cannot use mustard in any shape or bear it near her, so that she dare not apply a mustard plaster; and one young lady I knew who did not dare to pass a poulterer's shop. One would hardly believe these things, were not their reality placed beyond doubt; there is neither invention, nor imagination, nor exaggeration about them. I have known the presence of ipecacuanha in a room where there was no reason to suspect it at once detected by the oppression and asthma that it produced. I have known some incredulous people open an ipecacuanha bottle, unknown to the asthmatic, for the sake of experiment, to see if he would find it out, but always with the result of its immediate discovery. I have known the same with regard to other of these agents. Dr. Watson mentions an analogous anecdote with regard to the detection of the neighbourhood of hay. It is indeed in its intolerance of these and similar subtle and inappreciable emanations that asthma exhibits its most extravagant vagaries.

2. *Alimentary Irritants.*—Errors in the diet are a very fruitful source of asthma. Food may induce asthma in three ways : by being of the wrong quality; by being excessive in quantity; and by being taken too late in the day. In respect to quality, all foods generally acknowledged to be unwholesome and indigestible are apt to produce asthma, but there are some especially and above all others that have this tendency, and that quite out of proportion to their unwholesomeness. For a list of these, and for a discussion of the whole subject of the relation of food to the production of bronchial spasm, I must refer the reader to the chapter on the Dietetic Treatment of Asthma.

3. *Sources of remote Nervous Irritation.*—Various sources of irritation existing at, or applied to, parts of the body far removed from the chest, may act as exciting causes of asthma. In cases of hysterical asthma the source of irritation is uterine. In one case that came under my observation a loaded rectum would always bring on an attack; in another, the sudden application of cold to the feet would instantly induce it; and in more than one case I have known organic disease of the brain the apparent exciting cause of true asthma. These cases, then, show that sources of irritation affecting the organic nervous system (uterus and rectum), the cerebro-spinal (cutaneous surface), and the brain itself, are capable of acting as the immediate excitants of asthma.

4. Lastly, there are many examples to show that *psychical* stimuli —excitement, fear, or other violent emotions—are adequate to the immediate production of asthmatic spasm.

II.—ESSENTIAL CAUSE OF ASTHMA.

The essential cause of asthma—that in which the asthmatic differs from other men, which constitutes the asthmatic *tendency*, and renders the exciting causes operative—what is it?

I do not see that I can discuss this question, or arrive at clear

7

ideas respecting it, better than by endeavouring to answer the following questions :—

Is organic disease at the root of the asthmatic tendency?

Is organic disease *necessarily* present in all cases of asthma?

Is asthma, in its essence, a systemic or a local affection?

Is there necessarily in asthmatics some constitutional peculiarity, inherited, congenital, or acquired?

There is one circumstance in the history of asthma that is strongly suggestive of the idea that some organic injury of the lung is at the root of the asthmatic tendency: it is, that in the narrative of cases of asthma it will be so frequently found that the asthma dates from some disease that implicates the lungs, and in such a way as to imply injury of an organic nature, though apparently temporary, as, for example, whooping-cough, bronchitis, and measles. These diseases are, beyond a doubt, the commonest of all the causes of asthma : a large proportion (as much as eighty per cent.) of cases of asthma in the young date from one or other of them. In two of them a specific bronchitis forms an essential part of the clinical history. I think this fact does not admit of misinterpretation. I think this frequent association of asthma with an antecedent event implying organic, although apparently temporary, injury of the lung, must have a very important influence on our notions of the ætiology of the disease. A child reaches the age of ten years, and up to that time has never shown any tendency to asthma; it then has measles; and, although it perfectly recovers from the bronchial affection, from that forward it is liable to attacks of spasmodic asthma. From this I think we cannot but conclude both that this disease, by some change that it works in the organization of the lung, may leave behind it as a legacy a permanent tendency to asthmatic spasm, and that it may be the sole and efficient cause of the asthma.

There is another circumstance that strongly favours the view that the cause of asthma is organic, and seated in the lungs themselves; it is, the relative frequency of asthma in the two sexes. Purely functional nervous derangements are undoubtedly commoner in women than in men. Men, on the other hand, are much more exposed than women to sources of lung-injury, and their lungs are accordingly much more frequently the seat of organic diseases. Now, if asthma was primarily nervous and purely functional—if it were a simple neurosis we ought to find it commoner in women than in men; whereas, according to my experience, men are more frequently the subjects of asthma than women in the proportion of two to one.

In those cases in which the attacks are produced by some irritant admitted into the air-passages, we have no reason for thinking that the cause of the asthma is situated anywhere but in the lungs themselves; we have no reason for believing that in these cases there is any general constitutional vice of the nervous system, but every reason on the contrary for thinking that the mischief begins and ends in the lungs, and that, whatever it is in its absolute nature, it is something that renders the pulmonary nervous system unduly irritable and impressible.

This morbid sensitiveness of the pulmonary nervous system would appear to be due, in a large number of cases, to something that has organically damaged it, something that has damaged that surface to which its perceptive portion is distributed; for I think it will be found that in the majority of those cases in which the excitants of the attacks are stimuli admitted into the air-passages the original cause of the disease has been something organically affecting the bronchial mucous membrane—catarrhal bronchitis, measles, whooping-cough. In these diseases the bronchial mucous membrane is the seat of inflammation, often intense and prolonged, and in two instances specific: and it is probable that some organic although inappreciable change has been wrought in it, producing a morbid exaltation of its sensibility to which the tendency to spasms is immediately due, according to that law of the organization of the bronchial tubes to which I have referred in the chapter on the Absolute Nature of Asthma. At any rate, in those cases in which the tendency to asthma is manifestly dependent on organic bronchial disease (as in asthma accompanying chronic bronchitis), the provocatives of the paroxysms are pre-eminently stimuli applied to the bronchial surface —smoke, fog, cold, &c. If then this is so, the converse is probably true—if in asthma depending on organic bronchial disease the excitants of the attacks are stimuli applied to the bronchial surface, then, in those cases where the excitants of the attacks are stimuli applied to the bronchial surface the asthma probably depends on organic bronchial disease.

But is this always so? Probably not. In cases of ipecacuan-asthma the excitant of the paroxysm is something applied to the bronchial mucous membrane, but there is nothing in the history of these cases to imply that this surface has ever been the seat of organic disease. The same in cases of hay-asthma.

While, then, the induction of spasm by bronchial stimuli furnishes a *presumption* that the asthma is due to some cause that has organically injured the bronchial mucous membrane, it does not furnish a *proof* of it—in most cases it probably is so, in some not. And I think we may go a step further, and say that where the mucous membrane exhibits a *general* irritability, where a great number and variety of irritants are capable of producing the asthma, there the original cause is something that has damaged the mucous membrane; where, on the other hand, the membrane exhibits a *special* irritability, where the irritant is specific and single, there there is no such antecedent organic lesion. In the asthma of chronic bronchitis, for example, a multitude of irritants inhaled will give rise to the spasm: in hay and ipecacuan-asthma, on the other hand, the source of offence is single and specific. In the one case the cause of the asthma is something that has happened to the individual during his life, and the asthmatic tendency is acquired; in the other the cause is innate, and the tendency inherent.

But is it probable that there is some organic peculiarity in the lungs of *all* asthmatics? Certainly not. In a large number of cases there is not the slightest warrant for entertaining such a supposition. Take, for example, a case of emotional asthma, such as the following: A gentleman who has never suffered from any lung affection, and who is at the time in perfect health, is suddenly seized with difficulty of breathing, which proves to be spasmodic asthma, in consequence of extreme alarm from thinking that he has administered poison by mistake. His lungs were perfectly sound; there was no history of any pulmonary affection in his case; and he never suffered from dyspnœa under any other circumstances, either before or since. Moreover, the exciting cause was one not appealing to the lungs, but to the nervous system. In hay-asthma, too, there is generally, as I have just mentioned, no history of previous lung-disease, and in every part of the year, except in the hay-seasons, the lungs give the most positive evidence of their anatomical and physiological soundness.

What, then, *is* the cause of the asthma in these cases? I do not see that we can say anything more definite than that it consists in the asthmatic tendency itself; in that special irritability of the pulmonary nervous system (as in the case of ipecacuan-asthma), or that general irritability of the whole nervous system (as in emotional asthma, &c.), which constitutes the asthmatic idiosyncrasy with which the individual was born.

That in some cases a congenital asthmatic tendency does exist is strongly implied, I think we may say positively proved, by the undoubted hereditariness of the disease: in some families asthma is as much *the* disease as gout is in others. I have lately had under my care a gentleman whose father, paternal grandmother, and two paternal uncles, as himself, were asthmatic. Now, there is no doubt that what is inherited must be congenital—inborn.

But, Is any congenital peculiarity *necessary?* No; there appears to be no reason that a person may not *become* asthmatic; that the tendency to the disease may not be *acquired*, indeed, evidence as positive as can be imagined for believing that it may; that an asthmatic may at one time have differed in no respect from others, but that the tendency to his disease may have been engrafted on him by something that has happened to him. For example, the case of asthma as a sequela of measles, which I instanced just now. It is not conceivable that all the children whom this disease, or whooping-cough, leaves asthmatic, had any antecedent peculiarity. In no respect do they seem to differ from other cases, except that the disease from which the asthma dates, has generally been of unusual severity.

It would appear, then, that in respect to causation, all cases of asthma may be broadly divided into two groups:—

1. Cases in which the essential cause of the disease—that which

constitutes the individual an asthmatic—is some organic lesion, possibly not appreciable, either in the bronchial tubes, or in some part physiologically connected with the bronchial tubes.

2. Cases in which any organic lesion is not only inappreciable but non-existent, in which the tendency to asthma is due to something from within, not from without, in which the essential cause of the disease is a congenital, and possibly inherited, idiosyncrasy.

I steer, therefore, a middle course between those who say that asthma always has at the root of it some organic disease within the chest, and those who deny that genuine spasmodic asthma ever depends on organic lung-disease and maintain that it is always a pure neurosis. I think I have shown, on the one hand, that there are numberless cases in which the supposition of any organic cause would be purely gratuitous and in direct contravention of all clinical evidence and pathological reasoning; and, on the other, that we have every reason for believing that many cases, of the pure spasmodic variety, do really depend on some organic though inappreciable injury that previous disease has inflicted on the lungs.

CHAPTER VII.

CONSEQUENCES OF ASTHMA.

Tendency of asthma to disorganize.—The consequences of asthma fourfold:—1. Its direct results on the bronchial tubes; hypertrophy of the bronchial muscle; permanent bronchial contraction.—2. Results of obstructed pulmonary circulation: *a*. In the lungs (congestion, œdema, &c.); *β*. In the heart (hypertrophy, dilatation); *γ*. In the systemic venous system (venous stasis, œdema, &c.).—3. Emphysema: is pure asthma capable of generating it?—4. Acquisition of the asthmatic physique; its distinctiveness; its characteristic gait, physiognomy, and configuration; rationale of the asthmatic spinal curvature; pigeon-chest of young asthmatics.

ASTHMA never kills; at least, I have never seen a case in which a paroxysm proved fatal. If death did take place from asthma it would be by slow asphyxia—by the circulation of imperfectly decarbonized blood; and before this occurred I think the spasm would yield. When a case of asthma terminates fatally it does so by the production of certain organic changes in the heart and lungs; and it is on this tendency to the generation of organic disease that the gravity of asthma depends.

The consequences of asthma admirably illustrate two laws of our organization: one, that the workings and processes of life are so intimately bound together, so exactly fit and interlock, that one cannot go wrong without dragging the rest with it; the other, that healthy function is as necessary to healthy structure, as healthy structure is to healthy function. Without asserting that the perverted function of a tissue or organ is in all cases dependent upon some real though perhaps inappreciable perversion of its structure or constitution (which, though perhaps probable, is at present beyond our demonstration), we may safely affirm the converse—that no tissue or organ can long be the seat of peverted action without perversion in its structure or constitution inevitably following. Organs are made for action, not existence ; they are made to *work*, not to *be ;* and only when they *work* well can they *be* well. It is the universal law of organization that the function of parts shall be, if not absolutely coincident, at any rate indissolubly connected, with their nutrition. The very nutrition of organs is planned on the supposition of their being working machines, and in exact accordance with the work they have to do; so that their working can neither be suspended nor damaged without interfering with their nutrition, and therefore with their structure. Organs either misused or disused invariably organically degenerate.

If we examine the chest of an asthmatic who has but recently been affected with his disease, or whose attacks have been infrequent, we shall very likely find evidence of perfect anatomical soundness of all its organs; but if we examine him again in ten years we shall to a certainty, if the patient has in the interval suffered constantly from attacks of his malady, find evidence of organic disease of the lungs, and very likely of the heart. Now, why is this ? Why should organic disease be the inevitable sequel of that which is at first a mere functional and occasional derangement ? From the very law I have just above enunciated—that functional disorder cannot long exist without dragging in its train organic change.

The consequences of asthma appear to me to be fourfold : 1. The direct results on the bronchial tubes themselves of the inordinate action of their walls. 2. All those results of obstructed circulation, first pulmonary, then systemic, which the inadequate supply of air to the lungs induces. 3. That special result of the unequal and partial distribution of air to the lungs—emphysema. 4. The general effect of the disease on the physiognomy and build of the patient— the production of what may be called the *asthmatic physique.*

1. *Direct Results of the Asthmatic Spasm on the Bronchial Tubes themselves.*—Organic muscle obeys the same laws as voluntary ; its nutrition, and therefore its development, is proportioned to its activity ; and this evidently from the same final cause—that it may be equal to its work. No sooner is its activity exalted, or more work thrown upon it, than it immediately hypertrophies : witness the urinary bladder in stricture, and the gall-bladder in biliary calculus. The bronchial tubes in asthma afford but another example of the same thing, and their excessive action issues, from the operation of the same law, in a similar hypertrophous development. Accordingly, we constantly find, amongst the morbid appearances mentioned in the *post-mortem* examination of asthmatics, an undue conspicuousness

and thickening of the circular fibres of the bronchiæ.   One certain result of this hypertrophy of the bronchial muscle is a permanent thickening of their walls and consequent narrowing of their calibre; and one possible result is a greater disposition on the part of the hypertrophied muscle to take on a state of contraction.   To the former, perhaps, is in part due that slight constant dyspnœa which is so disposed to develop itself in asthma; to the latter, the increased tendency to and frequency of spasm which characterizes some cases.

Contraction of the bronchial tubes—a permanent diminution of their calibre—is another direct result of asthma.   A certain amount of narrowing is inevitably involved, as I have just stated, in the increased thickness of their walls, due in part to the hypertrophy of their muscular element, in part to the congestive tumidity of the mucous membrane, which is the almost invariable accompaniment of long-continued asthma.   Perhaps, too, as suggested by Dr. Williams, the very fact of an increase of the contractile element of the walls of the bronchiæ involves a degree of permanent passive contraction in excess of what is natural, just as the irritable bladder is a contracted bladder as well as a thickened one.   A certain amount, then, of thickening and a certain amount of contraction of the bronchial tubes, is fairly to be assigned to asthma, and has in it its sole and sufficient cause.

But we sometimes find in cases of asthma a degree of contraction far beyond what is thus explicable, amounting to complete occlusion. Now remembering how frequently asthma is complicated with bronchitis, how exactly such a condition of extreme contraction or occlusion is that which old severe bronchitis tends to produce, and how inadequate simple spasm seems to produce it, I am inclined to think that the asthma has nothing to do with it, that it is to be assigned wholly to the bronchitis that has complicated the case, and that cases of asthma in which it is found are always mixed cases.   This kind of bronchial contraction, converting the tube into a fibrous impervious cord or band, thickened and knotty, I believe to be always inflammatory in its origin.

Dilatation of the bronchial tubes is another morbid condition that has been found in asthma.   I think the most dilated bronchial tubes I have ever known were in a case of asthma.   But whenever I have seen it there has been bronchitis as well as asthma, and, for the reason I have just assigned in the case of contraction, I should attribute this also to the bronchitis and not to the asthma.   I do not see how bronchial spasm could possibly generate it, whereas I do see in the destruction of the vital and physical properties of the bronchial walls by severe inflammation the most rational explanation of its production.

And I may here remark in passing, that there are two circumstances that greatly impair the value and reliability of the specimens of the morbid anatomy of asthma found in our museums: one is, the looseness with which the word asthma is, and still more has been, used; the other, the extreme frequency with which, even in cases of true asthma, bronchitis has at some time or other existed.

2. *The Results of Obstructed Circulation induced by Asthma.*— Asthma is a state of partial asphyxia, and it therefore gives rise to an identical morbid anatomy, differing only from that of absolute asphyxia in its incompleteness, and in those ulterior changes for which in absolute asphyxia suddenly induced there is no time. When a man is drowned we know that an impassable obstruction is at once established to the passage of the blood through the capillaries of his lungs; within a minute or two the stoppage is complete. The pulmonary vessels, still filled from behind, become engorged with the blood that they cannot pass on; the right chambers of the heart become distended with the blood which they are unable to empty into the engorged lungs; and thus, the obstructing force propagated backwards, the cavæ and their tributaries become distended with accumulated blood in increasing quantities as long as life is prolonged. Meantime, the left side of the heart receives hardly any supply, and its action fails for want of its normal stimulus, while the right side becomes less and less able to contract on its bulky contents.

Soon, from these opposite causes on the right and left sides, the heart ceases to beat, and life is extinct. We open the body, and find—arteries, left side of the heart, and pulmonary veins empty; pulmonary artery, right side of the heart, and all the great systemic veins gorged with black blood. Now there can be no doubt that exactly the same thing takes place at every attack of asthma, but only to a degree that is compatible with life. If we could see into an asthmatic during a fit we should see a certain dose of the same deranged distribution of blood, and from the same cause—pulmonary capillary arrest from the shutting off of air. We should see pulmonary venous congestion, distended right heart, large veins full, and a scanty supply of arterialized blood finding its way to the left ventricle. All external manifestations are consistent with this:— the small and feeble pulse, the irregular and faltering systole, the turgid veins of the head and neck, the occasional hæmoptysis, the dusky skin. If all the bronchial tubes could be simultaneously so contracted as to be completely occluded the same result would take place as if a ligature were placed round the windpipe, the deprivation of air would be complete, and death would supervene. But such is not the case, all the bronchiæ are not simultaneously contracted, and their contraction does not amount to complete occlusion. The arterialization of the blood is lowered, not arrested, and life is maintained. By and by the spasm yields, air is freely admitted, the bar at the capillaries ceases, the pulmonary vessels unburden themselves, and all is well again.

But can such a state of things exist long, or exist often, without producing other organic changes? Certainly not. No tissue or organ can be long or often the seat of vascular disturbance without becoming more or less disorganized. I shall consider the changes that result from this stoppage at the pulmonary capillaries, that every attack of asthma gives rise to, in the order in which they occur—in the lungs, in the heart, and in the systemic venous system; that is, in those three segments of the circulation along which, in a retrograde direction, the obstructing force is propagated.

In the Lungs the first result is what is called venous congestion —a term in part correct and in part erroneous; for, while the congestion is congestion with venous blood the congested vessels are really branches of the pulmonary arteries. I am not aware that the exact seat of this congestion is determined, whether it is limited to the branches of the pulmonary arteries, or involves the capillaries as well. That will depend on the precise point of the seat of obstruction. If the capillaries are congested the seat of obstruction must be in front of them; if the capillaries themselves are the seat of the obstruction they cannot be congested—the congestion must be limited behind them. Now I am inclined to think that the exact seat of the obstruction is in the minute venules, just where the blood is passing from the capillaries into the pulmonary veins; and my reasons are these: The cause of the stoppage is the blood not being what it should, not being properly decarbonized: now, the capillaries are the seat of its decarbonization; it is not, therefore, until it leaves them and arrives at the ultimate pulmonary venous radicles that it becomes what it should not be—venous blood where it ought to be arterial. That point, then, where its defective arterialization must be first recognized, must be the point of its arrest. This would imply capillary engorgement. Whether the absolute capillaries *are* involved in the engorgement I cannot say, or whether it stops at the ultimate twigs of the pulmonary artery. It should be made the subject of careful microscopical observation, which I have not yet made it.

Indeed, I am not aware that the state of the vessels in chronic pulmonary congestion has ever been made the subject of microscopial investigation.

One result of this impeded circulation through the lungs which I believe will one day be demonstrated, is thickening of the walls of the ultimate arterial twigs analogous to that which Dr. Johnson has shown to take place in impeded circulation through the kidney, and produced in an identical way. This too, I regret to say, I have never, since the idea occurred to me, had an opportunity of verifying. Another result is, that the engorged vessels gradually lose their tone and yield to the distending force of the blood, so that the congestion becomes more and more considerable and of more and more easy induction. Another result is, that the serous portion of the accumulated blood transudes the walls of the vessels, and, escaping into the areolar tissue and air-cells, gives rise to œdema. From this accumulation of blood, and displacement of the air in the air-cells by serum, parts of the lung may undergo what has been called splenization, becoming quite solid, airless, sinking in water, non-crepitous, and black. And this is the state in which the more dependent parts of the lungs of those who have died of chronic asthma are often found;—a state not to be distinguished from that of the lungs in fatal chronic bronchitis, and which is, in fact, the morbid anatomy of slow asphyxia, however produced.

Hypertrophy and dilatation of the right side of the heart has long been a well-known and recognized complication of asthma. In examining the chest of an asthmatic patient we often find the heart's pulsation plainly felt, and even seen, in the scrobiculus cordis, while in its normal situation it can hardly be perceived. For this there are several reasons. One is, that during an attack of asthma the diaphragm is strongly and permanently contracted, refusing to ascend far even in expiration, so that the heart is drawn down lower than usual; another, that an emphysematous left lung may thrust it downwards and to the right, and also, by overlapping it, produce that undue resonance in the region of the heart's dulness and that indistinctness of the apex-beat beneath the nipple which are recognized signs of emphysema in this situation. But a third reason undoubtedly is dilatation of the right ventricle.

Although this last is the only cause I have seen assigned for this displacement of the heart's beat, I insist on the other two as adjuvant, because they are evidently sufficient of themselves to drive the heart down into the scrobiculus and transfer its pulsation thither without any dilatation of the ventricle. In cases of recent asthma, where there has been no time for dilatation or hypertrophy of the right ventricle to take place, and where, in the intervals of the attacks, the situation of the heart's beat has been perfectly normal, I have felt and even seen this pulsation in the scrobiculus very strongly marked at each fit, coming with the fit and going with the fit. Now, hypertrophy and dilatation of the right ventricle are not conditions that can come and go. It is evident, then, that a transference of the heart's pulsations to the scrobiculus may be produced by simple displacement of the organ, without any extension of its right chambers; and, therefore, when occurring during a paroxysm of asthma, this sign is not to be relied upon as evidence that the heart has organically suffered.[1]

But why should heart-disease be the legitimate sequel of asthma? Why should the stricture of the bronchial tubes tend to produce hypertrophy and dilatation of the right ventricle? The connection of these remote and apparently dissociated conditions is at once supplied by the law of asphyxia which I have just now referred to—that the

[1] Of the truth of this any one may satisfy himself by placing his finger on his scrobiculus cordis and taking a deep inspiration, when he will immediately feel the cardiac pulsations, which will continue as long as he keeps his chest at full distension;—he expires, and it is gone. Here we have the same conditions with regard to the situation of the heart that we have in asthma, only in a less degree—lung distension and flattening of the diaphragm; in fact, in asthma the parietes of the chest, diaphragmatic and costal, are in a state of permanent extreme inspiration.

shutting off of air from the lungs immediately brings the pulmonary circulation to a stand-still, and places in front of the right chambers of the heart an obstacle which they cannot overcome. This obstacle at the pulmonary capillaries provokes unwonted efforts on the part of the right ventricle, which of course becomes more or less hypertrophied. After a time the ventricle yields to the distending force of the accumulated blood, next, the auricle, and finally the great veins and the whole of the venous system; so that ultimately asthma may end in general venous congestion and dropsy, just in the same way as primary cardiac disease. But asthma may go on for a long time without any such results. It is surprising how severe the paroxysms may be, and for how many years the disease may continue (provided the fits are not prolonged and frequent) without the heart being in the least affected. It is only in cases of very long standing, and when the fits are tedious and leave a certain amount of permanent dyspnœa in the intervals (especially if there is some bronchitic complication), that these changes in the heart take place. As far as my experience goes, I should say that they never occurred as long as the recovery in the intervals was absolute. I cannot therefore agree with Dr. Todd (*Medical Gazette*, vol. xlvi. p. 1001) in the importance he assigns to evidence of dilatation of the right ventricle as a diagnostic sign of asthma. " I look upon this sign," he says, " as one of the most characteristic symptoms of asthma; and I consider its presence in any case where I suspect asthma as a clear confirmation of the correctness of those suspicions. In accordance with this view, one of my first steps in examining a patient whom I suspect to be asthmatic is to apply my finger to the scrobiculus cordis. If I find no beating of the heart there, my conclusion is a contingent negative. But if I find it beating there, and not in its natural position under the nipple, my conclusion is a certain affirmative."

Doubtless, in a case of suspected asthma, evidence of dilatation of the right side of the heart would strengthen the diagnosis; but the absence of it would go no way at all to negate the supposition that asthma existed. It would simply show that one of the results of asthma had not yet arisen, and it would establish a presumption that the disease had not been of long standing, that it was unassociated with chronic bronchitis, and that it had as yet inflicted no organic changes on the lungs. A patient's heart-beat may be in every way normal, and yet half an hour ago he may have been in the agonies of an asthmatic paroxysm. The positive evidence of heart-change in asthma is of some value; its negative evidence is worthless.

3. *Emphysema* is certainly the commonest of all the morbid changes that asthma tends to produce. I should say it was extremely rare to find the lungs of those who have long suffered from asthma entirely free from emphysematous inflation. The best examples of emphysema that I have ever seen have been in the *post-mortem* examinations of chronic asthma.

Adopting that view of emphysema so ably advocated by Dr. Gairdner—that it is essentially a compensatory dilatation, and implies the neighbourhood of non-expansible lung—I believe the mechanism of the production of emphysema by asthma to be as follows: The bronchial spasm shuts off the air; the shutting off the air produces capillary stasis—partial asphyxia; the congested vessels relieve themselves by the characteristic mucous exudation; the continued occlusion of the bronchial tubes, if the spasm does not yield, shuts up this mucus, and prevents its escape, and at the same time by barring the access of air, prevents efficient cough; so long as the spasm lasts, therefore, its escape is doubly prevented—by direct obstruction, and by the want of the natural machinery for its expulsion. The tubes affected by the asthmatic contraction thus become obstructed in a twofold way—at first narrowed by spasm, and then completely occluded by mucous infarction. As long as the spasm lasts the escape of the mucus is impossible. In the meantime, whatever may have been the length of the attack (and we know that it often lasts for days), the inspiratory muscles are making the most violent efforts to fill the chest, and are, in fact, keeping it in a state of extreme distension.

The length of time required for the removal of air from a lobule, from which communication with the external atmosphere is completely shut off by occlusion of its corresponding bronchial tube, I do not know; so I do not know if, in a single attack of asthma, any actual lobular collapse could take place, although, in a prolonged attack of some days I feel no doubt that it would. At any rate, the lobules whose bronchiæ are occluded cannot yield to the distending force of the inspiratory muscles; the whole distension of inspiration is, therefore, spent on those portions of the lungs whose communication with the external air is free; the open lobules have to expand for themselves and their occluded neighbours, and undergo an excessive inflation in proportion to the amount of lung that is non-expansible—in other words, become emphysematous. If we consider how complete the occlusion must be by this double process of spasm and infarction, how protracted asthma often is, and how violent are the inspiratory efforts that characterize it, I do not think we shall wonder at any amount of emphysema that is thereby produced, nor at its being one of the commonest organic changes to which asthma gives rise.

It will be seen, if the account I have just given is correct, that asthma produces emphysema just in the same way that bronchitis does. The two processes are essentially identical. In the one case the bronchial tubes are narrowed by inflammatory thickening of their walls and occluded by inflammatory exudation (muco-pus); in the other, they are narrowed by spasmodic contraction and occluded by the exudation of congestion (viscid mucus). The only difference is, that the narrowing and occlusion of bronchitis are generally of longer duration than those of asthma.

I think Dr. Walshe is quite right in his opinion that " the connection of emphysema with spasmodic seizures is certainly sometimes, possibly always, dependent on an intervening irritative or passive congestion of the tubes." That it is so sometimes I think is certain, because I think that congestion of the tubes is the immediate result of prolonged spasm. But is it always? If not, then emphysema may result from the spastic occlusion of the tubes without any mucous infarction. Is this possible? Is asthmatic spasm ever so complete and continuous as to produce without mucous exudation the results of plugging—lobular isolation, and collapse? This is a question that I think would be very difficult, at present perhaps impossible, to answer. One thing I feel strongly persuaded of, that it is not necessary that there should be any true bronchitis, anything actually inflammatory, in order that asthma should result in emphysema. I have seen emphysema developed in a case of asthma in which bronchitis never existed.

It is hardly worth while for me to describe the symptoms that mark the closing scene of those miserable cases of asthma that terminate in the production of these organic changes in the heart and lungs that I have just been describing. When once the right cavities of the heart have become dilated, and the obstructing force retrogrades upon the systemic veins, the symptoms are not to be distinguished from those which characterize a similar condition induced by chronic bronchitis. The cases differ alone in their previous history. There is the same rattling wheeze, the same choking cough, the same orthopnœa, the same abundant frothy expectoration (but in the case of bronchitis more purulent), the same venous regurgitation, the same choked-up breathlessness, getting ever worse and worse as the œdema and congestive solidification rise higher and higher in the lungs, the same general œdema beginning at the feet and gradually creeping up the trunk, the same cyanosis. The sufferings of this gradual choking out of life are most painful to witness till the increasing heaviness from the circulation of venous blood in the brain deepens into the insensibility which ushers in dissolution.

4. *Acquisition of the Asthmatic physique.*—Asthma is a disease that stamps on the body its own indelible marks. So characteristic and unmistakable is the physique of asthma, so plainly, so legibly does the asthmatic bear about with him the impress of his disease, that any one who has once observed it will never fail to recognize it, and would be safe in basing a diagnosis on its unaided testimony. In confirmation of this I may mention a circumstance or two that have occurred to myself.

I frequently meet in the streets of this city a distinguished savant, who is a great sufferer from asthma, and if I were to meet him at Pekin I should know him to be an asthmatic. The first time I saw him, I was walking behind him, but immediately recognized the characteristic configuration. So certain did I feel of it, and so curious was I to see if I could derive from his face any confirmation of my impression, that I overtook him, and as I passed saw at once who he was, from his resemblance to a photograph I had seen of him; and then I remembered what I had heard about his malady. This previous knowledge, however, could have had nothing to do with my impression, as at first I had no idea who he was, in fact, had never seen him before.

On another occasion, I was going down to Brixton in an omnibus, and sitting near me was a gentleman, whose figure and appearance very much struck me. He looked well in the face, was breathing without the slightest difficulty, and was engaged in animated conversation with his next neighbour. But I felt sure he was an asthmatic; he was exceedingly thin, his shoulders very high, and his back so rounded, that though quite a tall man, he sat lower, a good deal, than I did. He left the omnibus before me, and in walking his stooping gait and rounded back were still more conspicuous. When I left the omnibus, I asked the conductor " If he knew that tall, thin, stooping gentleman that got out at such and such a place." " Oh, yes," he said, "it is Mr. ———, of ———." " Do you know," I asked, "if he is subject to a complaint in his chest, that gives him fits of difficult breathing ?" " Oh, yes," he replied, "and has been for a long time—for years; sometimes he can hardly walk to the omnibus."

Here then are two cases in which I recognize the presence of asthma, merely by the changes in the physiognomy and configuration which it produces. I have done the same thing in several other instances. I often say to myself as I pass an individual in the street with the characteristic configuration, "You are an asthmatic."

What then is this unmistakable impress of asthma? How is it to be described? In what peculiarities does it consist? Partly those of the figure, partly those of the face. In configuration, the asthmatic is round-backed, high-shouldered, and stooping; but while the body is bent forwards the head is thrown back, and buried, as it were, between the elevated shoulders. There is no movement or pliancy in the body, but the chest is fixed and rigid, like a box, and from it the arms depend, hanging motionless, or swinging like two pump-handles, rather thrown back, and bent at the elbows. In walking, the legs seem the only part of the body that moves. From the roundness of the back, the asthmatic, for his height, always sits low. Those who have suffered from asthma long, are almost invariably thin, often to a degree amounting to emaciation; their limbs are attenuated and bony, every rib can be counted, and their clothes hang loosely on them. From the entire absence of subcutaneous fat the superficial veins are very conspicuous; though it is possible that venous obstruction, from impeded circulation through the lungs, may have something to do with their prominence—that it may be, in fact, slight general varix. The prominence and tortuousness of the veins is sometimes remarkable, especially in old asthmatics. The hands of an asthmatic are very characteristic; they are cold, blue, thin, and veiny. This blueness and coldness of the extremities is partly due, no doubt, to the feebleness, of the circulation in them, but in part, especially if there is some permanent dyspnœa, or the patient is at the time suffering from an attack, to imperfect decarbonization of the blood.

But the blueness of surface is not confined to the extremities, the complexion of the asthmatic is often distinctly cyanotic—a slight but perceptible duskiness. Where, however, there is no dyspnœa between the attacks, and the intervals are long, especially in young subjects, I do not think the complexion is perceptibly affected.

The face has generally rather an anxious expression, and often bears an aspect of age greater than the real age of the patient; even if not dusky it is always pale, and, like the rest of the body, is thin —the cheeks are hollow, and the lines of the face are deeply marked. The mouth is generally open, and the jaw rather hanging. There is a peculiarity about the eyes to which I would call particular attention, to which I often *have* directed attention among the patients at the hospital, and on the strength of which alone I have frequently diagnosed asthma; they are turgid, watery, and prominent. I believe this to depend, like the enlargement of the superficial veins, upon venous obstruction; the turgidity is that of the veins of the conjunctiva, the wateriness is due to an unusual amount of mucus and tears which the engorged mucous membrane and lachrymal gland pour out, while the prominence is due to the turgidity of the veins of the orbit. Wherever I find this appearance of the eyes in connection with chronic asthma I look out for dilated right heart.

The asthmatic's voice is often very peculiar; it is feeble, and slightly hoarse and rough; he speaks as a healthy person would speak if he were to expire as long as he could and then begin to speak—as if he were making use of the last breath in his lungs; and it is indeed to the small respiratory resource that he has for speech that this feebleness and roughness of the asthmatic's voice is due. His sentences are short, and frequently interrupted by a single dry cough.

Many of the external characteristics of asthma that I have enumerated, such as the gait, the dusky complexion, the eyes, the voice, will be seen at once to be those rather of chronic dyspnœa than of asthma, and I would so far qualify their value as diagnostic signs. Indeed, their value is rather generic than specific. In the purest cases of spasmodic asthma, in which there is no trace of dyspnœa in the intervals, they are the least marked, and are the most conspicuous in those which are complicated with some chronic bronchitis or bronchial congestion, so that I look upon their absence as a good sign, as a sign that the lungs are sound and unscathed; and it is because asthma seldom exists long without producing such changes as permanently embarrass the breathing, that these changes in the physiognomy and configuration come to be signs of asthma; they are just as much a part of its clinical history as those internal changes in the lungs and heart of which they are the sure sign and accompaniment. I have, however, seen the asthmatic physique very strongly marked in some cases where the lungs were organically sound; but these were always cases where the paroxysms were very long, lasting for days or weeks, so that the efficient cause was in continued operation for a long time; or else they were cases in which the asthma had been very severe in childhood, when the figure was forming, so that it got *set* in the asthmatic shape, and, although the disease afterwards quite disappeared, the figure never recovered itself. Such cases carry a certain highness of shoulders and roundness of back with them to the end of their days, however completely the asthma may be in mature life recovered from.

The degree of deformity of the back is, in some cases, truly remarkable; and (although I have not examined any of the spines of these cases after death) such as I cannot but think must involve some anatomical change in the bones or intervertebral disks. The curvature is always direct antero-posterior, never lateral, and involves the middle or lower dorsal vertebræ. In one case I have seen the angle made by the curvature almost as considerable as an angle of a hundred degrees. Now, it is certain that such a change in direction as this, almost a right angle, effected within the length of a few vertebræ, could only be produced by a great shortening of the anterior aspect of the column, involving a vertical shortening of the anterior part of its separate elements—vertebræ, or intervertebral disks, or both—converting the bodies of the vertebræ, or the disks of fibro-cartilage between them, into wedges, as shown in the accompanying diagram.

Fig. 3.

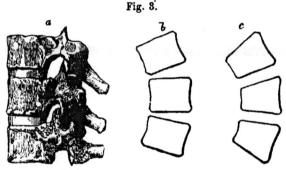

Diagram showing the change of form in the bodies of the vertebræ, or intervertebral disks, involved in the anterior curvature of asthma: *a*, natural shape; *b*, if the disks; *c*, if the bodies of the vertebræ become wedge-shaped.

The agency by which a disease affecting the air-passages produces this curvature of the spinal column was not very clear to me, and it was long before I arrived at what I believe to be its true explanation. It certainly was not a change of form having for its object the enlargement of the thoracic cavity, like the barrel-chest of emphysema; it was manifest that such a deformity must materially prejudice the size, the shape, and the movements of the thorax. It was equally certain that there was no spinal disease; that the curvature was the result of repeated attacks of asthma; that it was the permanent retention and constant aggravation of the asthmatic stoop which always exists during the paroxysms. But, beyond this, its nature and causation did not appear intelligible. At length I was guided to what appears to me to be its true *rationale* by the following considerations:—

1. Pressure produces absorption of the part pressed on; *e. g.*, the absorption of the sternum and ribs in aneurism.

2. In stooping—*i. e.*, in forward curvature—there is vertical pressure along the anterior face of the spinal column; *i. e.*, its elements exercise vertical pressure upon one another in their anterior portions.

3. The unsupported spine tends to fall forward—*i. e.*, to anterior curvature; the whole array of the muscles of the back are erectors of it.

4. When the muscles of extraordinary respiration are engaged in extraordinary respiratory efforts they cease to play their ordinary *rôle; e. g.*, the homo-hyoid muscle is ordinarily a depressor of the hyoid bone, but in asthma it is an elevator of the scapula, and powerless to depress the hyoid bone; the sterno-mastoid is ordinarily a rotator and anterior flexor of the head; in asthma, it is an elevator of the sternum and clavicle, and powerless to move the head.

I infer, therefore, that the muscles of the back, being engrossed during the asthmatic paroxysm with their violent respiratory labour, cease to act as erectors of the spine. The back is, therefore, unsupported, and obeys its natural tendency to fall forward. This, I am sure, is the true explanation of the asthmatic stoop; and we see, consistently with this view, that any effort to straighten the back is immediately attended with additional distress (because the muscles are temporarily withdrawn from their respiratory exertions), and that the stooping is always in proportion to the dyspnœa—that is, in proportion to the degree in which the muscles of the back are engrossed by the breathing. The back being, therefore, left thus to itself, and falling thus forward, the anterior parts of the bodies of the vertebræ and intervertebral disks are pressed together; and if the asthmatic state is continued long, and occurs frequently, this pressure is so protracted that it produces absorption of this part of the bodies of the vertebræ, or the intervertebral fibro-cartilages, or both; they become wedge-shaped, and the temporary stoop becomes a permanent curvature.

Now, I admit that I have never examined the spine, *post mortem*, in cases of this asthmatic deformity; and I merely offer this hypothesis as a reasonable explanation. In cases in which I have seen it there has not existed the slightest ground for believing that there was any spinal disease. In the most marked case that I ever saw (of which I have been disappointed of giving a figure, from the loss of a photograph I had taken and the subsequent death of the patient), the back was straight before the asthma came on, and the patient tall; but as the asthma became worse and the attacks longer and more

8

frequent, the stoop, which he always had during the attacks, went off less and less in the intervals, and gradually became more and more considerable, till it settled into a permanent deformity, which, though his legs were long, made him quite a short man.   No pain is experienced in the back in these cases (except an aching of the dorsal muscles during the asthma, from their violent respiratory exertion). Moreover, the curvature is never confined to a single vertebra, or to two or three, and is never angular; it is rounded and gradual, and involves a considerable portion of the back.   In such an absence of all evidence of spinal disease, and with an amount of curvature in some cases making some change of form in the elements of the spine a physical necessity, I do not see what explanation can be offered other than I have given.   If correct, it is certainly interesting; it has the interest of all facts which elucidate a *modus operandi*, and furnish the connecting links between associated but apparently diverse phenomena.

When my mind was engaged in thinking on this subject, a case of another nature occurred to me which confirmed my ideas, and seemed to show that mere loss of power on the part of the muscles of the back was adequate to the production of anterior spinal curvature.   A man in the prime of life, with an erect figure, who had never had anything the matter with his spine in any way, was seized with severe rheumatism in the muscles of the back, and the pain was so aggravated and rendered so intense by attempting to stand upright, that the muscles refused to perform their office; the unsupported spine bent forward as far as its elasticity would permit, and the back became round and the gait stooping, like that of an old man.   This went on for some months, without any decided curvature appearing; at length, distinct and gradually increasing curvature manifested itself, involving the seventh and eighth dorsal vertebræ, and to such an extent as to show that their bodies must have undergone some change of shape.   The patient recovered from his rheumatism, regained the power of supporting his back, and the curvature was arrested; but it has never disappeared.

If, then, loss of power of the spinal muscles, paralyzed by rheumatic pain, is adequate to the production of organic curvature in the way that I have supposed, why should not their paralysis, as erectors of the spine, from their being engrossed in their respiratory action, be attended with the same result?

In young asthmatics who have suffered from their disease in infancy I have observed a configuration of chest which I have seen, to a certain extent, in cachectic rickety children who have not suffered from asthma, but which I am not sure I have ever seen in children who have not suffered from any chest-affection.   I am not sure, therefore, what share in the production of the deformity ought to be assigned to the asthma, or what to the deficient strength of the bony parietes of the chest; or whether imperfect ossification and chest-mischief are both necessary for its production.   What inclines me to think that the latter cause is the chief one (or, at least, an essential one) is, that the deformity is just such as would be produced where there was an impediment to inspiration, and where violent but ineffectual inspiratory efforts were made by weak parietes—just such, in fact, as one sees in the inspiration of atelectasis or laryngitis.

In these cases, the upper part of the chest—above the fifth or sixth rib—is naturally shaped; but below that level, on each side of the sternum and along the margin of the false ribs, corresponding to the cartilages of the seventh, eighth, ninth, and tenth, the surface, instead of being convex and full, is excavated in two hollows. These hollows are bound internally by the lower part of the sternum, which stands forward between them in a ridge; and externally by the extremities of the ossified portions of the rib, which form a ridge on the outside. The situation of this flattening in of the thoracic parietes —its coincidence with the cartilages of the ribs—suggests the way in which it is produced, and explains how asthma might cause it. I take the method of its production to be this : when there is any impediment to the ingress of air into the lungs—from narrowed bronchial tubes, as in asthma, or any other way, the air cannot rush in so fast as the thoracic parietes are expanded, a partial vacuum is therefore formed in the chest, and the pressure of the air within it no longer balances that of the air without. This unbalanced external atmospheric pressure presses on the whole of the thoracic parietes equally, and drives in the most yielding ; in other words, the bony ribs, raised against it by the respiratory muscles, are able to resist it, but the soft cartilaginous portions are not. It must be remembered, too, that the diaphragm is attached along the margins of all the ribs below the fifth ; its strong contractions during the asthmatic paroxysm would tend therefore to draw them in, and, being

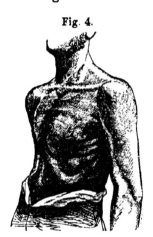

Fig. 4.

From a photograph of an asthmatic, whose disease dated from whooping-cough at three months old.

less opposed by their yielding cartilaginous portions, would concur in the production of this change of shape. This condition would, of course, at first only last as long as the paroxysm ; but if the attacks were frequent and severe at a time when the cartilaginous portion of the ribs was considerable and the figure forming, one can easily understand how the deformity would become permanent, and how asthma would in this way produce such a change in the form of the chest as I have been describing.

But the actual event to which I think this form of chest directly points—the particular morbid change that it immediately implies— is pulmonary collapse. One cannot but be struck, on looking at such chests, with their exact resemblance (except in the absence of what one may call the diaphragmatic stricture—the drawing in of the attachment of the diaphragm at each inspiration, as if a ligature were put round the body) to the shape of the chest in the inspiration of infants suffering from bronchial plugging, or its established result—atelectasis, or from croup, or laryngitis, or any affection that, preventing the ingress of air and the expansion of the lung, refuses to allow the parietes to follow the movements of the inspiratory muscles.[1] Pulmonary collapse would certainly be a more potent cause of this deformity than unaided asthma, because it is a more permanent condition and involves a more complete inexpansibility of lung, and therefore would more effectually resist the inspiration-movement of the softer parts of the parietes.

In so far then as this heteromorphism points to atelectasis, its occurrence in cases of asthma tends to confirm what I have already said of the tendency and sufficiency of that disease to produce this condition of lung. But remembering that it is only in cases that have become asthmatic young that this state of chest is well marked, and remembering how commonly asthma dates in the young from catarrhal bronchitis, from the bronchitis of measles, or from what has been called "whooping-cough with bronchitis," which is nothing more than whooping-cough in which the bronchitic portion of the malady has extended far and severely into the bronchial tree—remembering this, I say, one cannot but see it possible, that, at least in many cases, the pulmonary collapse may have been produced in the ordinary way, by mucous plugging of the bronchial tubes from the primary bronchitis, and not from the consequential asthma in the way I have suggested. I have seen this deformity strongly marked in cases where ordinary bronchitis had never occurred, and where the patient was entirely free from bronchitic complication or tendency; but the asthma dated from whooping-cough in infancy—and, in my opinion, no form of bronchitis has so great a tendency to generate collapse as that of whooping-cough.

Dr Gairdner, of Edinburgh, in his excellent papers on the " Pathological Anatomy of Bronchitis," alludes to this deformity of chest as an occasional permanent result of pulmonary collapse. "In rickety individuals," he says, " it is not only more marked, but apt to become permanent, especially when such subjects are affected with any considerable or persistent bronchitic affection. In such cases, the reversed movement of the ribs is stereotyped, as it were, in the form of chest called *pigeon-breast*, in which the sternum is protruded, particularly below, and the whole lateral region, including also the lower costal cartilages in front, flattened, or even at some points rendered irregularly concave."

One result of this collapse of the cartilages of the ribs is that they do not stand out from the sternum as they should; but decline from

[1] I have seen it strongly marked in the inspiration of laryngitis even in adults.

it at too acute an angle, narrowing and elongating the scrobiculus cordis.

Fig. 4, a very good example of this configuration, is taken from a photograph of an asthmatic who suffered from his disease from the age of three months. The condition has existed from his earliest recollection, and during his childhood was much more considerable, for since he has grown up his disease has nearly left him, and the shape of his chest has much improved.

I am of opinion that the occurrence of asthma once renders the subject of it more liable ever afterwards to a recurrence of it. It is very rare to hear of a person having a single attack; so rare that I am not sure that I have ever heard of a case. It might be said that a person who has had asthma once must have a predisposition to the disease, and therefore in him it will be likely to occur again, and since some attack must be the first, the first will be followed by the succeeding ones. But I do not think this is sufficient to explain the very common fact that a person may pass half his life before he has his first fit, but after it has once occurred will never pass a month without it; neither the fact that after asthma has once occurred causes will excite it that would not before; nor do I see why the same fact should not point to the same conclusion in asthma as it does in epilepsy and rheumatism. *So it is,* I feel assured, but *why* it is I cannot pretend to say. Is it that a certain nervous action having been once set going is, *ipso facto,* re-excited on the slightest provocation? Is it a case of mere vicious *habit?* Is it that the bronchial muscle becomes so hypertrophied by the asthmatic spasm that it becomes increasingly prone to take on a state of contraction

---

CHAPTER VIII.

TREATMENT OF THE ASTHMATIC PAROXYSM.—TREATMENT BY DEPRESSANTS.

Preliminary measures.—Ipecacuanha. Tobacco. Tartar-emetic.—Their *modus operandi.*—Their relative value and methods of administration.—Cases.—Value of tobacco in hay-asthma.—Cases.—Caution with regard to tobacco.—Importance of early administration of these remedies.—Practical observations.

THE treatment of asthma, like that of all paroxysmal diseases, naturally divides itself into the treatment of the paroxysm and the treatment in the intervals of the paroxysms, and although the last is the real treatment of the disease, while the treatment of the paroxysm is merely the treatment of a symptom, yet the paroxysm being in asthma, potentially though not essentially, the disease (for it is its sole manifestation, the only source of suffering, and the cause of those organic changes in the heart and lungs by which alone asthma threatens life), its treatment holds the first place in the therapeutics of the affection. If the paroxysms are mitigated the disease is rendered proportionally trifling—if they are prevented the disease is extinguished. The persistence of the asthmatic tendency is of not the slightest consequence as long as the fits are warded off, or indefinitely postponed; and thus the mere negative treatment of abstention from the exciting cause of the paroxysm may amount to a virtual and final cure.

The first thing to be done on being called to a patient in a paroxysm of asthma, is to ascertain if there is any exciting cause actually present and in operation, and if so to remove it. An undigested meal or a full rectum may, as peripheral irritants, produce bronchial spasm; the one I think through the pneumogastric nerve, the other through the sympathetic, and thus an emetic which relieves the one, and an enema (or any other means) which evacuates the other, may put a stop to the attack. I have previously mentioned a case in which the occurrence of an attack was entirely determined by the loaded or empty condition of the rectum: if the patient retired to bed without the bowels being relieved, he was sure to be awoke in the night with asthma; if they were moved before going to bed, he awoke at the usual time in the morning well. The relief obtained by an emetic is well known.

At once ascertain then, the condition of the patient in these respects, inquire what he last ate and when he ate it, and if his bowels are loaded; and if there is any source of offence in either situation—stomach or the lower bowel—secure its immediate evacuation. Ascertain, too, the state of the air he is breathing, if there is in it any known or unknown irritant, any of those subtle emanations of which asthmatics are so sensible, if there is a hay-field near, or ipecacuanha powder in the room, or dust, or smoke, and if so, let the removal from these influences be the first step taken. Inquire, too, if the patient has ever been seized with an attack in the same place before, if he has had any reason to imagine that that particular air did not agree with him, or if in any local peculiarities it resembles places that he has previously found offend his asthma. If so, get him away at once, never mind how difficult it is to move him, transport him to some place or some *kind* of situation known to agree with him; very likely before he has gone a mile or two he will be quite well; whereas, all treatment will be powerless as long as he is under the influence of the injurious air.

Let it be your first care, too, to place your patient in a favourable position;—get him out of bed and bolster him up in an arm chair, and place before him a table of convenient height, with a pillow on it, on which he may rest his elbows and throw himself forward. It is quite surprising, almost incredible, how much comfort this will give, and not only so, but how it will actually relieve the breathing and dispose the spasm to yield. Sometimes the patient's breath is so bad that he cannot sit; the same arrangements must then be made for him in a standing posture.

But if, as will probably be the case, the spasm persists in spite of these preliminary measures, and if no exciting cause can be discovered by whose removal the paroxysm may be at once arrested, our next step is to cast about for some remedy by which we may hope to cut it short. In our choice of this we shall be very much influenced by our patient's former experience. Few asthmatics suffer long from their disease without having discovered what particular remedy is most efficacious in their case, and in this respect different cases of asthma vary so much, and display such a caprice, that I really know of no other guide except the patient's experience.

Of all the different kinds of evidence on which we build our theories of the pathology of diseases, there is none more convincing, or that tells a plainer tale, than that which is derived from therapeutics. The success of a remedy given on certain principles proves the correctness of the principles on which it was given, and the known action of a medicine directly implies the nature of the pathological state that it relieves, as it shows that in any case of its successful administration the pathological state must have been such as that known action would antagonize or correct. This reflected evidence has all the force of the fulfilment of a prediction, like the re-appearance of Halley's comet at the exact time that its discoverer foretold.

My purpose in this chapter is to direct attention to the great efficacy and value, in the treatment of asthma, of certain drugs belonging to a class whose therapeutical action is very strongly marked, and about whose *modus operandi* there is no doubt, and which throw, therefore, a very clear light on the nature of the pathological condition that they relieve—the class of direct *depressants* or *contra-stimulants*. It is a class of remedies that exercises the most singular and powerful influence over the asthmatic condition, greater and more immediate than any other that I know, except, perhaps, mental emotion. As soon as their characteristic effect is established, the dyspnœa ceases—completely ceases from that moment; no matter how intense the spasm may have been, the moment the sensations characteristic of collapse are felt it yields, the respiration is free, and the patient passes from agony to ease. It is one of the most striking things to witness, in the way of a remedy, that can be imagined.

The three drugs of this class with whose use in asthma I am most familiar are, ipecacuan, tartar-emetic, and tobacco. No doubt they all act in the same way—by lowering innervation, depressing nervous vitality or irritability, or whatever we may call it, and enfeebling the contraction of the bronchial muscle, just as they weaken the heart's action, or relax the grasp wherewith a strangulated hernia is constricted, or relieve urethral stricture, or the spasm of colic.

With regard to their *modus operandi* in asthma I think a good deal of misconception very generally prevails; they are thought by some to act as emetics, by some as so-called expectorants. I believe they act neither as one nor the other, but as direct depressants, relaxing the spasm of the bronchial tubes in the way I have mentioned. In illustration of this I will just relate a case in which I had ample opportunity for some years of watching the effect of ipecacuanha.

The patient was a youth who had been asthmatic from his infancy. His attacks had increased in frequency till, at the time to which I refer, they occurred with tolerable regularity once a week. His asthma generally awoke him about four or five o'clock in the morning, and soon compelled him to sit up and wheeze in bed, or get out of bed and stand against some piece of furniture for support. In two or three hours he would be able to dress himself, and perhaps in the forenoon the severity of the dyspnœa would a little abate; but towards the afternoon and evening it would deepen, and towards bed-time get so intense that without an emetic there was no chance of sleep. The emetic would be taken, and in half an hour he would be perfectly easy, without the slightest trace of asthma. He would then take a light supper, go to bed, sleep like an infant, and have no more asthma till that day week. In this way he would have fifty attacks, or thereabouts, in a year; and cut them short at night with fifty emetics. If he did not take the emetic he passed a miserable, sleepless night, and was still bad the next day; indeed there was no definite end to the attack without it. I think *now*, that if he had taken it earlier in the day, or even in the morning on first waking up asthmatic, he would have cut short the attack equally well, and have saved himself a great deal of suffering. I never knew it fail. The dose taken was always twenty grains of the ipecacuanha powder; and, although he repeated it so frequently, it neither lost its efficacy nor did him any harm. It was clearly not as an emetic that it acted, but as a depressant, for the relief took place before the vomiting. About ten minutes or a quarter of an hour after swallowing the draught a sense of nausea would be felt, accompanied with a slight faintness, and dampness on the skin, and a profuse secretion of saliva which came from his mouth in a little clear stream. It was then that the spasm gave way, before a single act of retching had occurred; and his attendants would immediately know when the first sense of nausea was felt by the relief of the breathing that invariably accompanied it. Besides, the stomach was always perfectly empty; there was nothing of which it could be relieved.

The effect of *tobacco* is exactly the same, only the depression that it produces is more profound and amounts to actual collapse, and the relief, therefore, more speedy and complete. In those who have not established a tolerance of tobacco, its use is soon followed by a well-known condition of collapse, much resembling sea-sickness— vertigo, loss of power in the limbs, a sense of deadly faintness, cold sweat, inability to speak or think, nausea, vomiting. The moment this condition can be induced the asthma ceases, as if stopped by a charm. In one case in particular I have frequently watched its effects. In the case that I refer to the asthmatic fortunately never established a tolerance of the drug, and thirty whiffs of a pipe or half a cigar would at any time induce a condition of collapse. I have known him begin to smoke when his breathing has been so difficult that he could hardly draw his pipe; he would draw a feeble whiff or two, and then stop to recover his breath, and then another whiff, and so on. By and by he would lay down his pipe with a look of intelligence at his attendant, as much as to say, "it's all right now;" his face would become pallid and damp with perspiration, his limbs relaxed, his breathing long and sighing—but his asthma was gone. His object was to smoke just so much as to produce this condition, and no more, so that the moment he felt the sensation coming on he stopped. After this qualmy condition had continued for twenty minutes or half an hour, it would go off and leave him well—the attack cured. Sometimes, however, he would take a little to much, and then the operation of the drug would go on to vomiting, and sometimes he would overdo it altogether, and produce a deadly and protracted collapse, from which it seemed as if he would never recover. I have known his pulse hardly perceptible for nearly two hours, in spite of ammonia and brandy freely administered. It is this circumstance —the fear of this horrible and unmanageable collapse—that makes one so unwilling to employ tobacco; it is indeed a dreadful remedy, almost as bad as the disease; but the asthmatic is willing to undergo anything to get quit of his sufferings.

The following account, illustrative of the effect of tobacco, I have received from an intelligent patient long subject to severe asthma:—

"I have always found perfect relief from smoking tobacco in the attacks of spasmodic asthma to which I have been liable. In describing my own experience, I should say that no relief is felt till the poison gives evidence of having taken effect by its disagreeable consequences; and just in proportion to the sickness and faintness and other miserable sensations, is the relief of the difficult breathing. I never knew this remedy fail. As the use of tobacco was new to me it affected me very powerfully, and produced the most miserable prostration and faintness. The cure of the asthmatic spasm was very speedy, and frequently it was forgotten altogether in the horrors of a sensation known to all novices in smoking, so that I was often unconscious of its disappearance, or of the mode or time of its departure; the asthma seemed supplanted by another condition, and cold perspiration and fear of collapse closed the scene. I am not aware whether this was followed by expectoration, and the presence of mucus in the throat removed by the usual process—the common action of ' clearing the throat,' as it is called—which invariably appears when an attack of asthma spontaneously subsides, and which always accompanies the slower cure resulting from the mild use of ipecacuanha, which of late years I have preferred to tobacco, as my asthma is not of sufficient intensity to require so violent and distressing a remedy. I imagine these more natural and ordinary symptoms of recovery would always accompany the use of ipecacuanha, and that an increased dose would only accelerate the process of recovery up to the interruption by vomiting. The difference between the characteristics of these two modes of cure appears to me to be strongly marked and very important. I conceive this to arise from the intensity of the depression caused by the poison of tobacco, which cannot be the case in the use of ipecacuanha, as it is a simple emetic, and I doubt if the same kind of sensations and depression could be produced by ipecacuanha, even if its effect could be carried on and the medicine were not rejected by the stomach, which is invariably the case when the effect is increased to a certain point. I have not gone beyond the stage of perspiration and a feeling of sickness, and I have always found the cure to resemble the natural process of mucous discharge and clearing of the air-passages, only more promptly induced and more rapidly performed. I have frequently had short spasms of asthma produced by laughing, lighting a lucifer-match, or some other special irritant, from which I have recovered as rapidly as when under the influence of ipecacuanha, going through the stages of silent asthma, audible asthma, and the expectoration mentioned above, in about the space of ten minutes or a quarter of an hour. The distinction between these two modes of cure or relief is worthy the attention of medical men and their patients, as much distress and perhaps injurious results might be avoided if the ipecacuanha is found to be as efficacious as tobacco. My only doubt is whether tobacco might not be preferable in desperate and suffocating spasms on account of its speedy and violent action."

No doubt there is such a difference as that indicated above in the action of tobacco and ipecacuan. Ipecacuan, I think, could never produce such collapse as that caused by tobacco; but that it does not always act as an expectorant or emetic, but as a direct depressant, is shown by the case that I related just now. The fact is, ipecacuan acts very differently on different individuals: in some, producing vomiting with little more irritation than sulphate of zinc; in some, producing collapse to a considerable degree. Moreover, by relaxing the bronchial spasm, it renders free cough and expectoration possible, which were previously impossible from inability to get sufficient air into the lungs to effect them; so that the expectoration is the consequence of the relief, and not the relief of the expectoration.

In that mild but annoying form of asthma that accompanies the other symptons of hay-fever, and is known as hay-asthma, tobacco pushed *ad nauseam* gives more relief than any other remedy. In a relative of mine who is very much afflicted with this troublesome complaint, tobacco-smoking is the only thing that gives any relief. During the hay season and all the early hot summer weather, he suffers (besides the sneezing and running at the eyes, and tumid burning of the nose and throat, characteristic of hay-fever) from paroxysms of a wheezing dyspnœa of the true asthmatic type, coming on exclusively at night, so as almost to deprive him of sleep. During the rest of the year he never smokes, as it is disagreeable to him, and in other respects prejudicial; but during this season he is quite dependent on his cigar for any degree of comfort or alleviation of his symptoms. The following graphic account of the relief he finds from tobacco I cannot do better than give in his own words:—

"There is no remedy during a paroxysm of hay-asthma that has anything like the effect of smoking tobacco; and though this is especially the case in the latter stage of the attack, when the asthmatic element of the phenomena is most developed, still, in the earlier stage, when the lachrymation, sneezing, and faucial irritation are most distressing, tobacco-smoke has, in my case, a very marked influence in soothing and diminishing these symptoms.

"No doubt any of those medicines which Dr. Pereira has called 'cardiaco-vascular depressants' would produce a somewhat similar result; but none is of so easy application, or can be used so readily or pleasantly as tobacco. During the hay-asthma season—that is, in my case, from about the 15th of May to the 10th or 12th of July —I regularly smoke a cigar the last thing before going to bed, or perhaps more frequently after I am in bed. The effect is, that (excepting during the last fortnight in June, when I never get a night's rest) the sedative influence of the tobacco prevents the occurrence of any asthmatic spasm. If during this period I omit my cigar, I seldom sleep beyond four o'clock; usually three o'clock finds me awake hopelessly, though generally only slightly, asthmatic for the rest of the night; till, indeed, about nine o'clock, when almost always the asthma completely leaves me. This night-cigar is taken as a preventive. But tobacco will cure the asthmatic spasm when it is fairly on; only it requires a larger dose of the poison and in a stronger form. The sedative influence of the cigar will usually insure me a fair night's rest; but the powerful depression of strong shag-tobacco is necessary to cut short the spasm when it is established. Even when I do smoke my night-cigar I not unfrequently have to get up about three or four o'clock in the morning and smoke; and during the last fortnight in June this happens almost nightly.

"Distressing as are the sensations of collapse from tobacco-poisoning, they are an unspeakable relief when contrasted with the impending suffocation of asthma. I shall never forget an attack which I once had, and the joy with which I hailed the approach of collapse from tobacco-poisoning. It was late in July, many years ago. I had gone into Dorsetshire to stay with a relative in a country house. Immediately surrounding the house were grazing fields— not hayfields—and they had not been mown. In these fields was a grass—*Nardus stricta*, I think—still blooming luxuriantly; for it is a grass which cattle will not eat; and thus, though past the usual time for hay-asthma, I was accidentally surrounded by its most

potent cause—grass in flower.   The night came, and I had not been
an hour in bed when I was attacked with the most violent asthma I
ever experienced.   There were no cigars in the house, but one of
the servants had some rank shag-tobacco.   I smoked one pipe, then
another: and as my face blanched, and my pulse failed, and the
cold sweat stood on my forehead, miserable as were the sensations
of collapse, they were Paradise to the agonies of suffocation.   I
shall never forget those moments of relief.

"The story of this attack of asthma, by the way, is a very instructive one; and I may just add it here, in brief: I left my
friend's house the day after this paroxysm, and went to the sea-side,
where I was as usual perfectly well.   Two days after, I received a
letter from him asking me to return, as he had had the grass, in flower
about his house, cut down.   I did so, and remained with him a fortnight, sleeping every night as placidly as an infant.   The *Nardus
stricta* had given me the asthma: the scythe had cured it.

"To return to the tobacco.   A hay asthmatic should never smoke
tobacco but for his malady.   Smoking should never be to him a habit
or a meal, for it then ceases to be a medicine.   Indeed, to him it
should be as a deadly drug, for it is by poisoning that it cures."

Not long ago I was conversing on the subject of his malady with
a surgeon of some distinction in this city who is grievously victim-
ized with hay-asthma, and on asking him what he found do him any
good, he replied, "Tobacco; tobacco is the only thing; nothing does
me any good but smoking;" and he went on to tell me, that whenever he finds his asthma very bad, and that he shall get no sleep
without it, he immediately resorts to a cigar.   But the smoking does
him no good unless it produces a condition of collapse; the mere
sedative effect of it is of no use to him whatever; and having lost,
from the habit of smoking, an easy susceptibility to tobacco influence,
he adopts the following device to secure its more potent effect: he
fills his mouth with tobacco-smoke, and then, instead of breathing it
out again at once, as is usual in smoking, retains it in his mouth for
several seconds, perhaps a quarter of a minute, then takes another
mouthful, and so on.   In this way, he finds that the tobacco is more
rapidly absorbed by the mucous membrane of the oral cavity, and
that a state of collapse is speedily induced.   The moment the faintness and sickness come over him the asthma ceases, he turns into
bed, and has a good night.

The effect of antimony nearly resembles that of tobacco, and it
acts in the same way, but the nausea and collapse it produces are
long and tedious.

Of the three drugs, I should say ipecacuanha is the most man-
ageable, and entails the least suffering; tobacco the most speedy and
effectual.

There are one or two practical points on which I would add a
few words.

Remedies of this kind, given with the view of cutting short the paroxysm, should be given as early as possible; and for two reasons. First, because it is much easier to break through the asthmatic condition when it is but just established, while the longer it is allowed to go on, the more inveterate and uncontrollable it becomes, and the more difficult it is to arrest it; indeed, its giving way at all may depend on the earliness with which the remedy is applied. I have known treatment powerless after the dyspnœa has continued for some hours, which never failed if administered as soon as it declared itself. Just at starting, in the earliest stages of paroxysm, a very slight thing will determine its advance or retreat, and in proportion as it advances and deepens, in just such proportion do remedies become inoperative. The other reason is, that if the spasm *does* yield in spite of having been some time established, the recovery is not so complete as if the remedy had been applied immediately on its appearance. The longer the bronchial stricture lasts, the greater is the arrears of breathing and the resulting pulmonary congestion; and if this goes on unchecked and increasing for many hours, the disturbance of the vascular balance becomes so great, the capillaries of the lungs so loaded, that it is a long time, many hours, or perhaps even days, before that balance is restored, and the vessels recover their normal condition: and although the bronchial spasm may completely give way, there remains a certain amount of shortness of breath and an incapacity for exertion, and it is not until an abundant expectoration of mucus has taken place, by the pouring out of which the loaded vessels have relieved themselves, that the chest becomes clear and the breathing free. In asthma at once cut short there is no such accumulated congestion—no mucous exudation, and when the bronchial spasm ceases all dyspnœa vanishes. If on first awaking with the sensations of asthma the asthmatic nauseates himself with tobacco, or smokes his nitre-paper, or keeps himself in a standing posture, or in any other way cuts short the paroxysm, he will be throughout the succeeding day exactly the same, with the exception of the sleep he has lost, as if nothing had occurred; but if he suffers the fight between asthma and sleep to go on long, and then on the first remission of the dyspnœa lies back and goes to sleep, he will protract the asthmatic state, deepen the consequent pulmonary arrears, and not only postpone his recovery for many hours, but make it then slow and imperfect. I know an asthmatic who now never loses a day by his disease, in consequence of the promptitude with which he meets its first appearance in the early morning, but who formerly, from continuing to lie in bed and try to get sleep after the asthma had begun, protracted his sufferings through the day. He is attacked as often as ever, and at the same time—about three or four o'clock in the morning—but the moment he finds his asthma on him he takes measures to keep himself wide awake, stands leaning against a piece of furniture, and, if necessary, induces tobacco collapse, so that instead of a day's asthma he has half an hour's, and, as far as all the engagements of life go, has ceased to be an asthmatic.

It is a difficult thing for the asthmatic, I know, overwhelmed with sleep as he is, and generally with a peculiarly heavy drowsiness upon him, to leave his bed or light and smoke his pipe; but he *must* do it; he must rouse himself fairly up and adopt at once those remedies that in his particular case are most efficacious. In fact, the treatment of the asthmatic paroxysm should be so prompt as to be almost rather preventive than curative: in the treatment of no disease is the injunction "*obsta principiis*" of more vital importance.

One is sometimes asked—Which is the best form of tobacco to use, a cigar or a pipe? I think a pipe has the advantage of more certain strength; cigars vary so much, even the same sort. The tobacco that I generally employ is bird's-eye, as being a mild tobacco, and one by which you run little risk of inducing alarming collapse. *Shag*, or any other of the strong tobaccos, should not be used by the uninitiated, as the collapse they produce is apt to become protracted and unmanageable. For ladies and young children, a few whiffs of a mild cigarette are quite sufficient.[1]

Of ipecacuanha, I think the powder is better than the wine. I never give a very small dose, it is uncertain and teasing. I would say, always give such a dose as will be certain to secure its own prompt rejection. I never give less than twenty grains, however young the patient may be: it never does harm.

But ipecacuanha is a nauseous thing, and to those who have frequently taken it as an emetic it becomes almost intolerable. I have lately discovered that it may be taken very pleasantly and very efficaciously in the form of some strong ipecacuanha lozenges made by Messrs. Corbyn, of 300, Holborn. They are about four times the strength of ordinary ipecacuanha lozenges; three of them will produce prompt vomiting. They are very convenient, too, for keeping up a slight nausea; and for children they are invaluable. If vomiting is desired, they should be bitten and ground up in the mouth and swallowed at once.

---

[1] In an old number of the *Lancet* (vol. ii. 1837) I have met with the following notice of the beneficial administration of tobacco in asthma in the form of a tincture:—
"In disordered respiration tobacco obtained the well-merited confidence of the older physicians in cases where no organic alteration had occurred. It has, however, nearly fallen into neglect, from which state it will most probably revive, for it has lately been tried to a very great extent, and with no small success, under a false name. At the time that the *Lobelia inflata* was the subject of great panegyric, and that clinical lectures appeared in the periodicals, extolling its virtues in asthma, there was not a particle of it in the drug market. One firm, at the head of which was a shrewd, intelligent, practical man, had formerly had great experience of tobacco, and he proclaimed that his house was the sole mart for Lobelia; he made a spirituous tincture of the tobacco, which he supplied to the trade, pretty freely, and it became a great favourite of the profession. My own experience led me to its frequent employment; nor did I discover for some time the artifice which had been practised. It, however, induced me to place great reliance on an æthereal tincture of tobacco to mitigate the paroxysms of spasmodic asthma."

There is one circumstance that greatly detracts from the utility of tobacco in the treatment of asthma, that practically indeed almost destroys it. Our adult male population have so habituated themselves to its use that they have lost the susceptibility to its full influence, and cannot induce complete collapse by any amount of smoking. Now adult males constitute by far the majority of the subjects of spasmodic asthma; and thus the habit of smoking has rendered powerless, in a large number of cases, what I think may, without any qualification, be called its most potent remedy.

To the practical I need not apologize for these trifling hints, of which I know they will recognize the value.

CHAPTER IX.

TREATMENT OF THE ASTHMATIC PAROXYSM (*continued.*)—TREATMENT BY STIMULANTS.

Theory of the *modus operandi* of stimulants.—Illustrated by coffee.—Curative influence of violent emotion.—Its action analogous to that of stimulants.—It acts also as a "nervous derivative."—Cases.

ONE of the commonest and best reputed remedies of asthma, one that is almost sure to have been tried in any case that may come under our observation, and one that in some cases is more efficacious than any other, is strong coffee. To the question, "have you tried strong coffee?" the asthmatic is pretty sure to answer "Yes;" and he is also pretty sure to add that it gives him relief.

About the *modus operandi* of this remedy I was long puzzled; I could not make it out; and it is only lately that I think I have stumbled upon it. The *rationale* of its efficacy is, I think, to be found, on the one hand, in the physiological effects of coffee—the particular nervous condition that it produces—and on the other, in a feature in the clinical history of asthma which I have long observed, and of which I think the efficacy of coffee is highly corroborative.

This fact is, that *sleep favours asthma*—that spasm of the bronchial tubes is more prone to occur during the insensibility and lethargy of sleep than during the waking hours when the senses and the will are active. I have already referred to this in the chapter on the Clinical History of Asthma, in describing the phenomena of the paroxysm, and in explaining why the attack invariably (or almost invariably) chooses the hours of mid-sleep for its onset. Let me just refer to this subject again; for it is both interesting and important, as it explains a curious and very constant phenomenon in asthma—

the hour, namely, of the attack—is highly illustrative of its pathology, and furnishes the key to some of its treatment.

I think, then, that sleep favours the development of asthma in two ways—

1. By producing insensibility to respiratory arrears.
2. By exalting reflex action.

That sleep *does* exalt reflex nervous action there can be no doubt. It is a fact so abundantly inculcated by the history of disease as hardly to require illustration or proof. The phenomena of epilepsy, cramp, lead tremors, and other examples of deranged muscular action, all teach it. It is just as sleep comes on, just as the will is laid to rest, or during sleep, that these different forms of involuntary muscular contraction most commonly occur. Any one, to convince himself of it, has only to fall asleep sitting on the edge of his chair, in such a position that it shall press on his sciatic nerves. As long as he is awake his legs will be motionless ; but the moment he falls asleep they will start up with a plunge and suddenly wake him. As soon as he is awake they are quiet and still again, with no disposition to start, till he again falls asleep, and that moment they start again and wake him; and so he may go on as long as he likes. He changes his position, sits back in his chair, and they start no more. I need not explain what so clearly explains itself. I heard, some years ago, of a case of what might be called chronic traumatic tetanus, in which the source of irritation—the excito-motory stimulant— was extensive disease of the hip-joint. The moment the patient fell asleep he was seized with opisthotonos, which, of course, immediately awoke him. On awakening the tetanus vanished; on again falling asleep it reappeared; and this alternation of falling asleep and waking continued for weeks, if not for months, the patient getting no continuous rest, till he was quite worn out. As long as he was broad awake the tetanus never appeared.[1] Hosts of similar facts, illustrative of the same truth, might be cited.

Anything that exalts reflex nervous action increases, of course, the potency of reflex stimuli. Now, I have elsewhere endeavoured to show that the phenomena of asthma are, in almost every case, those of excito-motory action, and that the exciting causes of asthma are, in the great majority of instances, such as act by a reflex circuit. They would therefore, on the asthmatic's falling asleep, immediately acquire a potency they did not before possess, just as the pressure on the sciatic nerve did in the illustration I have given. Thus it is we see that the asthmatic may gorge himself with unwholesomes, and yet, as long as he keeps himself awake, suffer no consequential asthma ;—the irritant is there, the undigested food is in the stomach, but as long as he is awake, as long as the will is

---

[1] I was further informed, respecting this case, that, after everything else had failed, sleep was procured, with an immunity from the tetanic spasms, by putting the patient into the mesmeric state. In this way he got rest, and greatly improved; but what was the ultimate issue of the case I do not know.

dominant, it is inadequate to the production of reflex phenomena. But let him fall asleep, and in an hour or two the paroxysm will be established.

And not only will *sound sleep* determine, by this exaltation of reflex susceptibility, the production of asthma by its exciting causes, but a small dose of the same condition—sleepiness, drowsiness—will favour the supervention of asthma in a proportionate degree. Not only is drowsiness a premonitory sign of an attack, but a powerful predisposer to it; and the asthmatic knows that he yields to it at his peril. I have often noticed in asthmatics that the sleepiness that is so apt to come on after dinner will be accompanied by a slight asthmatic oppression and wheezing: as the drowsiness deepens, so does the asthma, and in this way it may settle down into an attack; but if the patient rouses himself, or if anything occurs to engross his attention so as to wake him up, broad awake, the asthma quickly vanishes. It is in this way, I think, that is to be explained the fact, that asthmatics can dine out late and unwholesomely with impunity, while if they dine at the same time and in the same way at home, asthma is sure to come on. At home they want that excitement which at a dinner-party keeps the animal functions in a state of exaltation and the mind vividly awake, and effectually banishes the least approach to drowsiness. Of the fact there is not the slightest doubt. I know an asthmatic who can with impunity dine out at seven o'clock, as dinner-eaters of the nineteenth century are apt to dine—shirk nothing from soup to coffee—walk home at eleven o'clock, a distance perhaps of four miles, with the wind of a deerstalker—go straight to bed, and get up the next morning scathless; but if he were to dine at home at six, or even at five o'clock, he would be wheezing at nine, and by four the next morning downright asthmatic.

I believe a certain amount of the curative influence of fright, or other strong mental emotion, is to be explained in the same way.

"But why," it may be asked, "all this round-about digression? What has all this to do with the curative influence of coffee?" I believe it is simply its explanation. For what are the physiological effects of coffee? They consist in the production of a state of mental activity and vivacity, of acuteness of perception and energy of volition well known to those who have experienced it, and to a certain extent very pleasurable, and which is the very reverse of that abeyance of will and perception which, in drowsiness or sleep, so favours the development of asthma. In sleep, will and sense are suspended; after taking strong coffee, they are not only active, but exalted. It produces rapidity of thought, vivacity of spirits, clearness of apprehension, greatly increases the working powers, and altogether intensifies mental processes. Not only is there no disposition to sleep, but sleep is impossible: the thoughts hurry one another through the mind; the bodily movements are energetic and rapid; and if the effects of the drug are pushed far, a very unplea-

9

sant condition is produced, something like that of delirium tremens, *minus* its hallucinations. Now, if the suspension of the will, or its depression, favours the production of excito-motory phenomena, and thus favours the development of asthma, is it unreasonable to suppose that its exaltation should prevent or cure it? It *must* do so—if not positively, at least negatively, by removing the predisposing condition. And bearing in mind this marked physiological effect of coffee —that this exaltation of the animal nervous functions is exactly what it produces—it certainly does seem to me reasonable to suppose that this is its *modus operandi*. And if of coffee, then of strong tea, and alcohol, and ammonia, and Indian hemp, and ether, and other stimulants of undoubted value in asthma.

To show that this is the *rationale* of the cure of asthma by stimulants I do not think it is necessary to show that it is only when the asthmatic is drowsy, or has been sleeping, that they do good. If anything that rouses the asthmatic to a state of wakefulness will put a stop to asthma that was creeping on him while he was sleeping or sleepy, *à fortiori* anything that carries him beyond a state of mere wakefulness—that gives him an active, not a mere passive wakefulness—will be still more efficacious, and will be adequate to the checking of an attack that, in spite of his being broad awake, was gaining on him.

The very frequency with which coffee gives relief makes it hardly worth while for me to narrate the history of any cases. I should think, from my own experience, that coffee relieves asthma in two-thirds of the cases in which it is tried. The relief is very unequal, often merely temporary, and sometimes very slight: sometimes it is complete and permanent. It is often taken in the morning; and patients will tell you, that previous to taking their coffee they are not fit for anything, can hardly move about; but that taking it is immediately followed by freedom of breathing, and an ability to enter at once on their daily occupations.

There are two or three practical hints with regard to the administration of coffee that are worth bearing in mind.

1. It cannot be given too strong. Unless sufficiently strong to produce its characteristic physiological effects it does no good, but rather harm; moreover, if given very strong it need not be given in much bulk, and quantity is a disadvantage—its effect is less rapid, and it oppressively distends the stomach.

2. I think it is best given without sugar and milk—pure *café noir*.

3. It should be given on an empty stomach; if given on a full stomach it often does great harm, by putting a stop to the process of digestion: indeed, so much is this the case that I consider coffee accompanying a meal, especially late in the day, so peculiarly apt to induce asthma, that it deserves to be classed among its special provocatives. I have mentioned elsewhere the case of an individual who never dared to take the usual after-dinner cup of coffee—it would make the simplest dinner disagree with him. But the same

asthmatic found in strong coffee, on an *empty stomach*, one of his most valuable remedies.[1]

4. For some reason or other, I do not know why, it seems to act better if given hot—very hot.

I adverted just now to the influence of mental emotion on asthma, and stated my belief that its *modus operandi* was, like that of coffee and other stimulants, by producing an exaltation of sense and will —an intense activity of the intellectual part of nervous action— and proportionately lessening the tendency to excito-motion; and this it does to a much greater degree than stimulant remedies, and its effects are, therefore, proportionately more sudden and complete. It was, indeed, the curative influence of violent emotion, and the observation that it and coffee-taking alike banish that condition in which asthma is most prone to come on, that first suggested to my mind the theory of the action of stimulants on asthma that I have just endeavoured to propound. I think, too, that mental emotion acts, if I may so express it, as a nervous derivative. There are many phenomena, both in health and disease, that seem to show that only a certain amount of nervous activity can be in operation at a certain time, and that if a nervous action of one kind comes into operation, another that had been previously going on is immediately depressed or arrested. Such is the explanation of the well-known experiment of the two dogs, one of which was taken hunting immediately after a meal, while the other was allowed to sleep. In the one that was taken hunting, digestion, on its return, was found hardly commenced; in the other, it was completely over, and the stomach empty. In the sleeping dog the whole vital dynamics, not being otherwise employed, were appropriated by the function of digestion; while in the hunting dog they were entirely taken up by its energetic locomotion, and drafted away, as it were, from that nervous superintendence of digestion without which the function cannot be carried on.[2] The power of strong emotion, or hard study, in retarding digestion, is

[1] Since writing the above I have received the following account, from an asthmatic gentleman, singularly confirmatory of my own observations: "I used to think," writes my informant, "strong coffee the best of all remedies. I remember one instance especially, only a pattern of many others, but more striking when told. With bent back, high shoulders, and elbows fixed on the chair-arms, I had been labouring for breath all the afternoon. About five o'clock I had two breakfast-cups of strong coffee. The hard breathing disappeared rapidly and completely. My sisters were dancing in the next room, and in less than an hour I was dancing with them, quite free from asthma. Of late, coffee has often had an opposite effect upon me. The after-dinner cup of coffee, to which I have been for several years habituated, now produces a sensation of stuffing of the chest, and incapacity of moving about. I believe this is because it stops digestion; and the reason I did not suffer for some years I take to be, that my originally most excellent and enduring stomach could stand it so long, and no longer. Coffee, on an empty stomach, I still deem a most valuable remedy. I do not share the prejudice against putting milk and sugar into coffee that is used as medicine, provided that it remain *café noir*, and be not made *café au lait.*"

[2] See Dr. John Reid's experiments, in Todd's *Cyclopædia of Anatomy*, vol. iii. p. 899; also those of Bernard and of Bischoff, in Müller's *Archiv.* 1843.

an analogous fact.   Just in the same way, I think, the extraordinary
activity and exaltation of thought and perception, that characterize
the state of mind that the taking of coffee, ether, Indian hemp, and
other stimulants produces, act as a nervous derivative in asthma,
and divert from the nervous system of the lungs that morbid activity
which engenders the spasm of the bronchial tubes.

The cure of asthma by violent emotion is more sudden and complete than by any other remedy whatever; indeed, I know few
things more striking and curious in the whole history of therapeutics.
The remedy that stands next in speed and efficacy—tobacco pushed
to collapse—takes time, a few minutes at least: but the cure of
asthma by sudden alarm takes *no* time; it is instantaneous, the
intensest paroxysm ceases on the instant.   This is a fact so little
known, as far as I can see, and yet so practically important and
theoretically interesting, that I think it will not be unprofitable if I
endeavour to impress it more deeply by the narration of some cases
of its occurrence.

CASE I.—A gentleman suffering an unusually severe attack, so
bad that he had been unable to speak or move all day, was suddenly
alarmed by the illness of a relative; he ran down two flights of
stairs and up again, and administered the restoratives he had
procured, and then observed, to his astonishment, that his asthma
was gone. This gentleman tells me, that on many other occasions
different forms of mental emotion have cured his asthma.

CASE II.—C. R., a confirmed asthmatic, states that when he was
suffering from an unusually severe attack a fire occurred just
opposite his house.   Previous to the occurrence of the fire he was
in bed, breathing with the greatest difficulty, and unable to move.
When the excitement of the fire was over, he found that he had
been standing in his night shirt, looking with others out of the window, and that he had forgotten all about his asthma.   His breath
was not quite well the rest of the day, but nearly so.   On another
occasion, when he was suffering from an attack, some sudden anxiety
arose about two of the members of his family being out late: the
alarm from which he suffered relieved his asthma, but not so suddenly
as in the case of the fire.   On another occasion, a sister of his was
seized with sudden illness that seemed to threaten suffocation; he
was suffering severely from asthma at the time, and was in bed; he
jumped out of bed in great alarm, and found then that his asthma
was perfectly cured.   He was sufficiently well to run for a doctor,
and continued well throughout the day.

CASE III.—Not long ago I was informed by a patient at the
hospital, who had suffered greatly for many years, that however
severe an attack might be, venereal excitement would almost
invariably cure it.   He told me also, that, when a youth, he had
been guilty of the practice of onanism, and that the unnatural excitement thereby produced had just the same curative effect on his asthma.
Indeed he pleaded this effect of it as a sort of excuse for the practice ;

and assured me that when his breath was very bad at night he used to
resort to it for the purpose of curing it.

I have known two or three cases in which sexual excitement has
had just the same effect.

CASE IV.—The following account of the curative influence of
mental excitement I have received from a medical friend, who has
suffered from asthma all his life : " On one occasion I was sitting
with fixed elbows on a sofa, breathing hard : a lady came into the
room whom I knew very well, and whom I had not seen for several
years. I got up to receive her, and sat down again on a music-stool ;
with no especial purchase, therefore, for the respiratory muscles,
and yet with comparative ease of breathing. This ease lasted for
about an hour, and then the difficulty of breathing came on again. I
attribute the temporary amendment to the diversion of nervous
energy. Just the same thing has happened to me more than once.
—On another occasion I was suffering a good deal at a farm-house.
I got on horseback with some difficulty, and an anxious hope that
the horse would go quietly, to fetch myself an emetic from a town
three miles off. The horse ran away with me. I pulled in, at first
weakly and almost despairingly, but the need of exertion brought
the power : after a run of about a mile I succeeded in pulling up
and was delighted to find my asthma gone.—Another time I was
breathing very hard, and a friend engaged me in an argument. At
first I could only get out a sentence in successive gasps ; but gradually, as I got excited, the hard breathing went off, and I could talk
fluently." [1]

From the foregoing observations, then, I think we may conclude—

That, since the abeyance of the will favours, in proportion to the
degree of that abeyance, the development of asthma, and since the
effect of strong coffee is to dispel such suspension or depression of
volition and restore the will to its wonted (or even an unwonted)
activity, it is by thus exalting the will, and so disfavouring the
development of excito-motory action, that this remedy relieves
asthma.

That the same interpretation applies to the relief of asthma by
all other stimulants whatever.

That thus strong coffee and mental excitement, although apparently so different, belong to the same category of remedies for
asthma.

[1] For additional cases of the cure of asthma by mental emotion, I must refer the
reader to Chapter II. on the pathology of Asthma.

CHAPTER X.

TREATMENT OF THE ASTHMATIC PAROXYSM (*continued.*)— TREATMENT BY SEDATIVES.

Their number and value.—Tobacco.—Chloroform: its varying efficacy.—Caution
with regard to its use.—Opium.—The objections to it.—Stramonium: its unequal
value.—Cases.—Its various preparations and modes of exhibition.—Practical
rules.—Lobelia.—Indian hemp.—Ether.

THE recognition of the nervous nature of asthma; of the paroxysmal character of its symptoms; of the fact that the air-passages
were in a state of spasm; that a part at least of its essential pathology appeared to be a morbid susceptibility to certain stimuli; that
many of its exciting causes were such as exalted nervous irritability;
that the subjects of it were commonly individuals of quick and
mobile nervous systems;—these, and analogous considerations, long
ago suggested the use of sedatives both for the prevention and alleviation of the asthmatic paroxysm.

The *modus operandi* of sedatives, both in the cure and prevention
of asthma, is doubtless by allaying nervous irritability; destroying
for the time that morbid sensitiveness of the pulmonary nervous
system that constitutes so essential a part of the disease. And
whilst, on the one hand, it is the nervous theory of asthma that has
suggested the use of sedatives, their efficacy on the other—the immediate and perfect relief that follows the use of some of them—
is among the best proofs we have of the correctness of this nervous
interpretation of the phenomena of the disease.

Of all the classes of remedies used in asthma, I think that sedatives constitute the most numerous. I wish I could say that they
excelled others in efficacy as much as they do in numbers. But
they are of very unequal power; for while one or two of them are
of very great value, others appear to be of little worth, and some
even prejudicial. Chloroform, for example, is, in my opinion, one
of the most valuable remedies for asthma that we possess; the inhalation of its vapour putting a stop to the asthmatic paroxysm more
speedily and more certainly than anything else I know. Opium, on
the other hand, I have found, as far as my experience has gone,
positively worthless.

Moreover, with regard to sedatives, asthma exhibits very strongly
its characteristic caprice;—stramonium smoking is, to some patients,
an infallible cure, while others might just as well smoke so much
sawdust, and not only receive no benefit, but experience no result of
any kind from it.

The principal remedies of this class are :—

I. Tobacco, in sedative doses; II. Chloroform; III. Opium; IV. Stramonium; V. Lobelia; VI. Indian Hemp; VII. Ether, in sedative doses.

Of some of these I have had very little practical experience. I will speak of those of which I have, and first of—

I. Tobacco.—I have, in a previous paper, spoken of tobacco as a depressant. But tobacco as a sedative is quite another thing. The dose is different; the physiological effects are different; the principle of the cure is entirely different. In smoking with the view of producing depression, the individual must be unaccustomed to the drug, or the tobacco very strong, or the dose very large; in smoking for sedation none of these is necessary. For tobacco to cure asthma as a depressant it must produce collapse; as a sedative it merely produces that composing and tranquillizing condition with which smokers are so familiar. As a depressant it renders spasm impossible by knocking down nervous power (doubtless by poisoning the nervous centres); as a sedative, by temporarily effacing a morbid sensitiveness to certain stimuli, and inducing a normal indifference and tolerance of them. Any one may experience the sedative effects of tobacco, and all smokers do habitually; but the production of its full depressant action is almost impossible in those who have long accustomed themselves to its use; in others, however, as in women and children, it is so easy, that the difficulty is to prevent sedation from running into depression. It is for this reason that it is necessary, in administering tobacco as a sedative only, to the uninitiated, the delicate, or the young, to give the very mildest form, in carefully measured quantities, and to insist on its slow and deliberate exhibition.

It is of the sedative use alone of tobacco that I am now speaking.

Asthmatics are very commonly smokers, and many of them find in the habit an almost unfailing antidote to their disease. But in almost all the cases that I have met with, it is rather as a prophylactic that it is used—to secure immunity when under dangerous circumstances, or to meet the first threatenings of an attack—than as a veritable curative to cut short spasm.

II. Chloroform.—One of the most powerful and speediest remedies which we possess for asthma, to which I should, perhaps, give the first place of all, is chloroform. It is, of course, a comparatively recent remedy; but its marked physiological effects early suggested its appropriateness, and the result has fully justified the trial. I have not had many opportunities of witnessing its effects personally, because when asthmatic patients consult one they are generally not suffering from the disease at the time; but in the cases in which I have witnessed it I have been very much struck with the completeness of the control which it exercises over the asthmatic condition, and with the absence of all danger in its administration, provided the asthma is of the uncomplicated spasmodic form. If the only source of dyspnœa is bronchial spasm, it seems to me that it may as safely be given to an asthmatic in the height of a paroxysm, as to a healthy person.

I shall not easily forget the first case in which I administered it. A poor woman was brought into King's College Hospital at the time that I was house-physician there, supposed to be dying by those who brought her in. She was quite unable to move, and could barely speak; but it was easy to perceive, from the violent action of the respiratory muscles and the loud wheezing that accompanied it, that the suffocation from which she was suffering was of the asthmatic kind. I at once administered chloroform. After a few whiffs the spasm began to yield, and before I had given her enough to make her insensible it had quite subsided and her breathing was free. In ten minutes after entering it she left the hospital—well.

Even in asthma with bronchitis I have known it, if carefully administered, of great service, by getting rid of the asthmatic element of the dyspnœa, and so putting a stop to one of the sources of suffering, and one of the causes of pulmonary congestion and bronchial exudation; and at the same time, by relaxing the constricted air-passages, facilitating the discharge of the accumulated mucous. In chronic bronchitis I have seen at least half of the dyspnœa vanish on its administration, showing how much of the symptoms were due to spasm. I think its usefulness in these cases has been overlooked, and that if carefully and tentatively given it might be tried in them without risk. Certainly for the time the patient is placed under much better circumstances, even as far as the bronchitis goes.

The sooner it is given after the commencement of an attack the better, for if the spasm has existed for some time it is apt to recur as soon as the influence of the chloroform passes off. The plan recommended by Dr. Russell Reynolds, of recurring to it at the first indications of an attack, is, I think, a very good one, for the spasm yields with much greater facility, and is cut short while it is in so incipient a state that the treatment is virtually preventive. He mentions the case of a young lady (*Lancet*, October 29th, 1853) who, by inhaling a few drops on her handkerchief whenever an attack threatened, at once averted it, and was thus virtually cured of her troublesome complaint.

Dr. Walshe says he has seen three results of chloroform inhalation, administered during a fit of asthma, and pushed to narcotism; —" Total relaxation of the spasm during the continuance of insensibility, with the immediate return of dyspnœa on the restoration of consciousness; gradual return of the difficult breathing as consciousness is restored; and suspension, or at least mitigation, of the paroxysm for the time being." The last effect he has found the rarest of the three; but, on the other hand, the temporary relief afforded by chloroform is sometimes more complete and more rapid than that afforded by any other agent.

As in other cases, so in asthma, the patient should never administer the chloroform himself. Dr. Todd's remarks on this point are so judicious, and enforced by so striking an example, that I cannot forbear quoting them. "In the administration of chloroform," he says, "I would give you this twofold caution: First, to give it gradually and cautiously, and not in a full dose, not to produce insensibility, especially if there be anything like blueness of the surface; because, though remedial to asthma, it will tend to increase the very consequences which are most to be feared from the circulation of venous blood. Secondly, to impress on your patient that he must never give it to himself, nor without the presence of a medical man. The following case was related in the papers the other day: A person who was in the habit of curing his attack of asthma by inhaling chloroform, when administering it to himself one day, and when in a state of half subjection to its influence, in order to produce the full effect placed his handkerchief on the table and buried his mouth in it; his insensibility became deeper and deeper, till at last he was too far gone to raise his head. He therefore continued inspiring it; his coma became more and more profound; and, a short time after, he was found in that position quite dead." (*Medical Gazette*, Dec. 1850.)

III. OPIUM.—To opium in asthma I have myself a great objection. I do not mean to impugn the correctness of those who profess to have seen benefit derived from it; all I would say is, that I am not certain I have ever seen it do good, that I have often seen it do harm, and that I should have antecedently expected, from its known physiological action, that it would be prejudicial, and tend to increase the very condition for which it is given. I have endeavoured to show that sleep favours asthma; that it does so on account of the ascendency that excito-motory action then acquires; that the heavier and more oppressed the patient is the intenser does the asthmatic spasm become; and, on the other hand, that the wider awake and more vigilant he is—the more exalted sense and will—the more readily does it yield, so that often simple rousing is enough to stop an attack that was gradually creeping on the sleeper.

Anything, therefore, that soporizes aggravates the asthmatic tendency. Now this is exactly what opium does. What we want in asthma is a sedative that, like stramonium, sedates but does not narcotize; or one that, like chloroform, goes much further, and produces universal muscular relaxation. And not only does opium act prejudicially by tending to exalt reflex action in proportion to the drowsiness and lethargy it produces, but, by lowering sensibility, it prevents that acute and prompt perception of respiratory arrears which is the normal stimulus to those extraordinary breathing efforts which are necessary to restore the balance.

But, beyond this, opium seems to have a specific tendency to excite involuntary muscular action, and induce a tendency to spasm. The exact explanation of this will depend upon the theory of muscular contraction that is adopted; and into this at present disputed physiological question I will not enter. If, then, I had been asked, antecedently to all experience, whether opium would be useful in asthma, I should have replied, on the strength of the spasm-theory of the disease, that it would not.

But I would not let any theoretical objection run counter to clinical evidence; and if experience said "give opium," no theory should prevent my recommending it. My own experience, however, coincides with these objections; and I am disposed to think that the frequency with which it is given in asthma depends upon an unthinking following of routine and a want of close and exact observation. Not only have I often seen asthma worse for it when given during the fit, but I have seen it brought on when it did not previously exist. An asthmatic gentleman, in whom I have often watched this, and who is frequently obliged to resort to opium on account of colic, never takes it without being rendered more or less asthmatic by it, however free from the disease he may have previously been.

I would say, then, prefer any other sedative to opium; and, unless there is some special complication that indicates it, never give it at all.

IV. Stramonium.—The smoking of the datura as a remedy for asthma was introduced in 1802, from India, by General Gent, and soon obtained, as new remedies are apt to, the reputation of being specific and infallible;—everybody with any shortness of breathing was smoking stramonium. Its use, however, has illustrated the general inapplicability of any one remedy to all cases of a disease, and the special caprice of asthma; and time has shaken it into its proper place, and assigned it its true worth;—that its original reputation greatly exaggerated its merits, but that it has undoubted though very unequal value, and will probably always maintain its place amongst the real remedies of asthma.

Perhaps no drug has been given with more contradictory results, and perhaps in no way is the caprice of asthma better illustrated than by its effects in different cases. In some it is *the* remedy; in the majority of cases, as ordinarily used, it seems utterly inoperative, and in some positively injurious.

"Sometimes," writes Dr. Watson, "it calms the paroxysm like a charm. The late Dr. Babington told me of a patient of his, who had been grievously harassed by asthma for a series of years, but who declared to him, after he had made a fair trial of stramonium, that he no longer 'cared a fig' for his asthma, which he could always stop in a moment. So, a Mr. Sills, in a collection of communications relative to the *Datura stramonium*, published in London in 1811, states that he had been a great sufferer from asthma; that the fits continued, with short interruptions, from thirty-six hours to three days and nights successively, during which time he had often, in the seeming agonies of death, given himself over, and even wished for that termination to his miseries. But, having at length discovered the virtues of stramonium, he uses this strong language : ' In truth, the asthma is destroyed. I never experience any ill effects whatever from the use of the remedy; and I would rather be without life than without stramonium.' "

Among several striking cases of the efficacy of stramonium, communicated by Dr. Gooch, of Croydon, I will quote the following : "Mr. L., 22 years old, for the last four years has had great difficulty in breathing, attended by wheezing and cough, which attack him suddenly, when in bed or at meals, disabling him from his business, and sometimes continuing more than a week. It occasionally seizes him so violently that he is unable to speak, and appears to be threatened with instant suffocation. He has had much medical advice, without receiving material benefit. He now smoked the thorn-apple, swallowing the saliva and smoke; by these means the fit terminates in a few minutes. He smokes every day, even when the fit does not occur. Sometimes it attacks him while dining in company; in which case he retires, smokes a pipeful, and returns to his friends breathing freely." I might go on quoting cases *ad libitum*, but must content myself with referring the reader to many very interesting and striking ones in the seventh and eighth volumes of the *Edinburgh Medical and Surgical Journal*, the twenty-sixth volume of the *Medical and Physical Journal*, and the various medical periodicals published at the early part of the present century.

In most of the cases that I have personally witnessed, it has given only temporary relief—mitigated rather than cured the spasm ; but, in a case recently communicated to me, its effects appear to be nearly as striking as in the cases I have just quoted. The patient was what is commonly termed a "martyr to gout," and suffered most severely from asthma. He could not walk, in consequence of the gouty state of his legs and feet ; and one of his amusements was to pick the chalk out of his fingers with a knife! "I remember," writes my informant, "one day, when I was at his house, he came home in his little hand-carriage, in which it was his wont to be wheeled about, and, on being helped into the parlour, he was in such a state from a violent attack of his asthma that he could not speak, but made signs to his daughter, by pointing to a cupboard, that she should reach him his pipe of stramonium. She lighted it, and, after he had taken a few whiffs, the breathing became relieved, and he was able to speak ; and, after a few more, the spasm and oppression so completely vanished that he could converse as well as usual."

On the other hand, one is always being disappointed with it; in a large percentage of cases it does no good at all, and in some has been said to prove injurious, and in a few instances fatal. Dr. Bree tried it in eighty-two cases; in fifty-eight of these it had no permanent effect, and in the remaining twenty-four it acted injuriously. General Gent, who was instrumental in introducing the practice, is said to have fallen a victim to it. Aggravation of the dyspnœa, paralytic tremblings, epilepsy, headache, and apoplexy, are some of the evils said to have been induced in some of the cases above referred to.

To what are these contradictory results to be attributed? Partly, doubtless, to the caprice of the disease, which behaves in the most irregular way to all remedies; but partly, I think, to the mode of preparation and drying of the drug. An asthmatic patient of mine informed me that while he received great benefit from stramonium grown and dried by a relative of his, that which he gets at the shops does him no good whatever. He sent me a specimen of this home-prepared stramonium, and certainly it was a very different thing, both in appearance and smell, from what one commonly sees: it had not lost its fresh greenness, nor the genuine solanaceous smell. I think, therefore, asthmatics would do wisely to grow and prepare their own stramonium. Part, too, may depend on the time at which it is administered; stramonium, like other remedies, will cut short an incipient spasm, while over one that has been long established it has but little power. The great thing is to give it in time; and for that purpose, since the patient in general is awoke from his sleep by the paroxysm, he should put his pipe, already filled, with the means of lighting it, by his bedside over-night, so that on awaking with the dyspnœa he might immediately use it.

My friend Dr. Buller, of Southampton, tells me that he has seen benefit from the inhaling (not the mere smoking) of stramonium smoke. "A year ago," he writes, "I met with an old asthmatic, who had cured himself and relieved many others by using *cold* stramonium-smoke. He smoked the stramonium as you do tobacco, then puffed the smoke into a tumbler, and then inhaled the cold smoke into his lungs. I am now attending an asthmatic lady, who could not inhale the hot smoke, but who inhales the cold smoke in this way with great relief."

The same plan of *inhaling* I find mentioned in a very interesting case in the *Edinburgh Medical and Surgical Journal*, as far back as 1811. The patient says: "The way in which I employ this remedy is thus: I fill a common tobacco-pipe with the stramonium cut in small pieces, and inhale the smoke as much as possible into the lungs, which causes heat and pain about the fauces and throat, and I am obliged to breath once or twice before I can inhale it again, when I draw in the smoke; and so on alternately till the herb is consumed, which occupies about half an hour, once a day. The saliva I swallow." Now this is introducing the drug in a different way, and certainly a more powerful one, than by simply smoking it, and one well worth trying. By ordinary smoking absorption takes place by the oral surface only; here it is introduced into the lungs themselves and absorbed by the respiratory surface, whose absorbent powers exceed those probably of any other surface of the body. Besides, it has the advantage of being applied to the very part affected.

There are several species of datura in use, of which that commonly employed in this country, the *Datura stramonium*, appears to be the least powerful. The *Datura ferox*, which was first introduced by General Gent, seems to be much stronger. The *Datura tatula*, from which what are called stramonium cigars are made, appears also to be stronger.

The seeds are much more powerful than the other parts of the plant; their analysis yields more than three times as much of the active principle, *daturia*. My friend Dr. Alexander, of St. Helena, where spasmodic asthma appears to be rather common, informs me that, while he has found the smoking of the leaves almost worthless, he finds the smoking of the seeds a most efficient and powerful remedy; and that whereas he was disposed before he tried the seeds to regard the reputation of stramonium as a myth, he has since their employment come to the conclusion that it is one of the most satisfactory of the remedies of asthma. He states, however, that the effects of the seeds are so powerful, that great care is necessary in their administration; they should be smoked in very small and gradually increasing quantities, and their effects closely watched. He has seen, on two or three occasions, alarming symptoms supervene on their use. I have not yet tried the remedy of smoking the seeds, but I shall certainly do so. I do not see why the leaves should not be steeped in a decoction of the seeds, dried, and then smoked, so as to administer by smoking a reliable preparation of an uniform strength.

Exhibition by smoking certainly appears to have some advantages; absorption by the oral surface, especially if combined with inhalation, is sufficiently rapid, and at the same time gradual and more easily regulated than by the stomach. One would rather either take or give any preparation of the *Solanaceæ* by smoking than by swallowing. One feels, with regard to such ticklish remedies, the full force of the *facilis descensus* and its alternative. Nevertheless, I frequently give the extract, and often with marked benefit. It should be commenced, I think, in quarter-grain doses, gradually increased to a grain, or a grain and a half. The Edinburgh preparation—an alcoholic, and not a watery extract—is the best and most reliable, the active principle, *daturia*, being very soluble in alcohol, but very sparingly so in water. The tincture may also be given in from ten-minim to twenty-minim doses every four hours, gradually increased till it occasions some obvious effect on the system.'

I may say, in conclusion, with regard to this drug, that its great value in some cases would, in spite of its too frequent impotence, always induce me to give it a trial in cases in which it had not been tried; that I do not believe it is attended with any danger except from the most egregious over-dosing; that, since the common fault is want of power, I should prefer the stronger forms, the *ferox* and *tatula*, giving them tentatively and carefully; that inhalation of the smoke and swallowing the saliva may be advantageously combined with the ordinary method of smoking, and that it cannot be given too early in an attack. I think it does more in the way of prevention than cure; I think I have seen better results from the long-continued practice of smoking a pipe of it the last thing at night, whether an attack of asthma is threatening or not, than by waiting until a paroxysm comes on. I have seen this nightly pipe, the last thing before going to bed, apparently keep the disease at bay for an indefinite time, as long as it was continued, but followed by its immediate reappearance as soon as it was left off. The stramonium seems to leave for some hours a state of nervous system in which the asthma is not likely to come on; and, since the attack is almost always at night, the use of the stramonium at bedtime conducts and guards the patient through the critical time. I should say, then, let this always be one part of its administration; and keep up the practice of smoking it the last thing at night for some months after the disease appears to have yielded, so as to completely break through the habit.

V. LOBELIA.—Of lobelia I can say but very little, and the reason I can say so little is, that, being doubtful of its really doing any good, I have for some time ceased to prescribe it. But I have lately heard of some successful cases of its employment by medical friends; and I am inclined to think that my want of success, and the want of success that has generally attended its use in this country, has depended upon not giving it in sufficiently large doses. I have never given it in larger doses than from fifteen minims to half a drachm; but I find that in America, where it is much more used than in this country, and has a high reputation as an almost unfailing specific in spasmodic asthma, they give it in vastly larger doses; they consider half an ounce a full dose, but recommend two drachms every two or three hours till some decided effect is manifested. In many successful cases on record it has been given in small antispasmodic doses;[1] but I believe, as I have said, its great success among the Americans, and in Dr. Elliotson's hands, and in many cases which I find scattered about in the journals, depends upon its having been given in doses producing the characteristic depressant action of the drug. In fact, that condition that a large dose produces is such as I should think no asthma could resist; it is almost identical with tobacco-poisoning—giddiness, faintness, sickness, cold sweat, and complete muscular relaxation. I should have the most perfect faith in its value in asthma when producing such symptoms as these; but they are not the symptoms one likes to produce in one's patients,

---

[1] "I have, for upwards of two years past, been afflicted with inveterate asthma, which deprived me of natural rest, and the spasmodic effects of which were frequent and most distressing. When I found these paroxysms coming on I took fifteen drops of tincture of lobelia, which invariably gave me immediate relief, although previously to my using this remedy the violent fits often lasted for hours." (London Medical Gazette, vol. iii.)

and cannot be considered devoid of danger. I see no objection, however, to Dr. Elliotson's plan of giving frequent small and gradually increased doses. He recommends ten minims every quarter or half hour, increasing each dose a minim till the disease yields, or the drug seems to disagree with the patient. If this last should be the case, and vomiting and headache come on, the medicine must be left off for a time, and continued when the headache, &c., is removed, not increasing the dose beyond the last given.

One circumstance that makes it the more necessary to be careful of overdosing a patient, and that strongly inculcates commencement with small doses, is that different individuals tolerate it in such different quantities. Dr. Elliotson states that in some instances a single minim produced sickness, while in other cases, on the contrary, sixty or even ninety drops were taken for a dose. He mentions a young lady who, being subject to spasmodic asthma, always carried with her ninety drops of the tincture in a small phial; this dose she swallowed whenever an attack of the disease came on. He mentions, also, the following extraordinary and almost incredible case: "A medical man, suffering from asthma, having failed to obtain his usual relief from his usual dose of the tincture, increased it to fifty-minim doses, which he took every hour for twenty-four hours. Experiencing but little relief, he added a minim to each dose till it reached seventy-five minims'; this he took for forty-eight hours, and the disease was relieved. His pulse was becoming intermittent, perspiration broke out over the body, and he became languid; small doses of ammonia soon restored him to his usual state. In the last four days this man must have taken twelve ounces of the tincture." (*Lancet,* vol. ii. p. 144.)

Another circumstance that makes it the more necessary to be careful not to administer this drug in undue quantities is, that different specimens of it differ so much in strength. Dr. Elliotson complains of this, and assigns it to faulty preparation. But the Americans say that the plant itself varies very much in strength, this difference depending chiefly upon the situation in which it has grown; that which has grown in damp situations being rank and strong, while that which has grown in dry places is almost inert. But I must not say any more on a medicine about which I began by saying I could say nothing.

VI. INDIAN HEMP.—The Indian hemp, *Cannabis sativa,* is much given in India as an anti-asthmatic, and among the natives has a great reputation. I can easily imagine from its physiological action that its reputation is well deserved. It is at once a stimulant and a sedative. I should be inclined to think it would act best in small stimulant doses. Given in this way it produces the same effects as coffee, only in a more marked degree—it exhilarates, imparts great activity and intensity to the intellectual faculties, and exalts the functions of animal life. In any case in which coffee is useful I should expect that Indian hemp would be so in a greater degree. I think in

large doses it might even do harm, from its hypnotic tendency. In
this respect there is the same objection to it as to opium. I can say
nothing of it from my own personal experience; I have never given
it, nor seen a case of asthma in which it has been given.

VII. ETHER.—Ether is mentioned as a remedy for asthma by
almost all writers on the disease. I have never seen but one case
in which it did any good, though I have given it in scores of cases.
In that case it acted, and always had acted, like a charm. I cannot say that in any other case I ever saw it do a particle of good,
and think I have often seen it produce a disagreeable oppression,
and even increase the spasm. Others speak well of it; but the
result of my experience is as I have stated it.

CHAPTER XI.

TREATMENT OF THE ASTHMATIC PAROXYSM (continued.)

Treatment of asthma by the inhalation of the fumes of burning nitre-paper.—
Cases.—Practical remarks.

AT a time when a more advanced pathology and physiology are
inducing us to discard much of our inherited therapeutics, when the
numerical method is giving us results so subversive of our faith in
particular remedies, when the tendency of the professional mind is
to trust more to treatment and less to medicines, and when the disposition to question the results of past experience has given rise to
a medical free thinking almost akin to medical scepticism, it is some
comfort to be able to fall back upon accessions to our *materia medica*
of unquestionable value, about whose worth the mind feels no doubt.
And when these remedies are those of a severe and intractable
malady the satisfaction is still further augmented.

The subject of this chapter is a remedy of this kind, of whose
beneficial effects I have lately met with several instances; and
although the treatment is not absolutely new, its effects are so
striking and its value so frequently unknown, that I think it worth
while to give in detail some of the cases which have come under
my observation in which it has been successfully employed.

This remedy consists in the inhalation of the fumes of burning
nitre-paper—bibulous paper which has been dipped in a saturate
solution of nitre, and dried. How or by whom it was discovered,
or exactly when, I know not; but I find from the references made
to it by different authors, it must have been in use for nearly twenty
years, and its great value and efficacy are now beyond question,
although for some time past it seems to have *hybernated*, and never

to have attained a general notoriety. Let me first briefly relate the cases that have come under my observation, in which it was successfully employed, and then offer a few observations on the method of administering it, and the *rationale* of its operation.

CASE I.—P. K. W., a young lady, aged twenty, who has had asthma ever since her fourth year, at which age the disease appeared with the symptoms of an ordinary cold; in a very brief time these passed into what was supposed to be a severe attack of bronchitis, but the *suddenness* with which all the symptoms disappeared at once made it evident that the attack was of a spasmodic rather than an inflammatory character. She was immediately taken to the sea-side, and for four months had no return of the asthma. From that time, however, the attacks became much more frequent, so that it was impossible for her to leave the house during the winter, and this for several years, and indeed one winter she was scarcely able to leave her room. As she advanced in years the attacks became more distressing; change generally produced temporary relief, but three weeks scarcely ever passed without an attack more or less severe. Of the results of treatment her father, who is a medical man, writes thus: "Of treatment I can say but little. In the earlier part of her life I gave her the benefit of consultation with a physician connected with one of the London hospitals, and subsequently with other medical men; but, to be candid, I must say that I cannot look back to any of their treatment, or my own, with a belief that it lessened the frequency of the attacks or mitigated their severity when they occurred. But, though she derived no benefit from any medicines, I must not omit to state that she has always (save in those attacks which resulted from inflammation of the mucous membrane of the bronchi) experienced very great relief from burning bibulous paper, previously soaked in a saturated solution of nitrate of potass, and then dried. The room became almost instantly filled with a dense smoke, and that which was pretty nearly death, or at least the greatest inconvenience, to others, was to her a source of the greatest comfort, always mitigating and sometimes completely relieving the spasmodic condition of the air-tubes. The most striking instance of its efficacy was during the worst attack of asthma that I have ever witnessed. My daughter, on the night to which I refer, had retired to her room with gloomy forebodings—the frontal headache, the tightness of the chest, the wheezing respiration, all foretold the coming attack. About seven in the morning the paroxysm was at its height, and as I entered her room the sight was indeed most pitiable: the livid, distressed countenance, the body thrown forward with the hands firmly pressing on the bed, the shoulders raised to the ears, the noise of the air passing through the narrowed tubes, so loud as to be heard in the lower part of the house, all showed too plainly the fearful struggle for life, and were the more distressing from the entire failure of every means which had been used to alleviate her sufferings. For a few

10

minutes slight relief seemed to follow the quick and regular passing of the hand along the course of the spine. I had left the room for a short space. Alone with her maid it seemed to both as if the contest could be continued no longer; in her agony she was just able to gasp out 'Try the paper again.' Taking a large sheet the servant quickly filled the room with a cloud more dense, if possible, than a London fog. Scarcely had two minutes passed, when, changing her position, she reclined her head on the shoulder of her attendant; two minutes more and she was lying back supported by her heap of pillows; and conceive, if you can (for I cannot tell you), my surprise and joy when, on entering her chamber within ten minutes of leaving it, I found her breathing as quietly, as noiselessly almost, as a sleeping infant. A change so sudden, so complete, I never before witnessed. You will not wonder that nitre paper has become an indispensable adjunct to the family medicine chest, or that my daughter should be loud in its praises and grateful for its benefits. The attacks have much diminished both in frequency and intensity of late; but the paper still maintains its high position as a remedial agent, and many have been the assaults warded off or repulsed by filling her room with its smoke when first she retires to rest."

CASE II.—G. T., aged forty-seven, has always had asthma, his first attack dating from cold in infancy. The frequency of the attacks is about once every three or four months, and their time of access about two or three o'clock in the morning. The only thing that he has found to do him any good is the inhalation of the fumes of burning nitre-paper, which, however severe his asthma may be, enables him to breathe easily. On the approach of a paroxysm he lights two or three sheets of this paper, which soon fills his room (rather a small one) with dense fumes. He describes the first effect as being somewhat oppressive and suffocating; but this is soon followed by a mitigation of the dyspnœa, and then its entire disappearance. This is invariably the result; and the relief is not temporary, but permanent—the attack is cured.

CASE III.—E. P., a lady, aged thirty-five, married, having previously enjoyed excellent health, and never suffered from any thoracic affection, was seized with what was thought to be severe inflammation of the lungs supervening on exposure to cold; but the urgency of the dyspnœa, the suddenness and completeness of its departure, and the repetition of the attack soon after, showed it to be asthmatic. From that time the attacks were frequent—every month or so. Every remedy was tried that could be thought of, but with no beneficial result. At length, happening to see in an American paper an account of an asthmatic who, having used all his tobacco, had on an emergency filled his pipe, in default of it, with the match-paper (paper soaked in a solution of nitre) with which he was accustomed to light it, and to his surprise had experienced more benefit from this than from his tobacco, and wished to know "the reason why," she was advised, by way of experiment, though little expecting benefit, to give it a trial. To her surprise she experienced great relief, and in her after-trials still more, because she managed it better than she had at first, and was more familiar with its manipulation. From that time she found it an unfailing remedy. Its effects were rapid and complete, and never failed. There was, however, one exception to its efficacy, and that was whenever the asthmatic attack was brought on and accompanied by bronchitis; in that case the relief it gave was trifling—it did indeed hardly any good ; the fact was that it only relieved the bronchial spasm—only put a stop to the asthmatic portion of the dyspnœa, while the bronchitic portion persisted; and, moreover, there was in the inflamed condition of the bronchial mucous membrane a permanent exciting cause that probably restored the bronchial spasm almost as soon as relieved. At first the paper was used only every month or so, as the attacks were rarer; but as the disease became more severe the attacks occurred more frequently, and at last the paper had to be resorted to every day. Always at night, before going to bed, she burnt it in her room; indeed without it she could not have gone to bed or got any sleep. It invariably had a marked sedative effect and sent her off to sleep in a few minutes, she could not resist the drowsiness that it gave rise to—she was quite overpowered by it, and was obliged to be watched lest she might fall forward or drop the burning paper on her dress ; when she felt her drowsiness overpowering her she would give warning, that the burning paper might be taken from her, and that she might put herself in a position from which she could not fall, as she had not power to save herself. Even by day, and when not previously sleepy, it would put her to sleep, as well as cure her asthma, in ten minutes : but if at all sleepy, as in the evening, she would be quietly asleep in three minutes. Now, we know that many remedies that relieve asthma are immediately followed by sleep in consequence of their removing that laborious dyspnœa which is the cause at once of the wakefulness and the weariness. But that this was clearly not the way in which the nitre fumes acted, but that they acted as a positive sedative, was shown by the fact that if this lady's asthma awoke her at night, and prevented her sleeping, the burning of the paper had the same speedy sedative effect. As soon as her asthma woke her she would strike a light and burn her paper, which she always kept by her bedside, and get immediate relief, and so quickly and suddenly would the sleeping come on, that though quite independent of her husband in the commencement of her operations she was always obliged to wake him that he might take the paper of her when the drowsiness overcame her. In three minutes after lighting the paper she would be sound asleep; sometimes her husband could hardly take the paper quick enough, so sudden were its sedative effects. Now here she was awoke *from* sleep to relapse again into sleep in two or three minutes ; there had been no accumulated want of sleep, no weariness

from protracted laborious dyspnœa.   So uncertain was the time at
which an attack might occur, and so certain was the effect of the
nitre-paper, that this patient never went anywhere without taking
some of it with her in her pocket.   If an attack came on at any
time, she would resort to it.   Sometimes when making a morning
call she would find her asthma coming on; she would bear the
increasing dyspnœa as long as she could, and then, when she could
bear it no longer, she would ask to be allowed to retire to some
room to use her remedy, and in ten minutes return to her friends
as well as ever.

CASE IV.—H. H., a gentleman residing in a country town, who
has suffered from asthma for twenty-five years.   At first it occurred
regularly every third night, but of late years has been less regularly
periodic; the usual time for the attack to come on is two o'clock in
the morning.   Of the effect of nitre-paper in his case this genleman
has given me the following account :—

"I certainly have great faith in the fumes of nitre.   I have used
it for twenty years, and *when the difficulty of breathing is purely
spasmodic* I am sure to get relief by its use.   I use it in the following manner: When I feel my breathing uneasy I burn a piece
of the saturated blotting-paper in my bedroom on going to bed, and
by lying high at head, I am almost certain of getting a good night,
and of leaving my room in the morning free from the paroxysm.   I
use *blotting*-paper, but a friend in London tells me that he uses
tissue-paper, which is thinner, and does nqt smoke so much.   I think
this is an improvement, but there is more difficulty in saturating it,
in consequence of its thinness."

This gentleman adds—"Some time since, I heard of a very bad
case at Sturminster Marshall.   I sent the poor man some papers,
and requested to be informed, in the course of a few days, what
effect they had upon him.   I inclose the poor fellow's answer ; he
is only a farm labourer."   The answer was, *verbatim et literatim*, as
follows :—

"June the 20, 1855.

"Honored Sir I have made a trial of your Goodness what you
sent to me Sir and I am Happy to inform your Honour that it is the
Best advice I ever had at all for I went to Bead at 7 at night and
never a woke untill 5 the next morning and that is more than I have
done for this 10 weeks past Honored Sir I do not know how to express my grattitude to you a nogh for your great and mercifull kind-
ness to me Honored Sir I return you Sir most Humble and Hartery
thanks for your goodness to me   Sir I remain your obedient and
oblided servant J CHRISTOPHER."

CASE V.—Even now, while I am writing, another case has come
under my knowledge.   It is that of a gentleman, an asthmatic from
infancy, but who has of late years enjoyed an almost perfect immunity from his disease in consequence of residing in London.   But

whenever he goes into the country he is sure to be assailed by his old symptoms, and cannot pass a night without asthma. Moreover, there is exhibited in his case that disposition to habitude which so often characterizes asthma—that tendency to maintain, like other periodic diseases, the rhythm of its recurrence when once it has been established—so that when once his disease has been excited by going into the country, it still continues on his returning to the place and to all the circumstances and conditions of life in which, before, he had been free from a trace of his disease. Two or three weeks ago, when in perfect health, he went into the country, and suffered from his asthma as usual. On his return it still continued —hung about him; hardly a night passed without its awaking him, and as it went on for several weeks without subsiding in the usual way he determined to try the nitre-paper. It was tried at once and was perfectly successful. He burnt two or three pieces of the paper in his room just before going to bed, slept without waking till about seven o'clock in the morning, and then awoke with his breathing perfectly free. He repeated it for several nights with the same effect. He then thought he would put it to its trial, so he took a late and not particularly wholesome supper, a thing very apt to bring on his asthma, then used his nitre-paper, went to bed, and had as good a night as ever. He then omitted it, and during that night his symptoms reappeared. He recurred to it the next night and for several following, and then on leaving it off suffered no return of his disease; the disposition to the nocturnal recurrence of the paroxysm had vanished—the spell was broken. He has not used it since, and probably will not till another visit to the country sets him wrong again.

I might multiply cases to almost any extent; hardly a week passes without my meeting one or more. Within the past week I have met with two, in one of which the nitre-paper was the only thing that did any good, in the other its efficacy was shared by stramonium. It has been suggested to me that if the nitre is dissolved in a strong infusion of stramonium instead of water, the result is still more satisfactory, but of that I have not made trial.

The value of nitre-paper in any given case is, in my opinion, in proportion to the purity of the asthma in that case—the cure it effects is only complete where the asthma is of the pure spasmodic type, and free from organic complications. In three of the cases that I have related, and others of which I have not preserved notes, it was of very little use when the attack was complicated with bronchitis. In such cases the dyspnœa is the result of two causes —the asthmatic spasm and the bronchial inflammation. The nitre-paper appeals to only one of them, and leaves the other undiminished; its effect is therefore but partial. Moreover, the bronchial inflammation is an abiding excitant of the spasm, and immediately relights it as soon as the effects of the nitre-paper fumes have passed off.

Let me, in conclusion, give a few practical hints with regard to the making of the nitre-paper. And this is not an unimportant point, for patients will find it more convenient to prepare the paper themselves, and unless it is properly made it will not produce its beneficial results. The object is to have as much deflagration of nitre and as little combustion of paper as possible. For that purpose the paper must not be very thin, or it will not take up sufficient nitre; nor very thick, or it will make the fumes too carbonaceous; but it must be moderately thick, and very porous and loose in its texture, so as to imbibe a sufficiency of the solution. The strength of the solution should be saturated at the ordinary temperature. If a saturate solution is made with warm water, and the paper is very bibulous, it becomes too much impregnated with nitre—too strong a paper, and burns too fast, with a sudden explosive flame. There should be no brown smoke in its combustion, but light, clear, white fumes. Those who have had a good deal of experience with this remedy tell me that they find the red blotting-paper, of moderate substance, the best. Some blotting or filtering papers appear to have a good deal of wool in them; they are loose, thick, and coarse. They should be particularly avoided, as they yield, on burning, a smoke of a particularly irritating and offensive kind, with a smell something like that of brown-paper smoke, only worse. The nitre-paper, when once made, should be kept in a dry place, and then will not be the worse for any amount of keeping; but if it gets damp it does not burn with sufficient freedom, and should then be dried before using.

The following is the way in which an asthmatic gentleman tells me he has been accustomed to make a paper that answers perfectly well: " Dissolve four ounces of saltpetre in half a pint of boiling water; pour the liquor into a small waiter, just wide enough to take the paper; then draw it through the liquor and dry it by the fire; cut it into pieces about four inches square, and burn one piece in the bedroom on retiring to rest at bedtime." I have tried this method of preparing the paper myself, and find that it burns perfectly well and is very efficacious; and I think *two* pieces are not at all too much to burn at once.

CHAPTER XII.

DIETETIC AND REGIMENAL TREATMENT OF ASTHMA.

Facts showing the connection between the stomach and asthma; illustrative cases.— Practical rules as to the quantity and quality of food, and time of taking it.— Special vitanda.—Summary.

IN no direction is asthma more accessible than through the stomach. Of all forms of prophylactic treatment, none, with the exception of change of residence, is more successful than that which is regimenal. This depends on the close relation existing between the stomach and the lungs. The intimacy of this relation is shown in asthmatics in various ways.

a. Asthmatics are generally dyspeptics. Not that they are apt to suffer from the severer forms of ordinary indigestion, but their stomachs are generally irritable, their digestion capricious and irregular, and their dietary restricted. It is very rare to see an asthmatic with a perfectly sound, strong stomach, about which he has never to think, and in the history of whose case dyspepsia finds no place. Sometimes the dyspeptic symptoms exist in a very aggravated form, and they are frequently such as to imply that the stomach disturbance is one of deranged innervation—that its sensibility, or its movements, or the nervous superintendence of its secretion is perverted. In these cases the stomach and lung symptoms are part of one morbid condition; the whole thing is deranged pneumogastric innervation, the dyspeptic symptoms being the manifestation of the gastric portion of this deranged innervation and the asthma of the pulmonary portion of it. The following is, as I interpret it, a good example of this association of stomach and lung disease :—

A little girl, living in the village of Selborne, in Hampshire, began to suffer, when about eight years of age, from extreme irritability of the stomach. It was intolerant of anything; the moment food of any kind was swallowed it was rejected. There was no pain, no tenderness, no feeling of sickness at any other time. The vomiting was not violent; it was the simple and immediate rejection of anything put into the stomach. Before the child had half finished her breakfast she would have to rise from the table and run to the garden. There an act or two of vomiting would empty the stomach, and she would return to the house quite well. The same with other meals; the same with any little thing, such as blackberries, that she might eat between her meals: indeed, her friends and playfellows used to know where she had been, and which way she had walked, by these vomited blackberries and other things at the side of the pathway. This went on for many years, and the only way in which she appeared to suffer from it was from weakness and extreme emaciation. All sorts of remedies were tried without any effect, and the only treatment that did her any good was the plan of feeding her with nothing but milk, in teaspoonfuls at a time, frequently. This small quantity of this bland material the stomach would tolerate, and in this way some nourishment was able to be retained. I heard nothing of her for some years, and then, upon inquiry, I was told that her vomiting had ceased, but that its disappearance had been accompanied by the appearance of another disease, spasmodic asthma, which had apparently supplanted it. With my previously-conceived notions about the pneumogastric pathology of asthma, this was particularly interesting to me, and this interest was increased by my further inquiries; for I found that not only had the vomiting ceased when the asthma appeared, but that when the vomiting had again appeared, as it had more than once, the asthma had ceased. In this way they alternated, the vomiting always coming on when the asthma was better. I regret to say that the intensity and persistence of the asthma have been such as to inflict on the lungs, by emphysema and thickened bronchial tubes, irremediable mischief, and to change the dyspnœa from paroxysmal to constant.

Now, I do not think that I am giving way to fanciful speculation in believing that the malady in this case was throughout one and individual—morbidly-exalted pneumogastric irritability, and that the supplanting of the vomiting by the asthma, the stomach contraction by the bronchial contraction, merely indicated the transference of this perverted innervation of the pneumogastric from its gastric to its pulmonary portion.

In another case of asthma, violent paroxysms of pain in the epigastrium, clearly dependent on cramps and irregular peristalsis, occurred at irregular intervals of two or three months apart. They were at first thought to be colicky, but were afterwards clearly proved to have their seat in the stomach, and, I believe, depended upon a strong hour-glass contraction, or spasm of the pylorus, through which the cardiac portion of the stomach was in vain endeavouring to drive its contents. It certainly so happened that when this patient was freest from his asthma he was most apt to be attacked with these paroxysms of pain, and *vice versâ*, and that he never had the two together. In this case, however, the vicarious relation of the stomach-cramp and the asthma is not so clearly marked as in the preceding, and I would not press that interpretation of the symptoms.

In the following case, however, I think this vicarious relation is indisputable. I will give as much of it as relates to this subject in the words of the gentleman who communicated it to me :—

" . . . . . . About three years since, the disease became very much modified; the attacks were less frequent and less severe, and till this period the case appeared to be one of genuine spasmodic asthma, unmixed, I think, with any other disease. At the time to which I have referred, my patient lost a sister, a year younger than herself (seventeen years), her constant companion in sickness and health. I mention this as it is somewhat curious that from that event the asthmatic attacks very nearly ceased, but in the place of them she has been subjected to attacks of *dyspepsia*, frequently causing her as much suffering and inconvenience as her previous asthma. During the past winter and (with an intermission of a few weeks in the spring and early part of the summer) up to the present time, this dyspeptic malady has rather increased than diminished. A leading symptom, as well as a most inconvenient and distressing one, is, that for many weeks together every particle of food, no matter of what kind, the moment it reaches the stomach, induces what, for want of knowing how better to describe it, I may call a *flatulent hiccough*. This is soon succeeded by an extraordinary generation of flatus, which continues frequently for eight or nine hours, and has not been amenable, I think, to any treatment that has been adopted; though I may just remark that I am now giving her strychnine, and I fancy the symptoms are somewhat lessening. It is remarkable that this large generation and accumulation of air in the stomach has never induced an attack of asthma, although previous to this change attacks of asthma were frequently brought on by indigestion."

Such cases as these are exceedingly interesting, and well worth close attention.

b. Another way in which this connection of the stomach with asthma is shown is, the frequency with which attacks of asthma may be traced to errors in diet—a debauch, a late dinner, a heavy supper. In many asthmatics the most scrupulous care is necessary in all that relates to food, and a late dinner or a heavy supper will at any time infallibly bring on an attack.

c. Another illustration of the same fact we see in the tightness of breathing that in some persons with asthmatic tendency follows every meal: as certainly as food is taken so surely, in an hour or two, does tight, dry, asthmatic oppression succeed. During an attack of asthma this tendency of food to embarrass the breathing is very much exalted, so that the sufferer is obliged absolutely to starve as long as the attack is on him. As the appetite is not affected in asthma this starvation adds greatly to the sufferings in this disease; but the intensity of the exacerbation of the dyspnœa that follows the taking of even a small portion of food is so terrible that the craving hunger is willingly endured. I have known more than one case in which, at each attack, the patient dared not suffer a particle of food to pass his lips for thirty-six or forty-eight hours. In one of these cases the attacks were weekly, and the patient had to starve himself from an early dinner on the day previous to the attack to breakfast on the day succeeding it.

d. Another example of the same thing may be recognized in those gastric symptoms that are so often premonitory of an attack, that constitute, in fact, its first stage—flatulence, hiccough, and such like.

In all these ways we see this one fact—that there exists between the state of the stomach and asthma a very close connection. From this fact we draw, on the one hand, instructive pathological teaching, and on the other, important practical rules. To these practical rules let me now turn.

One of the most important rules to be borne in mind in the dietetic treatment of asthma is the *time of day* at which food is given. The following case very well illustrates this point, and also the part that sleep plays in favouring the induction of asthma by food :—

A youth, residing in the country, had been subject to asthma from childhood. When quite young he ate and drank like other children; but as his malady became more severe he found that his attacks depended very much upon his previous day's eating; indeed, that that was the one circumstance which regulated them. If he ate late in the day (in other words, went to sleep soon after taking food) he was sure to be awoke the next morning at four or five with his asthma. At first he was obliged to give up suppers, and to make an early tea his last meal; then he was obliged to give up even that, and take nothing after an early dinner. He might drink, but could take no solid food. And for years two o'clock was the latest time at which . he could with impunity suffer solid food to pass his lips. He made a good breakfast at eight o'clock, always taking some animal food; and a good dinner at two, and from that time till eight o'clock the next morning he never took a mouthful. In this way he managed, in a great degree, to keep his disease at bay; but if he ever transgressed he knew the penalty he should have to pay, and which inexorably awaited him the next morning. He had a very good digestion and a ravenous appetite, and as evening advanced his hunger became so great that it amounted to a craving almost irresistible, but he dared not gratify it. Sometimes, not daring to trust himself, and yet knowing the painful price at which he would trangress, he used to make *vows,* that it might be impossible for him to eat. But on the rare occasions on which he yielded to temptation and ate supper, it was never till he had been asleep an hour or two that the dyspnœa came on; and if he did not go to sleep—as, for example, if he stayed up dancing half the night, or sat up reading, or took a very long walk—the asthma did not come on at all.

This gentleman has of late years almost completely lost his asthma; but if ever he gets it now it is after eating late the previous evening; a late dinner-party, or a supper, is always the *corpus delicti.* By going to bed later than usual, however, and thus throwing a certain number of hours between taking food and sleep, he is able to render his dinner or supper innocuous; so, when he has been dining or supping out he sits up a little later than usual, and no harm comes of it. He knows by his feelings when digestion is over and his stomach empty; and then he may go to bed in safety.

The simple explanation of these phenomena is this: The taking of food (either by its mere presence in the stomach, or by the process or results of digestion) acts as an irritant to the morbidly-irritable pulmonary nervous system. The affair is excito-motory; the food is the immediate or remote irritant, the nervous circuit involved is the pneumogastric, and perhaps in part the sympathetic; and, in obedience to the common law of reflex action, the potency of the stimulus is increased, or, in other words, the nervous irritability is exalted, by the condition of sleep. I need hardly recall to my readers' minds analogous phenomena in various diseased conditions—the frequency with which epilepsy affects the hour of sleep, or that debatable land between sleeping and waking; the restriction to sleep of the cramps and jactitations of those whose systems are impregnated with lead, and which cease the moment the sufferer from them is broad awake; the grinding of the teeth in children affected with worms, and various other similar phenomena. So, in the case of asthma, the food may be in the stomach, but unless the will is suspended and excito-motory action exalted by sleep no results follow.

Now, to what does all this practically point? To this simple rule, which of all the dietetic treatment of asthma is the most important —*let no food be taken after such a time in the day as will allow digestion being completed and the stomach empty before going to bed.* Of course the time at which the last solid food should be taken will depend upon what the bed time is; if ten or half-past ten, I would say let three or four be the dinner hour; after that take no solid food, or a mere scrap of bread-and-butter at tea. But I would rather insist on no solid food whatever being taken. As the day advances digestion becomes less energetic and rapid, and I am sure six hours is not too long to allow between the last meal and bedtime; a dinner is not got rid of so rapidly as a breakfast. Moreover, the digestion of asthmatics is often very slow.

But the rapidity of digestion, and therefore the time after dinner that sleep may be safe to the asthmatic, will depend upon two other circumstances—the *quality* of the food and its *quantity;* and these are two very important points.

With regard to the *quality* of the food there are two kinds of articles of diet that should never be given to the asthmatic—those that are *generally* indigestible, and those that are *specially* provocative of asthma. These are not necessarily coincident; for though, as a rule, it may be said that the foods that are found to be the most disposed to bring on asthma are those that are the most generally indigestible, yet there are some articles of diet that appear to have a special disposition to induce asthma quite out of proportion to, and in excess of, their general unwholesomeness.

With regard to the first, we should act upon the same rules as we should in ordinary indigestion; the food should be plain, well cooked, and containing the proper proportion of animal and vegetable elements. I am sure it is a mistake in asthma, as in other diseases in which it is desirable to give a peculiarly digestible aliment, to cut down the diet to too rigid and monotonous a simplicity—bread and mutton-chop, bread and mutton chop, in eternal repetition. The stomach of man requires a certain amount of variety, and wearies of, and refuses to digest pleasantly, anything, no matter what, that is offered to it incessantly over and over again. Bearing this in mind, and bearing in mind that as the asthmatic only eats twice a day, his food should be as nutritious as possible, the diet that I should prescribe as the best in a case of asthma would be, in detail, something as follows :—

For breakfast, a small basin, or breakfast-cup, of bread-and-milk, and besides this, an egg (two for a strong man with a good appetite), or a mutton-chop, or some cold chicken, or game. As a drink, if any is required besides the bread-and-milk, I think tea is better than coffee, cocoa better than tea, and milk-and-water better than either. For dinner (not before two or after four o'clock), let mutton be the staple meat, beef or lamb but rarely, pork or veal never. A little succulent vegetable and potato should be taken, and a little farinaceous pudding, or stewed fruit, or the fruit of a tart, should conclude the dinner. Only one helping of either meat or pudding. I believe, unless there is some special reason to the contrary, that water is the best accompaniment to an asthmatic's dinner. No cheese, no dessert. A great sufferer from hay-asthma tells me that a little boiled fish and brandy-and-water have the least tendency to bring on his asthma of anything he can take; he can take this when a dinner of butchers' meat would be certain to be followed by difficult breathing. With regard to the brandy-and-water I will not speak positively of its advantages in *hay-asthma*, but in ordinary asthma I do not like stimulus of any kind. With regard to the fish there can be no doubt that it is less of a diet, yields more readily and rapidly to digestion, than butchers' meat, and is, therefore, less provocative of any evil depending on prolonged and laborious digestive effort.[1] And here let me observe that butchers' meat is of all foods (with the exception of those particular articles of diet which are specially offensive to asthma, and to which I shall refer presently) that which is most apt to aggravate asthmatic dyspnœa, and it is because dinner is a meat dinner that it is necessary to take it so early. From any occasional late meal that convenience, or cir-

[1] In regard to this fact, common experience accords with Dr. Beaumont's observations. He found that while beef and mutton required from three hours to three hours and a half for digestion, most fish was digested in two hours, and salmon and trout in an hour and a half.

cumstances, may force upon the asthmatic, butchers' meat should always be excluded.

And now let me say a word or two about those particular articles of diet that have a special tendency to oppress and tighten the breathing of those liable to asthma. They are not the same in all cases; but those I have found have this tendency most commonly are the following: Anything in any way *preserved*, especially if strongly impregnated with antiseptics, whether condimentary or saccharine, such as potted meats, dried tongue, sausages, stuffing and seasoning, preserved fruits such as one gets at dessert, *e. g.*, preserved ginger, candied orange-peel, dried figs, raisins—especially almonds and raisins (a vicious combination). Cheese is bad, especially if old and decayed; nuts are worse. With regard to cheese, I remember hearing an asthmatic remark, that there was "as much asthma in a mouthful of decayed Stilton as in a whole dinner." Meat pies are very "asthmatic," and so, in a peculiar degree, for some reason or other, are beefsteak-and-kidney puddings. I have known more than one asthmatic condemn them as being very bad. Coffee, although of great benefit in some cases as a stimulant, is, from its indigestibility, especially if taken strong, and with sugar, so bad for asthma, that it deserves to be classed amongst its special provocatives. I know the case of a gentleman whose dinner making him asthmatic or not entirely depends on his taking, or abstaining from, the customary post-prandial cup of coffee. Heavy malt liquors, especially those containing a good deal of carbonic acid gas, as bottled stout and Scotch ale, are of all drinks the worst for asthma.

It will be seen that almost all the above fairly belong to the category of "unwholesomes." I believe their indigestibility depends on their impregnation with antiseptics; that which makes them "keep"—*i. e.*, opposes putrefaction—out of the body, opposes digestion in the body. The asthmatic should never touch one of them.[1]

But the *quantity* of food taken at a time is also very important. When asthma is brought on by eating (especially if it comes on independently of sleep), it is almost always after a large meal: a

---

[1] It is not always, however, as I have already stated, that articles of diet specially provocative of asthma are also specially indigestible; sometimes the contrary is the case, and they are of the most wholesome kind, as the following curious case, communicated to me not long ago by my friend, Mr. F. Bailey, of Liverpool, will show: "The child about whom I write to you is the member of a family in which the disease seems almost to be hereditary, for several of its members have suffered from it. The mother consulted me one day with regard to the propriety of the child's taking milk, for whenever he did, although perfectly well at the time, asthma was sure to come on. Her own medical attendant had laughed at the idea, but being in Liverpool she asked me my opinion on the subject. Of course I recommended that milk should not be given. The child is twelve years old, and very rarely has his asthma at any other time, except when he has taken a very severe cold. This will be one more instance of the sympathy existing between the stomach and lungs, and of the power of certain articles of food to produce asthma."

heavy dinner will inevitably be followed by asthma when a light dinner of the same articles of diet, and at the same time of the day, will as certainly not. And why is this? It is a very general belief that the true explanation· is a mechanical one—that bulk of food induces asthma by pressing upon the lungs through the diaphragm, and preventing the descent of the one and the expansion of the other. I do not believe this. Much less do I believe that the disposition of food in general to bring on asthma independent of its bulk, the tendency of recumbency to induce asthmatic breathing, and the relief that follows an emetic, have the same mechanical explanation, as is so commonly believed. I believe that a bulky meal is an asthmatic meal, because it is an indigestible meal; and it is an indigestible meal in two ways—because the demand on the powers of digestion will of course be in proportion to the quantity to be digested, and because beyond a certain amount, increase of bulk of food directly diminishes digesting power, by over-distending the stomach and so paralyzing its movements, and by being altogether in excess of the secreting powers of the gastric mucous membrane. If the mechanical were the true explanation of asthma coming on after meals, the tendency of food to induce it would be in direct proportion to its bulk, but such is not the case. An asthmatic may fill his stomach with arrowroot and gruel to any amount, but he will have no asthma; he may drink water *ad libitum*, but he will have no asthma. Moreover, in most cases, asthma does not come on immediately after finishing a meal, when its bulk is greatest, but an hour or so afterwards, when it has already been considerably reduced in bulk by the absorption of the more fluid portions of it. Again, the relief by an emetic is clearly not mechanical, as it comes on the moment the nausea is felt, before any vomiting has taken place; moreover, it affords relief even when the stomach has been previously empty and contains nothing to be vomited.

But although I cannot accept the mechanical explanation of the relations of food to asthma, yet, for the reasons that I have mentioned, the tendency of food to induce asthmatic dyspnœa depends very much upon its bulk. An asthmatic's meals should, therefore, always be compact and small. As a corollary to this, they should be of highly nutritious materials, for if he eats but little, that little must, for adequately maintaining the nutrition of the body, be rich in plastic materials: while, for the reason I have before mentioned, it should be very plain and digestible. We thus get the three qualities essential to the diet of the asthmatic—that it should be small in quantity, highly nourishing, and of easy digestion.

It is less necessary to bear these rules in mind at breakfast than at any other meal; indeed, at breakfast the asthmatic may do pretty much as he likes. I have known asthma brought on by every other meal, but I never knew it brought on by breakfast: I have never known breakfast followed by even that slight straitness of breathing (without any decided attack) that so commonly follows the taking of food in asthmatics. The tendency of eating to induce asthma is in direct proportion to the lateness of the hour at which the food is taken : it is slight after luncheon, worse after a late dinner, worst of all after supper ; but breakfast seems entirely free from it. I do not see any reason to believe that this depends on any increased disposition to asthma as the day advances, but rather on the diminution of digesting power which the stomach experiences as its resources are exhausted by succeeding meals, and which requires a night's rest for its restoration.

Breakfast is therefore the great meal for the asthmatic, and as he may at that time eat what he likes with impunity, and has had a long fast from the previous day's early dinner, he should eat as much as his appetite prompts him to, and of the most nutritious materials. He should take this opportunity, too, if any, of gratifying his palate, as the chances are that nothing he takes at breakfast will disagree with him. Of course there is a limit to this latitude, and of course his food should not be so indigestible as to become innutritious. Since, too, the interval from an early dinner one day to breakfast the next is so long, it is advisable that the breakfast hour be as early as possible : if the asthmatic rises at seven, let him breakfast at eight.

The rules, then, for the dietetic treatment of asthma, and the reasons for them, may be summed up as follows :—

1. The tendency of food to produce asthma is greatly increased by the state of sleep; therefore nothing should be taken after such a time as digestion and absorption may be completely over in—the stomach and small intestines, and even the lacteals, quite empty —before bedtime.

2. This long fast before sleep involves a long period of inanition ; therefore the asthmatic should break his fast early and heartily.

3. The quantity of food the asthmatic takes should be small; therefore it should be highly nutritious.

4. As a rule, the tendency of food to produce asthma is in direct proportion to its general indigestibility; therefore the asthmatic's diet should be of the simplest and plainest kind.

5. But there are some articles of diet that have a special tendency to produce asthma; therefore from these the asthmatic should exercise the strictest abstention.

CHAPTER XIII.

ON THE THERAPEUTICAL INFLUENCE OF LOCALITY.

Special curative influence of London air.—The air of great cities in general curative
of asthma. Exceptional cases.—Caprice of asthma in respect to the effect of local
influences.—Subtle and inappreciable character of the influences.—The asthmatic
tendency not eradicated by them.—Adequacy of locality to *develop* asthma.—Change
of air *per se* prejudicial.

I THINK I cannot better introduce the subject of the cure of asthma
by local influences than by relating the case that first directed my
attention to it.

D. M., a confirmed asthmatic from childhood, came to London at
the age of twenty. Previous to that time he had always lived in
the country, either in a small provincial town or the complete country, and had never been in any large town. From his infancy his
asthma had been gradually getting worse, its intervals shorter, its
attacks more severe. The intervals were rarely prolonged, but for
a year or two before he came to London they became less regular.
He had the characteristic physiognomy and physique of asthma ; he
was spare, rather high shouldered, and with a feeble circulation.
The only effect of change of air was, that at most places he seemed
worse than in the small provincial town in which he habitually resided and in which he was born. With the view of improving his
health he had been to many places near to where he lived, but none
did him any good, and from many he was obliged instantly to return,
as he could not breathe in them. He had tried all sorts of remedies
—stramonium, tobacco, opium, lobelia, ether, camphor, henbane,
squill, ipecacuan, tonics—in fact the whole list of ordinary asthmatic remedies: but nothing had done him good ; and nothing relieved
the paroxysms at all except emetics. He suffered an attack about
once a week, and it disabled him for two days, so that he was ill a
third of his time. His case was looked upon as a hopeless one; his
education was impaired; his prospects were marred; and he came
to London to pursue indefinite and preliminary studies, as it was
doubtful if he would ever be fit for any profession. No sooner,
however, had he arrived in London than his asthma ceased—completely, and at once—he had not another attack. And not only
had he no regular attacks, but he lost all asthmatic feelings; so that
after two or three years he said he had really forgotten what the
sensation of asthma was; he ceased to be an asthmatic. He could
take any liberties with himself, do anything he liked without fear,
eat what he liked and when he liked, go to bed and lie flat on his

back after a hearty supper; whereas in the country he had never dared eat after two o'clock in the day. He gained flesh; his looks improved; he was able to join in the business and pleasures of others; life became a different thing to him; for the first time he had a future. For fifteen years this effect has continued. He has had occasional reminders, just to show him that the tendency to asthma is not lost, and there are circumstances, to which I shall refer by and by, that show that it is living in London, and that alone, that keeps his malady at bay.

Such an occurrence as the following is, I believe, not uncommon: I have been told by one physician that he has known several such. An asthmatic resolves to come to London to get "the first advice;" and he comes to town over night that he may make his visit to the sacred regions of Brook Street or Savile Row in the morning.. But on waking the next day he is surprised, and almost disappointed to find his asthma gone; for he wanted the doctor to see him when his disease was on him, in order to form a correct judgment of it. So he waits till the next day, hoping he may then be able to show his doctor what his attacks are like; still, to his surprise, no asthma. He cannot think how it can be;—London—smoky, foggy, damp, dense London, the worst place in the world for breathing; he would have thought he would hardly have been able to live in it. He waits till the next day, and the next; at last he is tired of waiting and comes to the agreeable conclusion that his asthma has taken its final *congé*, and that, like the horse who died just as he had learned to live on a straw a-day, it has chosen to depart of itself just as he was going to get the best advice for it. But no sooner does he get back into the country again, than he is just as he was before he went to town. This is more vexatious than anything; so back he goes again to London. But again he is well. And then the light breaks in upon him. Now this I have been assured by one physician has happened several times within his own knowledge; and I believe that many cases of asthma have been permanently cured by London residence, from finding, on coming to consult some metropolitan physician, that London air was specific for them.

Since writing the above, the following apt and most illustrative case has come under my knowledge:—

G. C., a confirmed asthmatic, a native of a city in Scotland in which he resided, having been a sufferer for many years, came to London in 1838 for the sake of receiving the best medical advice. He took apartments in the centre of the city of London, somewhere near St. Paul's. His intention was to wait for an attack, and as soon as one came on, to present himself to his physician that he might witness it, and have a clear idea of the state he was in. He waited six weeks, much to his mortification, in expectation of an attack coming on, not only without experiencing one, but without any difficulty of breathing whatever; his health altogether improved, he slept well, and gained flesh. Being tired of waiting, he went back

11

to Scotland without having seen his physician at all, and, to his great disappointment, he had not been in his native city many days when he was attacked in the usual way, and continued to suffer just as before his visit to London. Subsequently, finding it necessary on matters of professional business frequently to visit London, he experienced the same result on all occasions as at his first visit— perfect immunity from his disease. To use his own expression, "he felt in London like a renewed man." On his first arrival in town he was in a miserable state; he could not move without feeling his shortness of breath distressingly, he got no rest at night, and was seldom able to lie down in his bed. But in London he could do anything—eat, drink, sleep. The consequence was, he gained flesh and strength, and went back to Scotland looking quite a different person. This was the invariable result. He used to joke about it, and say, that going to London was better than seeing a physician. Unfortunately, his professional engagements did not permit him to make London his permanent residence.

Some time after this (1850) a Scotch lady travelling to London to get advice for her asthma, heard of this case, and had her expectations raised that she might experience the same relief. On coming to London she took up her abode in Lombard Street, that she might have the most genuine city air, and to her great delight experienced the same happy results—her asthma ceasing from the moment of her arrival in town.

Now here we see, in these cases, confirmed and apparently incurable asthmatics suddenly and completely losing their disease on a change of residence—not experiencing a partial relief, a mitigation of their symptoms, but ceasing to be asthmatics altogether, becoming like other people. But we see something more. It will be remarked, that the cases I have mentioned have been cured by coming *to London*. And this is not from an accidental or purposed selection of cases; it is the rule. I believe that three-fourths or seven-eighths of cases of asthma would be cured by coming to live in London; indeed, I believe a larger percentage than this. I do not speak unadvisedly, or from narrow data; for years past I have had my attention directed to this subject, and have made a point of asking all provincial asthmatics "if they have been in London," and if they have ever had an attack of asthma when there. Their answer is almost invariable, indeed, I do not know that I remember a single exception; they all say, "No, never;" and some of them with surprise, as if they had never thought of it before; "Dear me," they say, "now you come to mention it, I remember that I never have." Of course, in speaking thus of this large percentage of cures by London residence, I am excluding the cases of natives or permanent residents in London who have become asthmatics while residing there. The following are a few striking examples of some of these cases of which I have taken notes, or of which I have been furnished with notes by my friends.

The Rev. Mr. V. was a martyr to asthma during the many years he was at Cambridge, as a boy (for it was his birthplace), college-student, and Fellow of King's in residence; but, however bad it might be, it was always quite well directly he got into London. "I have heard him say," writes my informant, Mr. Dyer of Ringwood, "that he has sat up night after night at Cambridge, 'living at the top of his breath,' unable even to speak; and in this state would accept an invitation to a dinner in town, well knowing he would be quite free of his disease directly he arrived."

R. D., aged twenty-nine, a solicitor living in the country, began to suffer from asthma at the early age of two, and is liable to attacks at the present time. Up to the age of eighteen he lived in the country; from eighteen to twenty-one in London; and from twenty-one to the present time again in the country. Whilst in the country, both before and since his residence in London, he has been in the habit of having an attack every few weeks; but during the three years that he was in town, he did not have a single attack.

Among many interesting cases that have been furnished me by my friend Mr. Macaulay, of Leicester, the following are illustrative of this fact. But I must mention that Mr. Macaulay's own experience has induced him to adopt an opposite conclusion, and to believe that the greatest number of cases of asthma would be relieved by a residence in a high and open locality, and that close confined situations are especially prejudicial. Although a large number of carefully observed and lucidly recorded cases, which I shall relate at a future part of this paper in Mr. Macaulay's own words, would appear to warrant his conclusions, I cannot say that I can agree with him; and indeed some of his cases, as the following, tell the other way. After expressing the above opinion, Mr. Macaulay goes on to say—"It is nevertheless impossible to predict, excepting by actual trial, what air will suit an asthmatic. The late Dr. John Heath, head-master of St. Paul's School, could not breathe at Rugby, and his life was apparently saved by his appointment to St. Paul's, where he never had an attack, although they returned upon him from time to time in various parts of the country. He lived in London until the age of eighty-two. It is rather curious," continues Mr. Macaulay, "that I picked up two more cases yesterday, in illustration of my position, that every patient may, if he tries perseveringly, find an *anti-asthmatic* locality, in which he will be able to breathe freely and enjoy his health. Speaking on the subject at the Infirmary yesterday to Mr. Paget, he mentioned the case of a Mr. P., some years ago living at Nottingham, in an open airy place called 'The Park,' on very high ground, who suffered severely from asthma for many years. Business compelled him to go to reside in London, and he took up his residence in *Thames Street*, in fear and trembling; but he soon experienced a very remarkable immunity from his old enemy, which, in fact, speedily disappeared. As long as he kept to Thames Street he was well; but whenever he went to Nottingham, to see his friends, he was sure to be attacked, and a return to Thames Street as certainly cured him." The other case I shall mention presently.

I could multiply such cases if it were necessary, for I have met with very many. Indeed it is the rule, as I mentioned just now, on putting to provincial asthmatics the two questions—Have you ever been in London? Did you ever have the asthma there ?—if an affirmative answer is given to the first, to receive a negative answer to the second. So that I always put the questions with the confident feeling of what answer I shall get, and rarely am I disappointed. I know many asthmatics who are wheezing about the country, passing suffering lives, and getting emphysema and dilated right hearts, who, if they would come to London, would enjoy perfect health. Some of them know it; but professional engagements, or family ties, or a dislike of London, prevent their migrating.

Now, are these remarkable effects of London residence on asthma to be attributed to anything peculiar and individual in London, *as* London, and that exist nowhere else, or to those conditions which characterize London as a thickly covered, densely populated, smoky city, and which are common to all other similar cities? This question is approximatively answered in favour of the last supposition by the fact, that the same results are observed in all our large, densely peopled, manufacturing cities, and that, as a rule, asthmatics are benefited by a change from a rural to any urban residence. The following are cases in point :—

A. B. was a gentleman of fortune, living in the neighbourhood of Glasgow. He had a fine estate and mansion within six miles of that city; but he had the asthma. He could not sleep a single night in his own house. He was quite well by day, but if he attempted to lie down and sleep at night, he was immediately attacked by his disease. In Glasgow, however, he was perfectly well, and every night of his life he went into that city to sleep. Even if he had a dinner party, and was surrounded by his friends, and however late the hour might be, he would always drive his six miles into Glasgow to sleep, and then out again the next morning.

The following case came under my observation a year or two ago: A gentleman, living at Knutsford, in Cheshire, constantly suffered from attacks of asthma. His medical attendant told him that he must go and live in a *back street* in Manchester—that that was the only place where he would be well. He did so, and was from that day completely cured. But if ever he went back again to Knutsford he was as bad as ever. Consequently he fixed his permanent abode at Manchester; selected one of the dirtiest, closest streets he could find, and has been perfectly well ever since.

"Some time ago," writes Mr. Macaulay to me, "I was called in great haste early in the morning, to see a little girl of delicate structure, aged nine or ten, who was reported in danger from inflammation of the lungs; she was residing on Charnwood Forest, supposed to be, and really being, the finest air in this county. Her father, a medical man, had applied leeches, given calomel, and used the hot bath, and with so much success that on my arrival the patient was *well*, and my friend was congratulating himself on the speed with which his prompt treatment had cut short the inflammation. But a few mornings after, a hasty message announced that the 'inflammation had returned, with greater violence than ever.' ' At what time ?' ' Exactly at half past two.' I was this time wide awake, and mounting my horse, rode the ten miles with all speed, and found the child, as I expected, in a violent fit of pure spasmodic asthma. In this case a change of air to the smoke of our town was of essential service. The fact nearest the truth," adds Mr. Macaulay, " appears to be, that whatever air the patient may be in, you should try the exact opposite,"—an opinion with which I entirely coincide.

Here, then, are three cases cured by residence in three cities— Glasgow, Manchester, Leicester, large manufacturing towns; and I have heard of so many similar ones that I am convinced that they are but particular instances of a general fact. And there is another curious fact, entirely confirmatory of this view—that it is as a dense smoky city, and not as London, that London cures asthma, and which carries us a step further in our search for the immediate therapeutic agencies at work, and their *modus operandi ;* and it is this—that those parts of London, and other cities, that have the city character most strongly marked on them, are those that are most beneficial to asthma—that it is in the most central, densest, smokiest parts, that the most striking results are seen. Take the following very interesting case as an example :—

E. P., a Scotch lady, aged thirty, who had been suffering from intense asthma for two years, determined to come to London, in part to consult Sir James Clark, but chiefly expecting to derive benefit from residence in town, in consequence of a case having come under her knowledge, in which a gentleman suffering from most severe asthma had been completely cured by residence in London. She had, in the previous summer, tried the effect of change of air, and had only discovered that the sea air was prejudicial to her, greatly increasing the severity of the paroxysms. On arriving in town she took up her abode in Lombard Street, that she might be in the densest part of the city; for that, from the history of the case she was acquainted with, was the part in which she expected to receive the greatest benefit. Her expectations were fully realized; she had not a single attack; she suddenly and completely lost them; regained her health and strength, and, from being so weak as to be quite debarred from walking, she was soon able to walk, with perfect ease, an hour at a time. She then made a tour in the west of England—Reading, Bath, Clifton, Leamington, and to the Channel Islands; but throughout this tour she was attacked with her asthma, and got no permanent freedom from it till she came back to London, where she immediately became quite well, as on the former occasion. She waited till her health was recruited by her residence in the city, and then returned to Scotland. She immediately became worse than ever, and passed a winter of most severe suffering. It was then determined that she should come and live permanently in London, as the only thing that afforded her a chance of the restoration of her health; and she again returned to the city with the same result as before—perfect cure, restoration to health and comfort in all respects. Soon after this she moved three miles farther west, to the neighbourhood of Cavendish Square, and there, although she enjoyed an almost entire immunity from attacks, she was not so perfectly well as in the city, into which she used frequently to go for short visits, for what she called " a dose of health." After being a twelvemonth here, in a state of very much improved health, she removed to the neighbourhood of Bayswater, and there her asthma began to reappear, and she had occasional attacks of the old spasmodic type. She was still, however, much better than anywhere out of London. Sometimes she would visit the sea-side or the country in expectation that the change would be useful to her, but she was always the worse for it. Thus we may say there were four degrees in which she was affected by local influences;—she was better in any part of London than in the country, but in its westerly suburbs she was decidedly asthmatic; in the city she was perfectly well; and in the intermediate situation between these last two her condition was intermediate. She used frequently to go for short sojourns in the city, and she would say that even a single day there would do her good. If she was suffering from her asthma at the time, she obtained an entire immunity from it as soon as she entered the city.

The following case, which I quote from Dr. Walshe,[1] is as striking an example of this particular fact as any that could be selected: " A man, one of the greatest sufferers from asthma I ever saw, lived in the neighbourhood of Chalk Farm, the pure air of Hampstead blowing across his house. I tried, I believe, almost every known remedy, in vain, for his relief. He was accidentally detained one night in the foul region of the Seven Dials; feeling persuaded he could not possibly survive till morning, so great was his dread of the close atmosphere. He not only lived through the night, however, but enjoyed the first uninterrupted sleep he had known for months. He took the hint; removed to Seven Dials for *the benefit of the air;* and when I last saw him, some six months after the removal, continued, though still a wheezer, perfectly free from serious dyspnœa."

I have seen just the same thing in numbers of cases. In the case that I first related it was strikingly shown. That gentleman, when he first came to London, took lodgings on the south side of the river, near Blackfriars Bridge; and a more smoky, foggy, dismal place

---

[1] " Diseases of the Lungs and Heart," second edition, p. 836.

could not well be imagined: there he was perfectly well. He next removed to Arundel Street, Strand; and there, next door to the mud and mist of the river, and in an atmosphere of smoke from the factories that cover its banks and the steamers that swarm on its surface, his breathing was perfectly free. The same in Surrey Street, close by. But when he moved to a clearer and more elevated part of the town—Woburn Place, Russell Square—his old symptoms frequently showed themselves, but immediately disappeared on his moving down to Carey Street, Lincoln's Inn, where he passed six months without, I think, an asthmatic feeling. He was afraid at one time that he would have been obliged to live on the south side of the river—the north side seemed to have lost its efficacy, the air of Arundel Street was too pure for him; and he actually took a bed-room in Stamford Street, on the Southwark side, and slept there two or three nights, by way of experiment. He found, as he expected, that he was perfectly well there. The level could have been but a few feet above the Thames, whereas in Arundel Street his room must have been 100 or 120 feet above the Thames level.

It was to some narrow *back* street in Manchester that the asthmatic from Knutsford was advised by his medical attendant to go, and it was in such a situation, the closest and smokiest he could pick out, that he found the locality that cured him.

A friend of mine once told me of an old lady who was compelled by her asthma to live in some wretched alley out of Smithfield—in no other part of London could she breathe; there she was well, but nowhere else, and her disease tied her to that foul district all her days.

Now, I am quite sure in my own mind that the localities that will be found beneficial in the largest number of cases of asthma are such as the numerous examples I have related would imply—large, low-lying, densely-peopled, smoky cities. But is this always the case? By no means. In some instances the very reverse is the fact —a low, damp, or smoky air is not tolerated, and the asthmatic is only well in some clear, open, elevated situation, as the following cases will show:—

"Asthma," writes Mr. Macaulay to me, "is *always*, more or less, a local disease—influenced, I mean, by locality—more than any disease I know excepting fen ague; so much so, that I am convinced a confirmed asthmatic has only to find out the exact spot that suits *his* case, and stick to it, to become well. This town [Leicester] is very bad for most asthmatic people, but the high ground in the immediate neighbourhood is almost universally salubrious in such cases. But towns, however close, are not alike to the same people. J. B. was a guard on the Manchester mail in the olden time (twenty years ago), and slept on alternate nights in Leicester and Manchester. He was seized here with asthma in the middle of the night and was unable to go out in the morning with the mail, remained very ill for some days, and then went to Manchester, where his wife and family resided, being, as was thought, unable to work. Before he got home he was *well*, and returned to his duties in a few days. But the first night at Leicester he was seized with asthma again, at one A. M., as violent as before. I then had him put upon the mail, and sent off, and by the time he had got three miles from the town the fit left him ; and so it went on for many weeks. At Manchester he slept soundly all night, but at Leicester he invariably had a fit, more or less severe. I then advised him to take a lodging on the high ground outside the town, one mile exactly from his then lodgings ; and he never had another attack, except once when long-continued immunity induced him, for convenience, to try his old lodgings, and then his disease made its appearance at the usual hour. I saw this man about ten years ago, and he had never had any more asthma, and was well.

"Captain M., a confirmed asthmatic, was travelling in search of health, and was seized with an unusually severe fit at an inn in this town. He suffered so intensely that I had him removed to a lodging on the high ground outside the town. The effect was not only magical for the moment, but he found his breathing permanently so much better than in any part he had tried before, that (without any tie or connection with the place) he stayed with us four years.

"Some years ago Mrs. T., residing in the centre of the town, was so worn down with attacks of asthma, and consequent loss of rest, that her medical attendant thought she must die. I was called in, and had her carried in a bed to the outskirts of the town ; and she slept all the first night so soundly, that her attendant was frightened. The asthma never returned as long as she kept out of the town.

"Very lately Mrs. U. consulted me for 'pain in her chest and difficulty of breathing.' As she was suckling a young child, and the stethoscope showed nothing but obscure dry *râles*, I did not take much notice of the matter ; but she got rapidly worse, and then a close examination of the symptoms revealed the fact that, although she was well enough by day, the evil she complained of always came on in the night, and generally about two A. M. She was immediately removed to the high ground to the south of the town, and remained there three weeks without any return of the paroxysms. She has just returned home *well*, but the permanency of the cure remains to be seen.

"Stagnant air is worst of all for asthmatic people. Mrs. P., living in a close back parlour, behind a shop, with high walls all round, and lighted from the top, is violently affected at times ; but in her own bed-room, which is large and airy, *at the top of the house*, she does much better. When this woman goes to a lodging on the high ground to sleep, she has no asthma. One more case illustrative of this point I will give you.

"Mr. J. B., of this town, has been asthmatic for twenty-five years past, his age being now fifty-four. His attacks had been severe and persistent for many years whilst he lived in the town, and a removal to the higher ground ten years ago was of very trifling, if any, service; but though he suffered most severely *his general health never gave way*. Two years ago, being in easy circumstances and a bachelor, he broke up his establishment, and went abroad to travel, in the hope of baffling the disease. He went to various places, and spent the winter in the neighbourhood of Paris, without any benefit. Returning to England in the spring, he spent some time in London, without being better. Three months ago he went to Brighton, and very soon experienced a marvellous alteration in his symptoms— his nights became more comfortable, and, in fact, his asthma disappeared; and he now writes to his friends that he is *quite well*, goes out hunting four days a-week, and cannot believe he is the same person who has lived for years such a life of suffering. It is rather curious that to this gentleman, though not a patient of mine, I had more than once given a confident opinion, in conversation about his painful malady, that he would some day stumble on a locality which would cure him."

This is the only case I have yet mentioned in which a sea-side air effected a cure. The following equally striking case is, in this respect, the counterpart of it:—

P. J., aged forty-two, of a healthy florid appearance, slightly made, and of an extremely nervous temperament, has suffered from asthma for the last thirteen or fourteen years. There had been only one case of thoracic affection in his family, and that was a case of asthma. He believes the original cause of his disease to be some obscure spinal affection, which he imagines he contracted from severe study while reading for the medical profession in London, as frequently before an attack of asthma sets in, he experiences a tingling sensation down the spine, with other symptoms of nervous disturbance, extreme irritability, &c. These symptoms sometimes continue for two or three days before the paroxysm comes on. When he is going to have an attack, his dyspnœa generally commences about ten o'clock P.M., and most frequently awakes him about two hours after falling asleep with the usual symptoms of asthma—a sense of oppression and suffocation, with intense difficulty of breathing. The attack may last for an hour or two, when the dyspnœa decreases and free expectoration ensues. He will sometimes have an attack on several successive nights, and more rarely on one night alone. He has tried almost every remedy in the pharmacopœia, with little or no benefit. Stimulants, sedatives, nitre-paper, stramonium smoking, have equally failed; but from *strong* coffee he thinks he has sometimes experienced a little benefit. He finds that by careful attention to his diet and digestive organs, generally he can obtain some degree of immunity from his attacks. But, nevertheless, in spite of every care, he suffers from asthma as long as he is in his usual residence, a dense, smoky, manufacturing town in Lancashire. About six years ago his sufferings were so great that his life was irksome to him, and he was persuaded to leave his profession for a short time, and try change of residence. Some time previously he had visited Blackpool, a small watering-place on the west coast, and found some relief. He accordingly gave up his practice and went to Blackpool, and there, to his great joy and comfort, found himself suddenly perfectly free from his disease. He remained there the whole of one summer, and then returned to his former place of residence; but his asthma returned too, and he suffered as much as before. Two years afterwards, he was again compelled to give up practice: again he tried Blackpool with the same happy result—every symptom of asthma disappearing, and he himself rapidly recovering both flesh and strength. He was again induced to commence practice, and again returned to his former residence, and, as before, his asthma returned with him. Nevertheless, he struggled on with his sufferings, occasionally visiting Blackpool for a few days; and if, when suffering from the most severe attacks of asthma, night after night, he went to Blackpool, his difficulty of breathing immediately left him, and he was able to eat and sleep well, and to enjoy life. Lately he has been again compelled to give up his practice and retreat to Blackpool, away from which place it appears impossible for him to live.

A third case of the curative influence of sea-side air on asthma came under my observation many years ago. The subject of it was a lady, the wife of an admiral; and so completely did the state of her breathing depend on her proximity to the sea that she used to take a house, one might almost say a cottage, on the shore, in a situation where the only other inhabitants were fishermen, and so near to the sea that in rough weather the waves broke against the walls of her house. In this amphibious residence she could breathe; she was never so well as there.

The following well-marked example of the reversal of the ordinary effects of town and country air in asthma, came under my observation about two years ago, among the out-patients of the Charing Cross Hospital:—

Matilda Brown, aged forty four, resident in London, emaciated, high shouldered, slightly cyanotic, with feeble voice, worn-out aspect, and extremities always cold—in fact presenting all the conditions and physiognomy of confirmed asthma. The disease is of four years' standing, and dates from an attack of influenza. She rarely goes more than a week without asthma, and as long as that only when the weather is very fine and clear; in such weather she has gone as long as three weeks, but very rarely. To secure such a result, however, she is obliged to be very careful as to what she eats; she does not dare eat beef, cheese, vegetables, particularly greens, or take porter or spirits of any kind; and of the most wholesome food, and that which agrees with her the best, she is obliged to partake in very small quantities. Last summer, after she had been some time under my care, and received but slight and temporary benefit from any treatment that I adopted, she went to stay with her sister at Canterbury, and immediately found a sudden and complete change in her condition. She lost all difficulty of breathing, breathed as freely and clearly as any one, and instead of being obliged almost to starve herself, as she was when in London, and abstain altogether from numbers of things, she might eat and drink what she liked, and when she liked, and might go to bed with perfect impunity immediately after eating a hearty supper of beef; she had not been at Canterbury a week before she could drink two pints of porter a-day. During several weeks that she was there she had not a single attack; and when she came home she was so much changed for the better that I should hardly have known her. She finds her breath always worse in London if her bowels are at all confined, and on account of this is obliged to take the greatest care in keeping them open; in the country, this is of no consequence. In all these points this case is exactly the reverse of the case of D. M., in which the *lædentia* were efficient in the country which in this case are efficient in London, and impotent in London which here are impotent in the country. In D. M.'s case asthma is certain to be brought on in the country by eating freely, by eating late, by many articles of diet, by constipated bowels; whereas in London he may disregard all these things. The two cases tell exactly the same story—the influence of air has just the same place in causation in both of them: it appears so to affect the condition of the nervous and muscular apparatus of the air passages, either immediately by its application to the bronchial surface, or by producing some general constitutional change, as to make them sensitive or insensible respectively to certain stimuli, so that in the one locality these stimuli inevitably produce bronchial spasm, in the other are impotent and cease to be felt as stimuli at all.

On returning to London this poor woman became as bad as ever, indeed worse—the attacks so severe, and the intervals so short, that she did not seem as if she could live under them much longer. Her dyspnœa became permanent; but that it was not from emphysema coming on, as I imagined, was shown by a second visit to the country being attended with the same beneficial results as the first; for had the dyspnœa had an organic cause it could not at once have yielded to change of air: and this, let me say, is an important point in a diagnostic point of view; no dyspnœa that is suddenly and completely removed can have emphysema for its cause. I have not seen this poor woman for many months, and I think she must either have died in London, or be living in the country.

I have now recited the histories of twenty cases, and I think nothing would be gained by multiplying them further. In one point they all tell the same tale—sudden and, in almost every case, complete relief, following change of residence from one locality to another. Beyond this point they cease to agree, and indeed offer the most opposite evidence. For while fourteen are only well while breathing the air of populous smoky cities (eleven out of these four-teen cases being cured by London air), seven are unable to breathe in cities, have been driven from them, and are obliged to take up their abode either in the country, or by the sea-side. But this general division into two classes does not anything like express the contrariety that exists between them; the city cases and the country cases differ among themselves in the most varied and irregular way; indeed, there is no end of the apparent caprice of asthma in this respect, the most varied and opposite airs unaccountably curing. Thus, the guard of the Manchester mail was well in Manchester and in the pure air of the elevated neighbourhood of Leicester, but in Leicester itself he could not breathe; whereas one would have thought that if Leicester was so much worse than its neighbourhood Manchester would have been worse still. In some of the cases other city airs, as Glasgow, Leicester, Manchester, have produced the same beneficial effect as London air has in so many others; whereas G. P. (Case 5[1]), who was always well in London, had asthma in Birmingham, Liverpool, Hull, in Staffordshire, at Darton, Darling-ton, and Newcastle; at the latter place all the time he was there. Take again the case of Captain A. B., which I have not yet related, from the report of which, made by a medical relative of the patient, the following is an extract: "With regard to climate, Guernsey is not what I could wish for him; it is damp, mild, and relaxing. He is only well in a dry bracing climate; either hilly country or sea-side suits him well; and he could break a fit sometimes in Guernsey by leaving home and going to sleep at the sea-side. His house in Guernsey is a mile from the sea, rather in a valley, very thickly wooded all round, and decidedly damp. In Paris, which is pre-eminently dry—at Bath, which is also dry, he is wonderfully well. London, too, agrees with him, at least the neighbourhood of Pall Mall. A bleak open country, where there are *no trees*, is always sure to agree with him; and a wooded country, especially if low, the contrary."

Here we plainly see what kind of air offends most—it is that of damp, low situations, abounding with vegetable life; and any air free from these conditions is beneficial, whether sea-side or dry inland. Contrast with this the case of D. M., who, though like Captain A. B., well in London, finds bracing inland airs such as Bath, the very worst of all for him. Contrast with it also the case of Lord ———, of which Dr. Ogier Ward recently told me, who was obliged, not long ago, to leave London at two o'clock in the morning and drive in all haste to Epsom, as the intensity of his asthma seemed almost to threaten his life. If Bath and London are both beneficial because they are dry, as Captain A. B.'s case would imply, why are London and Epsom, which are both dry, the one so prejudicial, the other so

---

[1] This case, being nearly the counterpart of some others, I have not narrated. Both it and the case which follows will be found in the Tables at the end of the volume.

beneficial, in the case of Lord ———? Again, I find, in notes of the case of the Rev. E. P., that Oxford and Sudbury agree with him, whilst London, Rugby, and Wales are prejudicial—what common characters unite, and what divide these localities? Again, Captain A. B. was well in London, Paris, and the sea-side: Mr. J. B. could not breathe in London and Paris, while Brighton cured him. Again, while I have cited three cases of cure by the sea-side I know other cases that cannot breathe near the coast.[1]

Often what one may call intrinsic eccentricities present themselves in the same case—an asthmatic stumbles across some remarkable exception to his general experience. Thus D. M. found, to his surprise, on more occasions than one, that Leamington agreed with him perfectly well, though it belongs to a class of localities in which he cannot possibly breathe. Some of the contrarieties I have met with have been very striking and special. Thus, a short time since Dr. Camps told me of the case of an asthmatic lady, who, on going to Holloway, became much worse, and was obliged to return to town. Opposed to this I find in my note-book the following case: "Louisa Uz, aged five, has had asthma ever since she was six weeks old. She goes to bed well, and is seized towards morning, and the difficulty of breathing is such, that the exertion makes the perspiration stream from her. The circumstances that chiefly bring on the attacks, are excitement, laughing, and exertion. *She has lately been living at Holloway for seven weeks, and while she was there she was perfectly well. No sooner, however, has she returned to Grafton Street, Soho, where she lived before, than the difficulty of breathing has come on again.* I have advised her mother to take her back to Holloway." But the most curious instance of contrariety in asthma was related to me lately by Dr. Birkett. He told me he knew the cases of two asthmatics, one of whom could only breathe in London, and the other could only breathe in Norwood; if they attempted to go, the one to Norwood, the other to London, they were stopped on their journey by their asthma, and could not proceed; and, what was very curious, they were both stopped at the same place— they could neither of them get beyond Camberwell Green, the one in his journey towards Norwood, the other in his journey towards London; there they were stopped, and had to go back. This seems

---

[1] The following case of the inability of an asthmatic to live near the sea has been communicated to me by my friend Dr. Theophilus Thompson: "Last Autumn and on several occasions I have been consulted by a professional friend living, or endeavouring to live, on the coast of Northumberland, who when at his own house is distressed with nightly paroxysms of difficult breathing. If he sleeps only five miles from the sea he escapes the attack, and he enjoys perfect immunity at Edinburgh; but walking for a short time on the pier at Berwick is sufficient to induce a paroxysm. Shortly after his visit to me he stayed for a time in Nottinghamshire, and was perfectly well, but in three days after returning to the Northumberland coast there was a fresh accession of the complaint, although the wind was westerly. However severely he is attacked at the sea-side the symptoms subside in a few hours after he comes inland."

almost like romancing; but the source from whence I derived the account is sufficient warrant for its literal fidelity.

Now, if this is so, if we find such an irregularity and inexplicability in the therapeutical influence of locality on asthma—if we find it defying all management and thwarting all expectation, what rules can we lay down for the guidance of those who are suffering in their present abodes from this dreadful malady, and have not yet found out where they can breathe in peace? Can we lay down any? None, I believe, with any certainty. It is impossible to predict what will be the effect of any given air—the cure is often an inexplicable surprise. This is strikingly shown in many of the cases that I have related. Thus, Captain M., after travelling about from place to place in search of health, stumbled across it on the high ground outside Leicester, and Mr. J. B., after an equally fruitless search, found perfect ease at Brighton. The only approximation to a rule, that I know of, is that referred to by Mr. Macaulay—that that air will probably cure which is the opposite of the air in which the patient is worse. Thus city asthmatics are benefited by sea-coast and country—country asthmatics by city air. P. J. found at Blackpool an air the very reverse of that of the smoky manufacturing town in which he was so bad. The first case that I narrated was well in London; worst of all in an air which I consider the opposite to this—the clear bracing air of high chalk districts; and in mild, low-lying places, and in provincial towns, his condition was intermediate. In the Scotch lady who was cured on coming to Lombard Street, the asthma reappeared and became more intense as the air she breathed diverged in its qualities more and more from the city air. I should therefore, on a provincial asthmatic asking my advice, make him try some close part of the city, or the river-side, or a back street in some large provincial manufacturing town that might be nearer his ordinary residence, and therefore more convenient to him. A London asthmatic I should expect to derive the most benefit from the pure air of some open and elevated inland situation, or from the sea-side at such places as Brighton and Ramsgate.

Some of the differences of air, or whatever it may be, determining the presence or cure of asthma, appear to be of the slightest possible kind, subtle, inscrutable, and arbitrary. I remember the case of an asthmatic in Dorsetshire, who could breathe perfectly well on one side of a hill but not on the other, and that quite irrespective of level. If his breathing was at all affected it immediately became easy when the summit of this hill, which was a very low one, was passed—a few yards would make all the difference to his breathing; he seemed suddenly to step out of an asthmatic into a non-asthmatic air. Dr. Ogier Ward told me lately of the case of a clergyman who could not sleep in a house his patron had built for him, while in his patron's house, close by, he was perfectly well. The only circumstance that could apparently account for this difference was, that around his patron's house was a moat which was immediately under the window of the clergyman's bedroom, so that the air he breathed was probably more humid. My friend, Mr. Macaulay, in writing to me on this subject, remarks: "It is surprising how slight a change of locality will affect asthmatics. Mr. C., aged fifty-four, has been asthmatic from his youth, and suffered at times severely; but for the last four years, during which he has lived in the same house, has had no attack. Last week he removed his residence about four or five hundred yards, to a higher spot, but more closely built round, and very near to the exit of a sewer; the third night he slept in his new abode he had an attack of asthma, and is suffering from a repeated attack at this moment." The change of locality here was only a distance of four or five hundred yards, but it was sufficient to light up the disease that had been in abeyance four years. Dr. Watson, in his excellent chapter on asthma, the best, and, for its length, the most complete treatise on the disease in print, gives some remarkable instances of this sensitiveness on the part of asthma to subtle atmospheric differences otherwise inappreciable. "A college acquaintance of mine," he says, "much tormented with asthma, is equally sensible to these inscrutable influences. Two inns in Cambridge are named respectively the Red Lion and the Eagle. He can sleep in one of them, and not in the other. Nay, he is thus variously affected within much narrower limits. He assures me that, when in Paris, he never escapes a fit of asthma when he attempts to sleep in the back part of Meurice's Hotel, and never suffers when he sleeps in a front room. Dover Street suits him; Clarges Street does not. He cannot rest in Manchester Square."

There are some cases that suggest to one's mind the idea, that the mere conditions of locality are adequate to the production of asthma in a person whose disposition to it was never before suspected, and who probably would never have had it had he not gone to such a locality. Whether this depends on certain localities being what may be called asthmatic places, having a special tendency to excite the disease in those who have a lurking predisposition to it, or whether the peculiarity is entirely in the individual, I cannot say. But certain it is, that some asthmatics appear to be asthmatic only at one place—never to have it before they go there, and never to have it after they leave. The relations of place and asthma appear to be in them the reverse of what they are in asthmatics in general. In most asthmatics there is only one place that cures, in all others the disease shows itself, while in these it is in one place, and only in one, that the asthmatic tendency is apparent. Such a case is the following; one of the many interesting cases that my friend Mr. Macaulay has communicated to me: "Mr. H., in his fortieth year, went on a visit to Spalding, in Lincolnshire, and was awoke the first night with intense spasmodic asthma; he stayed several days, being very ill with it, and recovered immediately on returning home. His health being perfect, no further notice was taken of it, and the following year he repeated his visit to Spalding, on which occasion he was seized, the first night as before, and with the same result. Two years after, he again went to Spalding, and was again attacked. He never went to Spalding again, had never any further attack of asthma, and died lately, aged sixty-three, of diseased kidneys." Now, certainly, there is every reason to believe that if this gentleman had never gone to Spalding he would never have had asthma, and his having a tendency to it would never have entered either his own or any one else's head. Another case, somewhat similar, that has lately come under my observation, is that of an old lady, now sixty-nine years of age, who, at the age of twenty-two, went to King's Langley, in Hertfordshire. She had not been there long —I forget how long—when she was seized with violent asthma, and her breathing became so difficult that she was obliged to hasten her departure. Immediately on her arrival in Holborn, her usual place of abode, she became able to breathe freely—in fact, quite well. And she remained quite well for years, and never had a repetition of her attack; but lately she has been suffering from chronic bronchitis and gout. She is now living, and has been for some years past, at Dorking, in Surrey. Now, if this old lady had never gone to King's Langley she would never have had her single attack of asthma. The case I have narrated of the Manchester guard looks very much like the same thing. He seemed well everywhere but *in* Leicester. In the pure air of its elevated neighbourhood, in the city of Manchester—a very opposite air—and in all the varied localities through which the coach road between these two cities passed, he was well: he had not left Leicester many miles, on the occasion of his attacks, before he was always well. If this man had always had his lodgings, as they were after the discovery of his asthmatic tendency, outside, instead of inside, Leicester, *he* too would never have been asthmatic.

Now, if this is so, it opens a very curious possibility—a possibility that there may be many healthy persons, who never have had asthma, and never may, but who would be asthmatics if their life had been cast in other localities, or would have had temporary attacks of asthma if they had visited such localities. A certain dose, so to speak, of the asthmatic tendency—a certain proclivity to the easy assumption of bronchial stricture, may lie latent in them, but wait the stimulus of some offending air to call it into activity; and if such stimulus is never applied, if such air is never breathed, the spastic contraction of the air passages is never induced, and the tendency to it never suspected.

But is the wonderful cure of asthma, thus wrought by change of place, permanent? Has the asthmatic acquired an immunity from all tendency to his disease for the future? By no means. The *tendency* remains, and attacks are only kept at bay as long as the patient resides in the locality curative in his particular case. The asthma recurred in the case of the Scotch gentleman as soon as he had returned to his native city.   Mr. P. J. returned from Blackpool again and again, in the hope that he was cured and could resume his practice; but he always returned to be as bad as ever.   Three times did Mr. H. visit Spalding, at the intervals of one and two years, and never escaped an attack.   D. M., though he has been living in London now fifteen years, all but perfectly free from his disease, suffers an immediate recurrence of it whenever he goes into the country.   Before he is many miles from town, while still sitting in the railway carriage, he feels a difference in his respiration, a dry tightness of the peculiar asthmatic character, to which in London he is quite a stranger; and if he attempts to sleep in the country he is sure to be aroused about three or four o'clock in the morning, and obliged to get up and stand an hour or two before he can breathe freely or dress himself.   He returns to town, and is as well as ever. This has happened not once, but dozens—scores of times; and *will* happen, in all probability, as long as he lives.   And so it is in all cases.   The disposition, therefore, is not eradicated, only suspended, and immediately shows itself on a recurrence to the original injurious air.

The mere fact of *change of air*, so beneficial in many diseases, not only does no good in asthma, but does positive harm—change, as change, is prejudicial.   It seems as if the stimulus of a new, strange air to the respiratory surface acts as an irritant.   On going to an unfavourable locality, it is generally during the first few days and nights that the asthma is the most intense; afterwards the patient becomes acclimatized, as it were, and the paroxysms become milder and rarer.   I have known, on several occasions, a patient, when perfectly free from asthma, immediately attacked on his return to the place that agrees with him best.   The attack is much milder than on going to a bad air, is soon over, and followed by perfect immunity.   I have known this occur over and over again, and have noticed it in more cases than one.   It clearly shows that it is *the change* that offends.   The following case, related to me by Dr. Birkett, appears to be explicable only on this principle.   A gentleman in a delicate state of health, but with no previously evinced, or even suspected, tendency to asthma, went to Leicestershire.   On arriving there he was seized with asthma, and was so bad that he was obliged precipitately to return.   On returning to town he at once became perfectly well.   But the general condition of his health made it desirable that he should go somewhere for change of air, and accordingly he went to Margate.   He stayed there some time perfectly well, and improving in every respect; but no sooner did he return to London, his usual residence, that he was attacked with asthma just as he had been in Leicestershire.   Now it could not be that London was an asthmatic air to him, for he had lived in it twenty-three years and never had an asthmatic symptom; and moreover, on his return thither, it had immediately cured the Leicestershire attack.

12

Lastly, the conclusions at which we would arrive are greatly complicated, and the constancy of the results in any given case often deranged, by what we must call, for want of a better word, the "caprice" of asthma. It undergoes such odd erratic changes, varies its type or habitude so unaccountably, that its behaviour to remedies cannot be counted on from year to year, and the air that is now intolerable may be well borne in a twelvemonth, and *vice versâ*. This I know is not the rule, but it sometimes is so, and quite upsets our conclusions—we find, to our surprise, that a certain change of locality has the very opposite effect to that which it had on any former occasion. Take, for instance, the following example. An asthmatic gentleman had been in the habit of going to Ryde for occasional visits, and he always did so at the price of increasing his asthma. On one occasion it was unusually bad, and became worse and worse night by night, waking him earlier each night, and obliging him to leave his bed first at four, then at three, and then at two o'clock in the morning, till, on the fourth night, he got no sleep at all. On the fifth day he was obliged to leave—it seemed impossible he could live there any longer. He was so disabled by the severity of his asthma that he could proceed no farther than Southampton that day. The following morning an attack of pleurisy developed itself, brought on probably by exposure in sitting out of bed for so many nights, and kept him at Southampton for a week. Then, being very anxious to pass a few days at Ryde, if possible, he determined to give it another trial. He passed the first night without asthma, the second, the third—in short, he had not the slightest return of it, and spent a month there without an asthmatic sensation—indeed, in much more complete immunity from the disease than in his ordinary residence, where he was accustomed to have an attack about once a-week. The following is another instance of the same thing. An asthmatic gentleman had been unable for years to sleep without asthma in a village about a mile and a half from the town in which he resided. Lodgings had often been taken for him there, with the view of improving his general health; but he never could sleep there in peace, and when his family migrated there in the summer he was obliged to stay at home. In the summer of 1846, he passed three months there without the slightest asthma; the tables were completely turned—instead of asthma driving him from the village, he had only to go there in order to be perfectly free from it if it threatened him in the town; even before he arrived in the village all trace of dyspnœa would leave him—the air that always before was poison to him was now his medicine, and it seemed as if he could never be asthmatic any more as long as he could resort to his country bedroom. How long this would have lasted it is impossible to say, as he was obliged at the end of three months to leave the country and come to London. It seems impossible to fall back, as an explanation of these eccentricities, on anything except the proverbial caprice of the disease. In such cases the difference must be in the individual, not in the air. We can understand how two places, however near or however much alike, may have subtle atmospheric or other differences, but the topical influences of the same place must be the same year by year.

There is one point that such cases seem to illustrate, and that is, the disposition to *habit* that characterizes asthma—to repeat that which has once been started, to continue the effect even after the cause has ceased—as we see sometimes apparently in epilepsy, and all nervous diseases that are of a "repetitive" type. Thus, in the cases I have just cited, the first visit to Ryde began with asthma, and it went on getting worse and worse; the second began well, and so it continued, and would apparently *ad infinitum:* the same with regard to the second case. It seems, as I have remarked in a previous chapter, as if it was a law of the disease to continue its present type and peculiarities, whatever they may be, till something occurs to "break the spell," and then to continue the acquired change, whatever that may be, till something else occurs, and so on. So that if an asthmatic is going on well the safest plan is to leave him alone, for there is no knowing what *cacoëthes* any change may set going. I have known an asthmatic go on well for months, as long as one day was but the repetition of another and all external conditions were preserved unchanged; but when something has occurred to put him wrong—as a visit to some asthmatic locality—it has been months before he has lost the asthmatic habit, and subsided into that immunity from the disease that he was before enjoying, although he may have at once recurred to the conditions in which he was previously so well.

Let me now briefly sum up the conclusions at which I have arrived, and which I think the cases cited in this chapter sufficiently establish :—

1. That residence in one locality will cure, radically and permanently cure, asthma resisting all treatment in another locality.

2. That the localities that are the most beneficial to the largest number of cases are large, populous, and smoky cities.

3. That this effect of locality depends probably on the air.

4. That the worse the air for the general health, the better, as a rule, for asthma; thus the worst parts of cities are the best, and conversely.

5. That this is not always the case, the very reverse being sometimes so—a city air not being tolerated, and an open pure air effecting a cure.

6. That there is no end of the apparent caprice of asthma in this respect, the most varying and opposite airs unaccountably curing.

7. That, consequently, it is impossible to predict what will be the effect of any given air, but that probably the most opposite to that in which the asthma seems worst, will cure.

8. That some of these differences determining the presence or

cure of asthma appear to be of the slightest possible kind, arbitrary and inscrutable.

9. That the mere conditions of locality appear to be adequate to the production of asthma, in a person whose disposition to it was never before suspected, and who probably would never have had it had he not gone to such a locality.

10. That, consequently, many healthy persons, who never have had asthma and never may, probably would be asthmatics if their life had been cast in other localities.

11. That *possibly* there is no case of asthma that might not be cured if the right air could only be found.

12. That the disposition is not eradicated, merely suspended, and immediately shows itself on a recurrence to the original injurious air.

13. That change of air, as change, is prejudicial.

14. That, from the caprice of asthma, the constancy of the results in any given case is often deranged.

CHAPTER XIV.

HYGIENIC TREATMENT OF ASTHMA.

Beneficial influence of sustained bodily exertion.—Cold shower-bath.—Value of tonics. —Avoidance of cold.—Regularity of life.—Inhalation of powdered alum; of nitro-hydrochloric acid vapours; of oxygen gas; of compressed air.—Galvanism.

IN concluding the subject of the treatment of asthma I would briefly advert to certain hygienic rules and plans of self-management, to which sufferers from asthma may with advantage subject themselves, and to certain tonic agents, whose employment, by elevating the standard of the general health and imparting to it a braced robustness, exerts a very marked efficacy in diminishing the tendency to that special nervous perturbation which manifests itself in the asthmatic paroxysm. The principal of these are : Sustained exercise; Shower-bath; Tonic medicines; Avoidance of cold; A rigorous regularity of life.

1. *Exercise.*—I have seen several cases in which prolonged bodily exertion has been of great benefit, indeed some in which it has been the best remedy to which the asthmatic could resort. This, at any rate, proves one thing—the compatibility of asthma with perfect organic health of lung; for if there were any structural defect in the organ—emphysema, bronchitis— or any heart-disease, it would be impossible to meet such extraordinary respiratory demands without embarrassment. It does not indeed show that asthma has *never* such organic diseases for its cause, but it shows that asthma *may*

exist without any organic basis, because it shows that in these cases such organic disease must clearly be absent.

This treatment is, of course, rather prophylactic than curative— it must be taken in the intervals of the attacks; but when so taken it seems to have a marvellous efficacy in keeping them off, and in giving to the asthmatic a lightness and freedom of respiration to which at other times he is a stranger.

Its rationale puzzles me. It may act in part by the vigour and activity that it gives to the function of the skin. The vicarious relation of the skin and lungs and the similarity of their excreta (carbonic acid and watery vapour being the principal constituents of both), we all know perfectly well; and it may well be that exercise, by increasing the amount of work done by the skin, throws less on the lungs, and gives that ease, and freedom, and sense of surplus power of breathing that I have mentioned. But I do not see how it can in this way prevent a tendency to spasm. I think it must thus act by the change that it produces in the blood. We know that each tissue is in proportion to the vigour of the function of which it is the seat, an excretory organ, that it depurates the blood of that particular material that is destined for its nutrition, that the action and nutrition of a tissue always go *pari passu*, and that if that action is feeble its nutrition is feeble, and it fails to withdraw from the blood that which it should. We know, too, that a blood rich in nutrient material, what we may call the *sanguis cibi*, the blood after a meal, is peculiarly offensive to the lungs of asthmatics, that its circulation in the capillaries of the lungs has a great tendency to irritate the pulmonary nervous system, and excite the bronchial tubes to spasm. In this way must, in a great degree, be explained after-dinner and after-supper asthma. If, then, a blood much charged with these recrementitious materials is the most provocative of asthma, that which is the freest from them must be the least so, and under no circumstances is the blood so free from them as after prolonged fasting and exercise, the fasting shutting off the supply of raw material, and the exercise drafting away, to supply the muscular waste, any unappropriated plastic store already existing in the blood. Whether this is, or not, the true explanation of the beneficial influence on asthma of prolonged muscular exertion, I am unable to offer any other.

The following cases are good examples illustrative of this point:—

CASE 1. " Of all remedies," writes a confirmed asthmatic to me, " there is none for me so complete and lasting as a day of severe walking exercise—five-and-twenty miles over hilly ground or across heaths. The strain must never be great. I begin slowly, almost saunteringly, and only increase my pace when it is pleasanter to do so than not. Towards the end of my day I can usually climb a hundred feet of cliff as fast as I can plant my feet, or run a mile or two to catch a train. Habitually I can never run or go fast up hill. In this matter of exercise it is of paramount importance not to overstrain. If I am 'winded' against a hill and stop at the top till I breathe freely, I can get up the next hill more easily, and so on. But if when the hill was surmounted I kept right on, I should get up the next hill worse, and so on. Rowing I consider bad, because the temptation to over-exertion is too great; and riding is most excellent, because exertion is sure, and over-exertion next to impossible. This habit of severe walking exercise, and such an arrangement of clothing at night as shall prevent the body being exposed if the breathing necessitates the erect position, I consider much the most valuable hints which my experience enables me to give to asthmatics."

CASE 2. The following I extract from an interesting case sent me by a medical friend: "For the last twenty years, in fact, ever since I can recollect, my father has been running the gauntlet of medical men in England and Scotland, without any sort of benefit, so much so that about eight years ago he gave this plan up, and took the treatment into his own hands—I ought to say *legs*, perhaps, for his only curative measure consisted in walking exercise; about twenty miles a day was, he considered, an average dose, and the result is that he is now comparatively free from attacks."

CASE 3. E. P., a clergyman, aged twenty eight, has suffered from asthma from the age of six years. With regard to remedies he states, that, while medicines directed to the relief of the chest have been useless, he has experienced the greatest relief from violent bodily exertion, such as boating and gymnastic exercises.

2. *Shower-bath.*—I think it is a law without an exception that nervous affections are less prone to occur in proportion to the general bodily vigour, and what, for want of a more definite term, we must call the *tone* of the nervous system. Anything, therefore, that corroborates and invigorates renders asthmatics less prone to their attacks. In this way the shock of the cold shower-bath, or sponge-bath, or sea-bathing, is often of great service to asthmatics. By raising the standard of the general health they also tend to prevent those humoral derangements which are often the exciting cause of asthma.

3. *Tonics* have the same value, and for the same reason. Of all tonics in asthma I think quinine the best, and next to quinine, iron. Whether the special value of quinine depends at all on its antiperiodic power I cannot say, or whether the periodicity of asthma is one which quinine would not be likely to control. The tonic that I commonly order, and from which I think I have seen the best effect, is a combination of quinine, iron, and a mineral acid.

4. *Avoidance of cold.*—Exposure of the external surface to cold is apt to induce asthma in two ways—immediately and directly, or remotely through the intervention of bronchitis. Some asthmatics are at once conscious of an asthmatic tightening of their breathing if they venture out of doors with their chests imperfectly covered, or if their feet get damp and cold. I am acquainted with the case

of an asthmatic lady whom a walk of two minutes in her garden will
render asthmatic if her chest is bare.   This is evidently not from
the respiration of cold air; for, under identical circumstances, the
mere fact of her chest being covered will entirely prevent the occurrence of the asthmatic breathing; the same result as immediately
happens if her feet get damp and cold.   In such cases there is
clearly no time for the production of the asthma *viâ* bronchitis.
But is it certain that there is in these cases no vascular disturbance
of the bronchial mucous membrane, and that this is not the link
between the cold and the asthma?   Until lately I felt no doubt that
the asthma was, in these instances, a mere reflex nervous phenomenon, but of late I have seen some cases, not asthmatic, that have
shown me how quickly—how immediately, indeed—cold to the surface and extremities may derange the vascular balance of the
bronchial mucous membrane, and which suggest, therefore, that
even in these asthmatic cases the vascular condition of the bronchial
mucous membrane may be the link between the external cold and
the bronchial spasm.   One of these cases is as follows: A gentleman is liable to slight chronic inflammation of his trachea and larger
bronchi, which shows itself by sternal pain, slight tracheal tenderness,
short husky cough, dryness and hoarseness of voice, and the expectoration of little pellets of viscid mucus.—From these symptoms,
from the whole history of the case, and from the result of treatment,
I feel no doubt as to the seat and nature of the affection.   This
gentleman assured me that all his symptoms may be induced *in a
few minutes*, by walking out in damp weather with his feet imperfectly protected.   I have seen other cases nearly as striking.   It
would seem, then, that the inmediateness with which asthma may
supervene, on exposure to cold, does not prove that the vascular
condition of the bronchial mucous membrane has nothing to do with
its generation.

But the most frequent way in which asthmatics suffer from cold
is by its producing catarrhal bronchitis.   In these cases the asthma
is not immediate; it is accompanied by all the signs and symptoms
of bronchitis, and is proportionate to the intensity of the bronchitic
affection, of which indeed it is but a complication, and without which
cold never produces it.

There is yet a third way in which cold generates asthma—by its
direct application to the bronchial tubes, by the inspiration of cold
air.   I have lately had under my care a lady, of whose asthma this
appears to be the one sole cause.   Whenever she breathes cold air
the wheezing immediately comes on, and no amount of warm clothing makes any difference.   If a fire is kept up all night in her
room she sleeps uninterruptedly till the morning, quite free from
asthma, but if it goes out her dyspnœa shortly wakes her.   A re-
spirator is a perfect cure.   I should mention that she has no symptoms of bronchitis.

The practical rules that I draw from these facts are: That asthmatics should wear flannel next their skins, that they should vary the amount of their clothing in proportion to the temperature, that they should immediately change wet garments, avoid cold after perspiring, and take all other precautions for precluding catarrh.

5. Lastly, there is one general rule, which, trifling as it may seem, is perhaps exceeded in importance by none, and by attending to which the asthmatic may do more to evade his attacks than by any other. It is, to establish a rigorous unformity of life, to make one day the exact counterpart of another, and to avoid irregularities of every kind. Asthma often seems as if it were lying in ambush watching its opportunity, or on the look-out for some loophole through which to make its attack, and there is hardly any change of life or habit of which it will not, as at were, take advantage—change of air, change of sleeping apartment, alteration of meal hours. I have already referred to this subject in speaking of the tendency to *habitude* which characterizes asthma, and I would only now enforce the great importance of the asthmatic's guarding himself from all possible sources of offence by tying himself down to a life of monotonous regularity.

In concluding this chapter I would just mention some methods of treatment which I have been informed have been employed with advantage, but of which I can say nothing from my own personal experience.

Inhalation of Powdered Alum.—I have heard of two cases in which this treatment has been successfully employed; but I very much suspect they were rather cases of chronic bronchitis than asthma. That the local application of an astringent might do good to a congested and tumid mucous membrane is intelligible; but that the application of alum could relieve muscular spasm I cannot believe.

Inhalation of Nitro-hydrochloric Acid Vapour.—The inhalation of nitro-hydrochloric acid diluted with aqueous vapour I have also heard recommended; but I should imagine that this would act in the same way, and be appropriate for the same kind of cases, as the alum, and I should be very chary of using it during a paroxysm of asthma. The way in which my informant had used it was this: Nitro-hydrochloric acid, a teaspoonful, in a quarter of a pint of water, to be raised to a temperature of 150°, and inhaled in an inhaler for a quarter of an hour three or four times a-day.

Inhalation of Oxygen Gas.—I am not sure that this has ever been tried. I have no distinct recollection of ever having heard of a case in which it has; and I am not sure the idea did not spontaneously occur to my mind from its own inherent reasonableness. The great thing that is wanted in asthma is oxygen: it is because it stops oxygenation that the shutting-off of air by the bronchial spasm produces the distressing sensation that attends it, and the violent efforts for its relief; it is because oxygenation is suspended that the capillaries refuse to transmit the blood, producing pulmonary congestion, and a condition of partial asphyxia. If, then, instead of a scanty stream of the dilute oxygen of which the atmosphere consists, a more concentrated form could be supplied, its concentration might make up for its tenuity, and, while spasm might still persist, those results which alone make it important would be suspended; the blood would be oxygenated and freely pass on, the vessels would unload themselves, and the congestion, the distress, and the effort would cease. I regret to say, that from the necessity of a special apparatus, and from my not having had, since the idea occurred to me, a case in actual spasm on which I could try it, I cannot confirm my anticipations by the results of my own experience.[1]

Another plan of treatment which *has* been tried extensively, and which, I think, is the same in principle as the oxygen inhalation, is the *respiration of compressed air.* At the hydropathic establishment at Ben Rhydding, in Yorkshire, and at Montpellier, and Nice, this treatment has been in operation for some time, and from the accounts that I have heard from intelligent eye-witnesses of its effects, as well as on its own merits, I should think very favourably of it. The patient is placed, in a sitting position, in an air-tight chamber, into which additional air is forced under gradually increasing pressure, till the required condensation is attained; at this point it is maintained for a certain time, according to the prescribed length of the *séance,* and then gradually lowered. If the pressure is that of two atmospheres, every cubic foot of air will of course contain the oxygen and nitrogen of two cubic feet at the ordinary pressure, and the ordinary volume of air breathed will therefore contain twice the quantity of oxygen. It is manifest, therefore, that an asthmatic whose contracted bronchi allow him to change in respiration only half the usual amount of air, will, on breathing such an air as this, have the balance exactly restored, and be respiring the same amount of the atmospheric gases as a healthy person in a natural atmosphere. In this way, and in this way only, do I think it would act; it would alleviate the conditions engendered by the spasm, but I should very much doubt its having any power to destroy or diminish the asthmatic tendency. It would be well, I think, if this treatment could have a more extended and regular trial, and if its results could be subjected to an enlightened scrutiny.

There is one agent that has long been recommended in asthma, against the employment of which I would, in concluding this chapter, earnestly caution my readers; it is *galvanism*—the passing galvanic shocks through the chest. I object to it both on theoretical and practical grounds. What idea could have originally suggested it I am at a loss to imagine, unless it were the paralysis theory of the disease—that asthma depended on loss of power of the bronchial

[1] Since writing the above I have received the notes of a case of a medical friend, who has tried the inhalation of oxygen in his own person with great advantage.

muscle, or the muscles of the thoracic parietes. I have known it
do great harm; I have known it bring on an attack in a patient at
the time free from asthma, and I have known it aggravate existing
spasm; but I have never known it do any good.

CHAPTER XV.

PROGNOSIS OF ASTHMA.

1. Indications derived from the actual condition.—The influence of age in determining prognosis.—Presence or absence of organic complications.—2. Indications
derived from past history, *e. g*, *a*. Length of attacks. *b*. Frequency of attacks. *c*.
Completeness of recovery. *d*. Persistence of expectoration. *e*. Cough. *f*. Indications derived from exciting cause.—General conclusions.

IN a disease whose tendency is so little generally understood as
asthma, and which is so alarming and distressing in its manifestations,
the ultimate issue of the case is often a subject of the most painful
anxiety to the sufferer and his friends; it is therefore a matter of
some importance that the physician should be able to detect the tendency of the disease in any given case, and to form something like
a definite prognosis.

Now this prognosis must be based partly on the actual condition
of the patient, and partly on the previous history of his case. As
far as relates to the *actual condition*, the circumstances by which
our prognosis will be influenced are the patient's age, and the presence or absence of organic mischief in the heart or lungs. As far
as relates to the *previous history* of his case, the circumstances influencing the prognosis are the duration of the attacks (rather than
their severity), their frequency, the completeness of the recovery
between them, their apparent tendency, that is, whether they appear to be getting more frequent and more severe, or less frequent
and lighter, and lastly, the length of time the asthma has existed.

*I. Circumstances connected with the actual condition of the
patient.*

1. *Age.*—The influence of *age* in determining the tendency of
asthma constitutes a very constant and characteristic feature in its
clinical history. In young asthmatics the tendency is almost invariably *towards recovery*, whereas, in a person who is attacked with
it after forty-five the tendency is generally towards a progressive
severity of the disease, and the production and aggravation of those
complications by which asthma kills. In no disease, in my opinion,
does the question of age affect prognosis more, and in none is better
shown the power of youthful organisms to repair, in the intervals of
health, the injuries of disease, and to resist the tendency of func-

tional to the production of organic mischief; or, on the other hand, the loss of this power in the advance of life, and the proportionally greater tendency of occasional and recurrent derangements to produce permanent and irreparable injury.

To the young asthmatic under fifteen one may almost safely predict, barring organic disease, a favourable issue of his case, and tell him he will most likely gradually "grow out of" his complaint. I can call to mind, at the present time, four or five cases of individuals who have thus grown out of their malady, and are now perfectly well, but whose childhood was rendered one of great suffering by asthma. In asthma commencing from twenty to forty, age tells much less in favour of the patient, and the prognosis is, as far as age goes, doubtful; but if the lungs are entirely free from any organic complication, if there is no emphysema and no tendency to bronchitis, the patient has, under proper management, a very fair chance of recovery. Above forty-five the recoveries are, I believe, few indeed; the tendency is, as I said just now, generally towards a progressive severity of the disease, and the prognosis should always be guarded, if not absolutely unfavourable.

Now, why is this? Why, *cæteris paribus*, should age have such a determining influence on the tendency of asthma? Partly for the reasons that I have mentioned;—that in the young the powers of repair are great, in those advanced in life feeble; that in the young the pulmonary congestion, that always accompanies asthma, completely vanishes in the intervals of the attacks, the capillaries recover their tone, and the nutritional balance of the lungs is regained; whereas in the old the engorged capillaries are slower in recovering themselves, and the pulmonary congestion hangs about the patient some time after the asthmatic spasm has disappeared, manifesting itself by a profuse mucous exudation, and a certain thickness of breathing and incapacity for exertion. If the attacks are frequent, this pulmonary congestion never entirely vanishes, and thus is produced a kind of spurious chronic bronchitis, with a tendency to aggravation by each attack, which is one of the worst and commonest complications of the asthma of the old. Another complication of asthma—dilated right heart—is much more apt to occur in the old than in the young, and for the very reason that the dyspnœa in the old is so apt, by the generation of this spurious bronchitis of which I have been speaking, to pass from the occasional and intermittent form characteristic of pure asthma, and become continuous and permanent. As far as I have seen, the right side of the heart never becomes dilated by asthma, however severe the dyspnœa may be during the attacks, if the intervals between them are considerable, and the recovery in those intervals complete. It is a continued and not an occasional and transient arrest of the pulmonary circulation that dilates the right side of the heart. It is from this fact that we see dilatation of the right side of the heart, venous stasis, and general dropsy, so much more common as a result of chronic bronchitis than of asthma.

But this greater disposition in asthma to produce organic change in the old than in the young is not the only circumstance which imparts to age its determining influence on the tendency of the disease. In asthma, as in all other constitutional disorders, we have in the young much more room for hope from those changes in the type and build of the constitution which in them are so marked and striking; whereas in the old the constitution is set and fixed, and we have but little to hope on this score. Indeed, the existence of a constitutional peculiarity in a child is of itself almost a presumption that he will one day lose it; while in an old person it furnishes a presumption equally strong that it is fixed and indelible.

Again, in an old person the probability is that the asthma had existed longer than in a young one, and, as I shall show presently, the chances of recovery from asthma (as is the case in almost all diseases, are in inverse proportion to the length of time that the disease has existed.

But there is a special reason, depending on the nervous nature of asthma, that makes us sanguine of recovery in the case of the young; and which explains at the same time the greater frequency of pure nervous examples of the disease in the young than in the old. What, for want of a better name, we must call "nervous irritability," is much more marked in the young than in the old. It appears continuously to diminish from birth forwards. Sources of irritation that in the young are adequate to the production of the most violent nervous phenomena, in mature life are powerless to produce such effects. The cutting of a tooth, for example, will send an infant into epileptic convulsions; one never hears of a fit from the second dentition. A young child will grind its teeth, or even be violently convulsed, from the presence of ascarides in its rectum; but one never sees such results from worms in the adult. And thus the diminution of nervous irritability, as childhood passes into youth and manhood, may make an attack of asthma less and less prone to occur on the supervention of its exciting causes, and less intensely spasmodic when it does occur. I believe, indeed, that this diminution of nervous irritability is the true explanation of that gradual recovery of young asthmatics which is so common, so almost universal.

Lastly, age influences unfavourably the tendency of asthma, not only because it is more apt in advanced life to engender organic disease, but because it is also more apt to have organic disease as its cause. The causation of asthma in youth and age is indeed very different. In age there is commonly some appreciable organic basis for it; in youth much more rarely.

2. The other circumstance in the actual condition of an asthmatic determining the tendency of the disease in his case, is *the presence or absence of organic diseases in the respiratory and circulatory organs.* This is the most important of all the points affecting the

prognosis, and is, of itself, sufficient to turn the scale. Its exact value is this: if the heart and lungs are perfectly free from organic disease, recovery is possible; if they are the seat of such organic disease as tends to engender bronchial spasm, and as is in the given case the actual cause of the asthma, recovery is *impossible.* The cause is incurable, and therefore its consequence.

II. *Circumstances in Past History.*—A very important one of these is the *length of the attacks.* I have just now stated that one of the ways in which repeated attacks of asthma damage the lungs is by the production of permanent pulmonary congestion. At each attack, the shutting-off of air by the narrowed bronchules suspends the normal respiratory changes of the blood in the capillaries; this produces capillary arrest, and this, engorgement of the whole pulmonary circulation, capillary and venous. Now this pulmonary congestion, as is the case in all derangements of vascular balance, congestive or inflammatory, becomes formidable and intractable in proportion to the length of time that it has existed. If the attack is short, and speedy relaxation of the bronchial tubes quickly re-admits a free supply of air, the vessels are at once relieved, the blood passes on, and the transient congestion leaves no trace behind it. But it is very different if the attacks last several days, or even weeks, as is sometimes the case. Then, the capillaries and venules, long distended, never completely recover themselves, their *tone* is lost, and the pulmonary congestion, manifested by chronic dyspnœa and expectoration, is permanent. This pulmonary congestion, involving as it does the bronchial tubes, and occluding them with mucus, becomes, in its turn, a source of bronchial irritation, and thus tends to excite and keep up the asthma which has caused it. The length of the attacks, therefore, has an important bearing on the prognosis, because it has an important influence in determining the production of that particular damage of the lung which is the commonest way in which asthma becomes hopeless.

The *frequency* of the attacks is another point bearing directly on the prognosis, and for the same reason and in the same manner as their duration. The more frequent they are the worse the omen. If the intervals are so short that the lungs have not time completely to recover from one attack before the occurrence of another, the omen is very bad, because the mischief of each attack being engrafted on some portion of that of its predecessor, the organic derangement is accumulative, and the case one of progressive disorganization.

Another point that should be carefully ascertained is the *completeness of the recovery* between the attacks. I always ask a patient, "Is your breathing in the intervals of the attacks perfectly free from any shortness or difficulty whatever?" If he says "Yes," then I know that his attacks leave no permanent vestige on his pulmonary circulation, that it recovers itself absolutely, and that the disorganizing tendency of asthma does not, in this case, furnish any ground for alarm. But if he says "No," I am sure that the mischief which the attacks inflict persists, I confidently expect to find other evidence of organic disease, and I form an unfavourable prognosis.

Especially do I draw an unfavourable inference from the *persistence of expectoration*. Spitting is one of the worst signs in asthma. In fact, what is called "humid asthma," is neither more nor less than asthma complicated with bronchial inflammation or congestion.[1] Wherever there is chronic expectoration, we may be sure that the lining membrane of the air-passages is the seat of organic change. Indeed, the mucous exudation is a positive evidence of, and in its quantity a measure of, that loaded condition of the bronchial vessels which it is its purpose to relieve. A certain amount of expectoration after each attack, of a thick gelatinous mucus, like pellets of very thick arrowroot, is common, almost universal, especially in the morning succeeding the attack (indeed the most transient fits of asthma, lasting only a few minutes, are generally followed by the expectoration of a pellet or two of this mucus, with whose discharge the little attack appears to terminate), and from such an expectoration, if it lasts only a few hours, or even days, no harm is to be inferred; it is when it never completely ceases that it becomes ominous. Wherever there is mucous exudation there is cough; *chronic cough*, therefore, is a very bad sign in asthma, and tells just the same tale as the expectoration.

There is one prognostic sign, common to all disease, and which should not be disregarded in asthma; it is, the *direction* that the disease appears to be taking. Is it becoming more, or less, intense? Are the attacks becoming more severe and more frequent, or milder and more distant? One often derives from this source a most valuable indication of what the upshot of the case will be. The loss and the acquisition of the asthmatic tendency is generally a gradual process, and the future of a case often but a reflection of its past history. If a patient can tell you that his attacks have mitigated in severity, and are getting less frequent, you have, especially if he is young, one of the most hopeful auguries of his ultimate recovery. Such a case would probably get well of itself without any medical interference. If, on the other hand, the disease is *gaining* on him, you have what must be considered a very bad sign, and one which, unless some speedy and great change is induced by some of those means which control asthma, will leave but very little hope.

There is yet one more circumstance, to which I have not yet referred, that will very materially affect our prognosis; it is, our ability or not to *detect the exciting cause* of the attacks, and the controllability of that exciting cause. If the exciting cause is clear, single, and such as may be prevented, nothing is simpler than the treatment of the disease, or more certain than a favourable prognosis. We

---

[1] By an unfortunate looseness of nomenclature the term "humid asthma" was formerly, and is even now, applied to cases of simple chronic bronchitis that have nothing specially asthmatic about them.

hold in our hands, as it were, the key of the disease, and by shutting off the exciting cause we may indefinitely postpone a repetition of the attacks. If the attacks never occur but as the consequence of this exciting cause, and its recurrence is permanently prevented, this preventive treatment amounts to an absolute and final cure. If, for instance, which is not uncommon, there is some particular locality where the asthma is sure to come on, and in no other, we have simply to say, " Avoid that place and you are cured." Or if, which is much commoner, there is one place, and only one, where the patient never has any attacks, we may say, with almost equal certainty, " Stick to that place and you have seen the last of your asthma." Or if, again, the asthma never comes on but as the result of some error of diet—eating something known to disagree, or eating largely and late in the day—the patient's cure is certain if he will only keep himself within strict dietetic rules, and he may safely and positively be told so. If, on the other hand, the exciting cause is not to be detected, or, being detected, not to be prevented, the omen is bad : for, in the one case we are debarred from adopting any preventive treatment, or in any that we may try we are hitting in the dark ; and, in the other, the prevention of the attacks is manifestly impossible.

If, then, an asthmatic were to present himself to me and seek my opinion as to his prospects, I should, having ascertained his age, and carefully scrutinized the condition of his chest, put to him the following questions: How long do your attacks last ? How often do they occur ? Do you lose all traces of shortness or difficulty of breathing between the attacks; or is the breathing always a little difficult ? Do you habitually cough and spit ? Does the disease appear gaining on you, or the reverse ? Is the exciting cause of the attacks clear; and can you undertake that it shall not recur ?

If the patient is young, the chest sound, the attacks short, the intervals long; if there is no permanent shortness of breath, no cough or expectoration ; if the attacks are getting milder or rarer, and if the exciting cause is clear and such as may be obviated, then a favourable prognosis may be given.

If the patient is old, the lungs damaged, the attacks frequent and severe, the breathing never quite free, coughing and spitting constant, the disease apparently gaining ground, and the exciting cause occult or irremediable, then, *quoqd* all or any of these circumstances, there is no alternative but to give an unfavourable prognosis.

APPENDIX.

A.

NARRATIVE CASES.

SCATTERED throughout this work are the partial histories of a large number of cases, scarcely under a hundred. But they are all partial, some of them fragmentary, some so short that they cannot be called "cases" at all. Indeed I have as a rule purposely confined myself, in the text of the chapters, to those points in cases I might be quoting which were illustrative of the subject under discussion, partly for brevity's sake, partly that the attention might not be diverted from the point I wish to enforce by the narration of irrelevant detail.

But I am anxious that this purposed brevity should not preclude my giving the reader, as far as it can be given in writing, a faithful picture of asthma as it actually occurs. With this view I have related in full, in the following pages, the history of eleven selected cases. I have chosen them from a large number, on account of their diversity, their varied interest, and their instructiveness. They will be found to illustrate almost all the points in the clinical history of asthma, and many in its therapeutics, to which I have directed attention in the preceding chapters, and I would especially commend them to the reader's careful perusal. Let any one who wants to get a living and faithful picture of a disease, read cases. It is vain to attempt, by linking together pathological phenomena in a general description, to convey that simple and life-like impression which every case observed or well told conveys. There is the same difference between an actual case of a disease and a general description of it, however faithful and careful, that there is between a real human face and a Greek ideal; the ideal may be complete and faultless, but there is a want of that rugged force and those self-consistent irregularities and imperfections that add so much to the general effect, and that stamp on the whole thing an individuality not to be forgotten; and there is no *life*. So is it with disease: and I frankly admit that in Chapters III. and IV., where I have endeavoured to give as forcible and close a portraiture of nature as I could, I have utterly fallen short of (what I must necessarily fall short of) that living picture of the disease which the reader will find in the following cases.

In all those instances in which these cases have been communicated to me in the first person, I have preserved that form, as being more animated, and as giving the very words of the narrator.

CASE I.

HAY ASTHMA.

First manifestation in childhood.—Progressive development in advancing life.—Annual progressive development of symptoms as the season advances.—A day at the worst season.—Symptoms.—Hints for management of cases, &c.

Before entering upon the details of my symptoms, I should premise that I rejoice in exceedingly good general health, far above the average of people, and that I am a member of a large family, all of whom enjoy a singular immunity from constitutional disease; the only exception, which perhaps may be mentioned, being a slight tendency to asthma in two other of us, especially in the æstival form, and an unusual amount of irritability of the mucous membrane of the nose, leading to continuous paroxysms of sneezing when once a sneeze occurs, this peculiarity having affected in a marked degree both my father and grandfather. I should add that at the present time I am thirty-four years of age, and, as is pretty generally the case with those who suffer as I do, am of fairish complexion, with thin delicate integument, and of a mobile nervous temperament.

I well remember the first attack of those symptoms which, now more developed and regular in their appearance, I recognize as my annual "hay-fever" torment. I was a little boy, eight years old; it was in the month of June, and I was one of a hay-making party. I was at the play-work of hay-making with my young companions, surrounded by new-mown grass, when I was suddenly seized with all the eye and nose symptoms of hay-fever—profuse lachrymation, swelling of the conjunctivæ and lids, with intense ecchymosis, well-nigh blinding me, and ceaseless sneezing. I recollect that I was taken into the house by my elder companions, and speedily recovered.

It was, however, about the fifteenth year of my age, before I was conscious of my annual infirmity—before I understood that at every early summer I was liable to sneezing fits if I ventured into the country; but from that time till the present this tendency has been abiding, has manifested itself every year, and has always governed my habits and residence during the month of June, and part of May and July. I have said I was eight years of age when I first suffered from hay-fever symptoms; I was fifteen before they became established as an annual recurrence; the liability was obviously intensifying as I advanced in life. I had not, however, then become liable to one of the most distressing elements of the complaint—asthma; for I think I must have been full twenty years of age before that symptom was one of those which combine to constitute this singular complaint when fully developed. In my case, the malady was not established in all particulars and to its full force till about my twenty-fourth year: since then it has remained pretty much *in statu quo*.

I am now usually first attacked by sneezing and lachrymation about the middle of May, though this is much determined by the nature of the season; the warmer the weather, and the more advanced the vegetation, the earlier does my malady show itself. It usually lasts till the end of the first week in July (when it leaves me very suddenly), though this also is determined by the rapidity and shortness of the hay-making season; for in a hot dry season, in which the hay is rapidly made and carried, my immunity from trouble occurs a week or ten days earlier.

As in my youth, sneezing and lachrymation were the first, and for a long time the only symptoms, so every summer do the same phenomena first show themselves. The asthmatic element only appears when the causes of the complaint are in fullest operation, namely, towards the end of June. Thus it appears that the malady increased with my age from a greater predisposed tendency within myself, while it increases as each season advances by the greater development of the exciting (extraneous) cause.

Perhaps the best idea of my case would be gleaned from a faithful account of the manner in which I pass the twenty-four hours in any day towards the end of any June. There is an unhappy sameness in my condition every day about this time. As to my lesser ailment earlier in the month and in May, lop off the asthmatic element, and reduce the other symptoms in degree, and the same description will do.

Say it is the twentieth of June, the weather, as it usually is then, warm and bright. I get up at nine o'clock, weary with a short night, feverish and irritable, and with this I am headachy, and without appetite from the tobacco smoking to which my asthma has compelled me the night before. The bright light of the morning, and the irritation of my razor on my upper lip, which is then almost ticklishly sensitive, are enough to start off the sneezing, which, when once established, goes on in a long paroxysm. I always try to stave off these first morning sneezings; one sneeze starts a paroxysm, and one paroxysm starts another, and so on throughout the day, and any effort to prevent this at first is worth any sacrifice of time and trouble. The way I prevent, or endeavour to prevent, the sneezing is this: directly I find it coming on I seize my pocket handkerchief and continuously blow my nose, inspiring wholly by the mouth, and pinching the nostril while I do so: added to this I close my eyes, or seek a dark place, and then in a few minutes the tingling and irritation of the nose pass away, and *that* paroxysm of sneezing is frustrated.

The sneezing and the fight against it are the continuous and constantly recurring trouble of the day. If the sneezing gets once established, then the lachrymation and inflammation of the conjunctivæ speedily follow; and added to this, intense irritation of the fauces and soft palate, the latter being principally on the posterior or nasal surface; indeed it often seems on bad days as if the back of the soft palate had been sprinkled with cayenne pepper—the itching is terrible. As the day advances the conjunctival symptoms become more marked, and frequently by three or four in the afternoon (having to employ my eyes all day), the conjunctivæ become so œdematous, especially from the cornea to the inner canthus, that the eyes can be scarcely closed, and this is only relieved by complete rest in a perfectly dark room. As evening comes on and the light fades, and one's nervous system becomes less irritable (as it always does with the advancing day), the general symptoms become greatly palliated. But then the asthma gives warning of its approach by the first slight sense of thoracic constriction, and that curious, never-failing, subjective symptom, *itching of the chin*, which all asthmatics so well know as the accompaniment and forerunner of their sufferings. All these symptoms increase as the evening goes on, at the season I am now referring to—the end of June—and would be very distressing were it not that I am able to palliate, and always do palliate, them by smoking cigars. This cigar-smoking is an immense comfort; it does not prevent the asthma coming on in the night, in the worst season, but it mitigates the present tendency, and enables me to get to sleep, smoking as I do a cigar the very last thing, and often after I am in bed.

But asthma at night is *the great* trouble of the victim of hay-fever, and it is mine. By the aid of my cigar I get through the night pretty well early in the season, but by the middle of June I seldom pass beyond four o'clock, often three, before I am awoke by a sense of suffocation, and then, wretchedly sleepy from continuous broken nights, oppressed with asthma, unable to lie down, uncomfortable from having smoked on the previous night, I am condemned to a still stronger dose of the poison to enable me to get relief. For a few breaths I can breathe easier by taking one long deep inspiration; it seems to burst open the contracted bronchial tubes, but they soon contract again, and re-set themselves at a diminished calibre. Another thing gives temporary ease—coughing and expectorating the little clear pellets of stiff mucus that constantly form in this state : after the cough and spitting some half-dozen respirations are tolerably easy, but the ease is transient. What *does*, however, give me real and continued aid in this nocturnal distress, is smoking strong tobacco in a pipe until I am approaching a condition of collapse—a failing pulse and a damp sweating skin are always accompanied by marked alleviation of the sufferings, the relaxation of the contractile tendency affecting the bronchial as well as the other organic muscles. Time, too, comes to my aid, for under any circumstances this asthma vanishes by about seven in the morning, and a refreshing sleep follows, unfortunately but too short, on account of my daily occupations, which soon recall me to their performance, weary and worn out as on the previous morning.

The amount of asthma I have at night very much depends on the sort of day I have had previously, and how I have conducted myself gastronomically. As one sneeze begets a paroxysm, and as one paroxysm begets others, so does a sneezy day beget a night of asthma. The excitement of the sneezing act seems to render the bronchial muscles peculiarly irritable, and liable to take on spasm; the same is the case with violent laughing; indeed, much laughing, especially just after dinner, will often bring on asthmatic spasm at once. A quiet day without much sneezing (when that rare luxury *does* occur), is often followed, even at the bad season, by an almost unasthmatic night. One's stomach has a good deal to do, as well, with the amount of asthma— more than would, *à priori*, be expected. A late unwholesome meal—a late dinner with beer or port wine (two terribly asthma producing beverages), always augments one's trouble. A moderate *fish dinner*, enough for nourishment, with brandy and water, very weak, makes for me the best meal in the bad season, and it should be taken not later than five o'clock, and nothing solid after. When I recommend brandy and water, I do it as a help to digestion and a supporting stimulant, and I think, moreover, that its relation to asthma is not altogether negative. Alcohol, free from the matters which are associated with it in beer and wine, if properly diluted, does more good than harm in my case, even when the spasm is on me.

These rather discursive remarks have applied to my condition as I am now annually in London. The country I never face in the grass-flowering season, and have not for years. I have long ago determined for myself beyond all dispute, that this—the grass-flowering—is the cause of the malady. We Londoners are, however, situated in the valley of the Thames, the largest hay-field in the world, and though removed somewhat from the close proximity of the immediate cause, still we, if hay-asthmatics, get enough of it to bother us sadly. But when the hay around the metropolis is carried, the unspeakable relief—the consciousness that one *can* breathe, *can* sleep, *can* go to the country if one wishes, without the miserable torture of the previous weeks—is almost worth the past suffering. But the recurrence of the season brings it all over again inevitably—it never misses.

I find I have omitted one or two little matters in the narrative of my case, which I must now put in at the end, though perhaps rather out of place. The itching of the chin, which I have mentioned, is purely subjective; scratching gives no relief; for the time being it may mask the underlying sensation, but leave off the scratching and there is the itching still. When the influence is strong upon me, the whole skin of the body becomes irritable, especially down the middle of the back; there is a tendency, too, to the development of urticaria-like wheals, more particularly about the forehead and lower lip, upon rubbing the surface; scratching seems to bring them up rapidly, almost like erectile tissue. I never have them at other seasons. It is a great point, too, to keep the skin warm: it is very susceptible at this time of change of temperature; and sudden cold (there are many cold windy days in June) will start off sneezing, which nothing can resist. A warm, slightly perspiring skin is most salutary. The cloudy, cold, blowy days that are very common about hay-making time are the very worst.

As to medicine, I can say but little. The only one I ever tried was *arsenite of potass*, in the usual solution and in ordinary doses. I took it three years ago, at the suggestion of my friend, Dr. Martin of Rochester, who had found it of marked benefit among his own patients, one of whom herself told me that she takes it annually with the greatest advantage. I took it for a month; it seemed certainly to reduce the severity of the symptoms, but nothing more, and it acted as a general tonic; at last it upset my stomach and bowels, and I gave it up. I have never since tried it.

Of course I have met with many sympathizers and fellow-sufferers—for hay-fever is really a very common complaint, increasingly so, I think—and many remedies have been suggested to me. I will only mention three, because they are the only ones respecting which I have reliable evidence.

A country gentleman in Kent, an old and very intelligent man, tells me that he has had hay-fever all his life; he cures, or all but cures himself, every year with *hydrocyanic acid*. When the season is sufficiently advanced for the complaint seriously to bother him, he shuts himself up in a darkened room for a couple of days, and liberally doses himself with his drug, taking as large doses as are safe. It quite cures him for the time, and renders him far less liable to the malady for the rest of the season. Perfect dependence can be placed on this statement, I am sure, and it would be worth while to try the plan with those who can afford (which I cannot) the sacrifice of a couple of days.

The continued use of *strychnine* during the afflicting season is almost an absolute cure with many persons. I have a lady friend who takes it every year, and while she does so has perfect immunity from the malady; but it is a fearful remedy, and once nearly cost my friend her life.

A cruise in a yacht is an absolute specific, because it removes the sufferer from the cause of his suffering. I know of many noblemen and gentlemen of wealth who are afflicted with hay-fever, and who take to their yachts every early summer, and remain afloat till the hay is all carried. They thus escape the complaint altogether. Unfortunately I cannot afford the money or the time to do this myself; but if even at the worst season I happen to be near the sea, I take a day's boating, and am well all the time. I can, moreover, walk with perfect immunity on Ryde pier, when I could not go a quarter of a mile on the other side of the town without being at once *hors de combat.*

One point more. The grass or grasses that are most obnoxious are meadow grasses, such as *Holcus, Anthoxanthum, Alopecurus, Phleum, &c.;* whereas the grasses that grow on heaths and sandy places (*Agrostis, Aira, Festuca, &c.*) are less potent. On walking over such places as Ascot-heath, the New Forest, Poole-heath—regions of the "Bagshot-sand" formation, inimical to the growth of meadow and pasture grasses—I suffer nothing comparatively. I expect that another day we shall discover what are the offending grasses, and I suspect also we shall find that they are some species that have increased of late years, both in proportion to other grasses and in area of distribution; if so, that will explain the more general and more severe development of hay-fever which appears to have recently occurred. One curious fact as to grass species is this, that they are strictly European, for hay-asthmatics who are very bad in Europe, never suffer at the Cape or in India.

CASE II.

Dating from measles.—Partial cure in Egypt; complete at Jerusalem; Jaffa invariably prejudicial.—Local influences in England and Scotland, and in different parts of London.—Provocatives and remedies.—Inhalation of oxygen.—Interesting family history.

I am a native of Aberdeen, a town from its position much exposed to cold east winds and sea fogs.

The first attack of an asthmatic character that I can remember having experienced, was when I was recovering from measles, at the age of eight or nine years. This attack was speedily relieved by the application of a mustard poultice to the chest.

I can remember having occasional fits of dyspnœa at night from this time till the period when, on commencing the study of medicine, I recognized them to be asthmatic. At that time I believed them to be the consequence of catching cold, but since I studied the malady, I frequently could not account for them in this way. Sometimes their origin seemed purely nervous, from mental causes and the like, sometimes arising from indigestion, and sometimes from unknown atmospheric or terrestrial causes connected with particular seasons or localities.

In the year 1852, I went to reside in Alexandria, Egypt, which is in several respects a locality which could scarcely be recommended as a residence for an asthmatic patient, having the sea nearly surrounding it, while the great brackish Lake Mareotis, for several months in the year little else than a salt marsh, is not far distant. The climate is not excessively warm, the common summer temperature being 83 degrees, but the air is frequently loaded with moisture, especially in autumn, giving rise to heavy dews as soon as the sun sets. In winter and spring, heavy rains fall, and there are cold winds, felt all the more that few houses have fireplaces. In the course of my practice I had daily to be in the harbour, sometimes in rough weather. I was frequently out at night when my clothing and hair were saturated with the heavy dews; yet during the three years I resided there I very seldom indeed had an attack, never a severe one, though other persons who had never suffered in England, were severely affected in the winter season.

I may here mention an anecdote illustrative of the nature of the complaint, and the causes which may produce an attack.

On one occasion I had to spend the night in the house of a patient, a house having a very bad repute on account of the severe remittent fevers which had attacked successive inhabitants of it, under an attack of which my patient was labouring. In the course of the night I lay down for an hour or two in another room, and was there attacked by asthma. I found that a gentleman who resided in the house suffered from asthma when he slept in that room, but in no other in the house. In my case, of course, want of rest and anxiety may have contributed to bringing on the attack.

In November, 1855, after a short visit to Scotland, where I again suffered slightly, I went to reside at Jerusalem. In crossing the Continent on my way thither I had an attack at Basle, and a very severe one at Lucerne. On both occasions the hotel I slept in was close to the water. At Fluelen, at the other end of the Lake of Lucerne, I did not suffer, nor in crossing the Alps by the Pass of St. Gothard, though I performed the journey from Fluelen to Milan without stopping, occupying about twenty-eight hours, almost entirely by *diligence*.

The climate of Jerusalem is in many respects very different from that of Alexandria. The city is placed at an elevation of 2300 feet above the sea, but though well situated for drainage, is exceedingly filthy; and to this cause I am disposed to attribute the great prevalence of ague and fevers of a remittent type. The climate is, on the whole, dry; but in winter there are generally heavy rains and occasionally snow, as occurred during the winter I spent there. Affections of the lungs are very common in winter, and I had a patient, a Jewish Rabbi—originally, I believe, from the Crimea —who had severe attacks of asthma. In Jerusalem I was considerably exposed on several occasions—at one time having been caught in one of the heavy showers of winter, and as thoroughly drenched as if I had been dragged through a river; on another occasion, having to travel for fourteen hours continuously on horseback, on a very cold Christmas eve, and moreover, having a good deal of anxiety during the whole time of my residence in the country. From the peculiar construction of the houses there I was also exposed to sudden changes of temperature in passing at night through the open air from my sitting-room to my bed-room. I remained in Jerusalem from the end of November to the end of May, with the exception of the month of April, and during that time was perfectly free from asthmatic attacks.

The month of April I spent at Jaffa, and here I suffered almost nightly. I should observe also that, during two nights I had previously spent there on my arrival in the country, I suffered from these attacks.

Jaffa lies on the sea-coast, and the house I resided in was outside the town, in the midst of a luxuriant orchard of orange and lemon trees, which were flowering at the time, and it is possible that their powerful fragrance, and the dampness arising from the profuse watering they undergo, may have had something to do with my attacks. On my return to Jerusalem my asthma at once disappeared.

I left Palestine in the end of May, again suffering slightly on passing through Jaffa. On my way home I spent some days in Alexandria, and a fortnight in Malta, in neither of which had I any attack, though in the latter my sleeping apartment was in a very confined situation. My next attacks occurred in Aberdeen, one of them being the most severe I had yet experienced. I then went to reside in Yorkshire, where I remained for nine months, in an elevated bracing locality, where I tried some of the appliances of the so-called "Water-cure." Of these and other remedies I shall afterwards speak. During my residence in Yorkshire I had occasion to pass through Lancaster twice, and both times, in the same hotel, had severe attacks.

In July, 1857, I came up to London. The first night I spent at an hotel in the Strand, where I was quite well. I then had lodgings in Hemingford-terrace, Barnsbury, where I was attacked almost nightly; but on removing to Percy-circus, Pentonville, I found myself quite well, and continued so for a month, when I again visited Aberdeen, where I had several slight attacks. On my return to London I resided in Brompton for about six weeks in October and November, and there also suffered occasionally. I then removed to my present residence in Cannonbury, where, with the exception of an attack produced by accidentally inhaling a little chlorine, I have remained for nine months, almost altogether free from my old enemy.

With regard to the causes of the attacks, I have found them to follow a heavy meal; certain dishes, such as plum-puddings; certain beverages, as bitter ale, especially Bass; some kinds of wines, and whiskey; and I have found port wine relieve an impending attack apparently brought on by whiskey punch: Brandy and gin do not act like whiskey, nor does sherry relieve as port does. Mental anxiety or irritation has also been a cause. Exposure to cold when heated, as in getting out of bed in a cold night, I have found a frequent cause. During the attack, the feet and surface generally are cold, but not invariably so; the pulse is small, weak, and slow; the face pale and anxious, the pupils contracted. Inspiration is short, and expiration greatly prolonged and laborious, and accompanied by sonorous râles. The attack ceases on the expectoration of pellets, and what seem to be casts of the air tubes, composed of a rather tough, gelatinous, transparent grayish substance; and most frequently also there is profuse perspiration. Considerable debility is felt after a severe attack.

As to remedies, I have found nothing so efficacious as a very strong hot infusion of coffee, and this with me has never lost its effect, though I have for years been in the habit of drinking coffee at breakfast. When taken during an attack, it gives almost immediate relief, followed by deep sleep and profuse perspiration. I have occasionally found relief from the common prescription of morphia and ether. The inhalation of the fumes of nitre I have also found of service, and on the theory that it is the oxygen evolved which is the active agent in this remedy, I have tried the inhalation of the fumes of chlorate of potass in the same manner, and this in one most severe attack gave instantaneous relief, at a moment when I feared I should be unable to draw another breath. I have also tried with considerable benefit, both in my own and other cases, the inhalations of diluted oxygen gas.

I spoke of the water-cure. On one occasion, when well, I had myself put in a "pack," but this at once brought on an attack. I have found, however, that a gentle douche applied to the spine and the chest has warded off impending attacks, being followed by an expectoration of the substance above described. The habitual use of cold bathing, summer and winter, has, I am convinced, a good deal to do with my present immunity from attacks. There is another remedy little known in this country, and here, unfortunately, associated with hydropathy, which I believe to be well deserving of investigation, I mean, the compressed air-bath of M. Taburié. On this subject I would refer to the works of Bertin and Pravar, where very striking cases are recorded. I have seen something of this remedy, and am inclined to think very favourably of it. With regard to depressing remedies, such as tobacco (stramonium I have never tried), I have found them in my case generally do more harm than good. On one occasion I nearly poisoned myself smoking tobacco, and without any relief to the asthmatic attack. Much I think depends on the character of the attack, whether the nervous system is in a depressed or an excited state. On one occasion when in Egypt, I tasted a little whiskey after dinner. This at once brought on dyspnœa. As pipes were being handed round, as is customary there, I took one, though no smoker, and smoked a little of the mild tobacco used there. The relief was immediate, but I felt very giddy and faint, and had considerable nausea. In other instances where the cause of the attack seemed to be a depressing one, tobacco has been useless. Mustard poultices to the chest I have found a very useful adjunct to other treatment. They seem to act not only locally, but generally, and increase the tendency to perspiration produced by other remedies. I remember one attack, a good many years since, apparently induced by immoderate laughter, which disappeared after ten or twelve hours with the usual expectorations, in consequence of the effort of climbing up a steep highland road.

I have found quinine very serviceable in the debility consequent on the attacks.

One remaining point of interest I would mention in connection with my case. The medical history of my family seems to indicate a morbid sensibility of the nervous system. My great-grandfather on the mother's side, and my aunt on the father's side, had asthma. One of my brothers suffers from it. My father suffered for many years from general neuralgia, ending in paralysis. One of my brothers when a young man had attacks of spasmodic dysphagia or spasm of the pharynx, another has had epileptic fits, and several of the family have had sleep-walking.

<hr>

CASE III.

Disease congenital.—Change of type.—Cure by London air.—Effect of position.—Coffee.—Prolonged exercise.—Mental emotion as a cure.—Clothing at night.—Food and sleep.—Medicinal remedies.

E— D—, æt. twenty-six, a physician, slightly under the middle height, rather spare, rather pale, and a little stooping. Has resided (1) at Kirby Moorside, a richly cultivated wooded valley; (2) Whitby, a bleak and rocky seaboard; (3) London; (4) Oxford; and (5) London again. His first asthmatic symptoms appeared when he was a month old, and must therefore be assigned to a congenital proclivity to the disease. His first attack at this early age was characterized by great difficulty of breathing, wheezing, and no cough. It was soon succeeded by others, and he became a confirmed asthmatic. Throughout his infancy and childhood the paroxysms occurred about once a month; in these there was seldom any fever, but the lips were livid, the chest distended, and the pulse quick and weak. The disease was probably inherited, as his grandfather was bowed down with asthma for many years before his death; there appears, however, to be no other history of asthma in his family. The attacks have occurred of late years with no regularity whatever; he has gone as long as two years on two occasions without an asthmatic symptom, except on occasion of change of place, which always brings the attacks on. The time of their occurrence is *always three o'clock in the morning*, and their provocatives, in by far the greatest number of cases, atmospheric; sometimes they have been brought on by exposure to cold, and sometimes by other causes, as, for example, by a *fit of laughing;* they are generally preceded by no premonitory symptoms, unless perhaps a feeling of unusual security. The only pathological associations of the paroxysms are *neuralgia* and *paroxysmal sternutation.*

The following is an account with which this patient has furnished me :—

" Looking back over the six-and-twenty years during which I have lived and been asthmatic, I see that the asthma has in some degree changed its character. In my childhood it came in fits, in violent abrupt paroxysms which began suddenly, lasted two nights and two days, and ceased in the sound sleep of the third night; then I was well, could take violent exercise, and join in the out-door sports of other boys, until another brief abrupt fit laid me up. For ten years I have scarcely had one of these well-defined fits, except as a welcome to a new or unfavourable place during the first days of my stay there. I have been constantly liable instead (during the uniform course of life in one place) to be for many nights (on two occasions, for many weeks) unable to lie flat in bed. This has not generally interfered much with my comfort or activity of mind or body during the day, but my ordinary breathing is not what it used to be in the intervals of the early severe attacks. I have not the capacity for exertion or violent exercise; and any little thing, such as a meal, or laughing, sets me wheezing.

" All my earlier attacks came on, as far as I can remember, about three o'clock in the morning. They began invariably with cough, as well as difficulty of breathing. I never awoke at once, but remained in a troubled half-sleep, fancying the sound of my own cough to be some other noise, and the effort of coughing to be some other struggle. These fancies were very distressing. One of the most painful was an anxious doubt whether I was really myself. Up to my eighteenth year I never got up on account of the fit; I sat up during the day, and went to bed at night. My father was a physician, and for that reason I had no idea of following what I *felt* to be best, but of doing what was ordered me. I remember when I was a child, when I had passed the evening comfortably propped up on a sofa, how I dreaded to be taken off to bed, and sometimes feigned sleep that they might leave me a little longer in quiet. The attacks generally lasted two days and two nights, and went off during the third night. I could generally tell whether I should be able to rest in bed or not when I had an attack already. I could seldom or never predict an attack.

" The first change in my malady was *when I went to London* in my nineteenth year. *For two years I remained perfectly free from asthma.* I lived for a year and a-half in Bloomsbury-square, and afterwards near Eaton-square. Soon after I went to London I had an attack of bronchitis, preceded by extreme sensitiveness to bad air or dust, but neither before nor during this attack had I the slightest symptom of asthma. The bronchitis was not extensive, it produced little difficulty of breathing, and that little of quite a different kind from the asthmatic.

" *Effect of position.*—Often when I have been lying flat in bed, with my head on the pillow, breathing hard, and coughing frequently, I have drawn myself further up in bed, put my arm across the pillow, and rested my head on my hand; the coughing has ceased, the breathing has become gradually better, I have slept and waked well. The pillow supports the chest, and the sensation of its pressure on the ribs is wonderfully comforting. The elbow is fixed between the pillow and the head of the bed. This is a constrained position, and I am obliged to change from the left arm to the right at least every hour now, when I am accustomed to it, and I used to need change much more frequently. But very often the effect of this position is so speedy and great that I slip down unconsciously into the natural sleeping posture before I have needed change once, and do not awake till morning. The head rests most comfortably when the hand is laid flat against the ear, with a silk handkerchief between.

"*Effect of coffee.*—I used to think strong coffee the best of all remedies. I remember one instance especially, only a pattern of many others, but more striking when told. With bent back, high shoulders, and elbows fixed on the chair-arms, I had been labouring for breath all the afternoon. About five o'clock I had two large breakfast-cups of strong coffee. The hard breathing disappeared rapidly and completely. My sisters were dancing in the next room, and in less than an hour I was dancing with them, quite free from asthma.

"Of late, coffee has often had an opposite effect upon me. The after-dinner cup of coffee to which I have been for several years habituated now produces a sensation of stuffing of the chest and incapacity of moving about. I believe this is because it stops digestion; and the reason I did not suffer from it for some years, I take to be, that my originally most excellent and enduring stomach could stand it so long and no longer. Coffee on an empty stomach I still deem a most valuable remedy. I do not share the prejudice against putting milk and sugar into coffee that is used as a medicine, provided that it remains *café noir*, and be not made *café au lait*.

"*Prolonged exercise.*—Of all remedies there is none for me so complete and lasting as a day of severe walking exercise—five-and-twenty miles over hilly ground or across heaths. The strain must never be great. I begin slowly, almost saunteringly, and only increase my pace when it is pleasanter to do so than not. Towards the end of my day I can usually climb a hundred feet of cliff as fast as I can plant my feet, or run a mile or two to catch a train. Habitually I can never run or go fast up hill. In this matter of exercise, it is of paramount importance not to overstrain. If I am 'winded' against a hill, and stop at the top till I breathe freely, I can get up the next hill more easily, and so on. But if, when the hill was surmounted, I kept right on, I should get up the next hill worse, and so on.

"Rowing is bad, because the temptation to over-exertion is too great, and riding is most excellent, because exertion is sure, and over-exertion next to impossible.

"*Mental emotion as a cure.*—On one occasion I was sitting with fixed elbows on a sofa, breathing hard; a lady came into the room whom I had known very well, and whom I had not seen for several years. I got up to receive her, and sat down again on a music-stool with no especial purchase therefore for the respiratory muscles, and yet with comparative ease of breathing. This ease lasted for about an hour, and then the difficulty of breathing came on again. I attribute the temporary amendment to the diversion of nervous energy. Just the same thing has happened to me more than once.

"On one occasion I was suffering a good deal at an isolated farmhouse. I got on horseback with some difficulty and an anxious hope that the horse would go quietly, to fetch myself an emetic from a town three miles off. The horse ran away with me. I pulled in, at first weakly and almost despairingly; but the need of exertion brought the power. After a run of about a mile I succeeded in pulling up, and was delighted to find my asthma gone.

"Another time I was breathing very hard, and a friend engaged me in an argument. At first I could only get out a sentence in successive gasps; but gradually, as I got excited, the hard breathing went off and I could talk fluently.

"*Clothing at night.*—One thing which I must speak of as a successful measure, or rather as a preventive measure, and which I hold of the greatest importance, is so to envelop the body during sleep that if one is obliged to rear up by asthma, one shall not catch cold from exposure. I know that a cold so caught will not manifest itself by the ordinary running at the nose, but I feel assured that it will often complicate with bronchitis what would otherwise have been mere spasm. What I do is to wear always in bed a double-breasted well-fitting jacket, made to fasten close round the neck, and *pantaloons à pied*, both of flannel, and of such thickness as to afford about the same protection as an ordinary suit. This and walking exercise I consider much the most valuable hints, which my experience enables me to give to asthmatics.

"*Food before sleep.*—Suppers I consider on the whole bad, unless after a long day of much exertion and little food. I fancy I am more likely to rest well in an unfavourable place with a supper than without, *provided I take a nap in a sitting posture before I go to bed;* and I have no doubt the attack which always awaits me in certain places is much worse if I go to bed directly after supper than if I avoid supper or sit up afterwards.

"*Medicinal remedies.*—The attacks are little relieved by anything but emetics—Ipecacuan in Ɔj or Ʒss doses—but most of all by pretty large doses of calomel, which commonly act both as an emetic and a purgative. The emetics are generally followed by a short sleep, and I awake well."

CASE IV.

Sudden production by emotion.—Twenty-four years' asthma in India.—Effect of hay first noticed in this country.—Auscultatory signs.—Treatment.—Prognosis.—Observations.

Mrs. A., a native Hindoostanee lady, forty-four years of age, has had spasmodic asthma for twenty years—*i.e.*, since she was twenty-four, when it came on one night suddenly, when she was in a state of great distress from the sudden loss of her husband. She never had any such attacks before: she has been liable to them ever since. She has been accustomed to attribute this first attack to cold, but it does not seem to have been preceded by any bronchitic symptoms, and the principal reason for her thinking she had cold seems to have been the expectoration that succeeded the attack. The attacks always come on in the evening about nine or ten o'clock; they last that night, the following day, and the next night; the second morning they pass completely off. The first night she gets no sleep at all, and sits up, generally leaning forward on something. Towards morning the expectoration commences, and there is a sensible mitigation of her symptoms, but the dyspnœa continues throughout the day; she, however, gets snatches of sleep in the sitting posture. The second night is much better than the first, and she is able to lie back and get a little sleep; the dyspnœa gradually and insensibly passes off in the morning, and the attack is over. The expectoration continues, however, for a day or two, and indeed may be said never completely to leave; she spits a little every day, and has for years, especially in the morning. When the attack is on her she feels as if a cord bound her heart and a heavy weight rested on her sternum. She cannot bear anything tight round her; but if she attempts to put her dresses on she cannot make them meet by some inches; when the difficulty of breathing goes off she recovers her usual size. The attacks are usually preceded by a drowsiness and lethargy, and chest constriction.

There is no regular interval for these attacks; they are quite irregular, and occur from a fortnight to six months apart. The longest interval she ever had was three years; for that time previous to last October she had no attack: in October she had. Since she has been in this country (three months) she has had two attacks—one in June, the other in July. The attack in the end of June seems undoubtedly to have been brought on by hay, the smell of which is peculiarly oppressive and offensive to her. Once in two months appears the commonest interval.

The principal provocatives of attacks are heat, dust, smoke, certain foods, such as sweets (meat not), beer, a late dinner or a supper. The other day she dined out late, and hardly had any sleep at night. She ordinarily dines at three, and after that takes nothing but a *little* soaked toast in some tea at seven o'clock; but even after dinner at three, she feels, beginning about half an hour after, and lasting till digestion is completed, a certain amount of tightness of breathing, though slight. After a late dinner or supper this is so increased as to constitute an attack. She never feels it after breakfast.

In India she is never so bad in the rainy season; never laid up, only a slight occasional tightness. The hot season is the worst.

Auscultatory signs, such as show that remarkably little injury has been inflicted on the lungs; the configuration of the chest is good, no emaciation, no hyper-resonance; good chest movement, air enters everywhere, producing nearly normal respiratory murmur; no moist sounds; the patient says, however, she is frequently troubled with *râles*. Resp. 16; pulse 84. Respiration deliberate, easy, with good post-expiratory rest.

Until very lately this patient had tried no remedy whatever for her disease, but of late she has been taking, at the instance of a native *savant*, gr. viij of some powder three times a day, and she thinks with a mitigation of her symptoms. What it is I do not know; it does not nauseate or purge.

Treatment.—I have ordered the trial of the nitre-paper, stramonium-smoking, strong ipecacuanha lozenges, and, from the connection of her symptoms with digestion, I have ordered her to take no solid food after three o'clock, but a little soaked toast at six. Cold shower-bath every morning if possible—*i.e.*, if she can bear it.

Prognosis.—From the undamaged condition of the lung, and the three years' interval that she has lately had, I should be inclined to think this a case in which some good may be done, and to make a favourable prognosis.

Observations.—One of the principal points of this case is that the patient is an East Indian, and that the disease, occurring in India and in a native, has all the most characteristic features that it possesses in England—the sensations, the provocatives (dust, candle-smoke, hay-effluvium), all just the same. It is a case I should be rather sanguine of London curing; but the lady finds it inconvenient at present to try London residence.

CASE V.

Cause, whooping-cough at three months old.—Progressive development of the disease.
—Cure by coming to London.—Tendency not destroyed.—Description of an attack.
—Treatment; ipecacuanha, tobacco, emotion.—Freedom from organic mischief.

I am thirty-five years of age, five feet five inches in height, exceedingly
thin, rather high-shouldered, with my head set back, and with a curiously
shaped chest, which I have had ever since my earliest recollection. It is
not ordinary "chicken breast," for the sternum is flat and the upper part
of the chest quite well shaped, but below, on each side, in the situation of
the cartilages of the ribs, it is flattened, and even drawn in; so that below
and to the inside of each nipple is a hollow in which you might almost lay
your hand, the deepest on the left side.

A brother and a sister suffer from asthma. If inherited, the only source
from which it can be derived is from my paternal grandmother.

Up to the age of twenty, I suffered horribly from asthma; at that age I
lost it suddenly and completely from coming to London, and have only had
occasional reminders of it since, and that chiefly from going into the country.

My asthma commenced at the early age of three months from a violent
attack of whooping-cough, which I had so badly, and which left me in such
a suffering and miserable state, that it was long before my parents expected,
and still longer I think before they hoped, that I should live. For the first
ten years of my life my attacks were occasional, at long and irregular intervals; I used to go for months without one. Even at this time, I remember
that they always came on in the early morning, and that they were very
severe. At this time food had no tendency to make me asthmatic. I
could eat a supper and be as well as usual the next day. Moreover, I
remember that my usual breathing was perfect; I never had any asthmatic
sensations except at these distant and severe attacks, never after food, or
after running. The attacks at this early age were frightfully severe, fully
as bad as at any period of my life.

At about ten years old a change took place. The attacks became frequent, regularly periodic, and milder, perhaps I should rather say shorter.
From this age till fifteen, they came on at first about once a month, then
once a fortnight, then once a week, and latterly at this interval with great
regularity, appearing every Monday morning. They awoke me about five
o'clock, and went off about nine; for the rest of the day my breath was a
little short on exertion, and I was disposed for some hours to spit little pellets of a pearly viscid mucus; but I was able to get about and follow my
usual occupations and amusements. I then went on through the accustomed
interval to the next attack, when exactly the same thing was repeated. I
cannot say that during this time my asthma was a source of much *suffering*
to me. I had four or five hours wheezing sitting up in bed once a fortnight,
or once a week; and of that, not above an hour or two was severe dyspnœa;
it always went off spontaneously, never required any remedy. About this
time the tendency of food to produce asthma, and the influence of the stomach over it, first showed itself, and I was obliged to forego suppers.

At fifteen another change took place; the attacks ceased to leave me in the
morning, and continued throughout the day. At first, by absolutely starving myself all day, they would subside spontaneously towards evening; but
soon they showed a disposition to continue on through the night, and it was

found necessary to take an emetic to cut them short. This, however, never failed. Every attack could be curtailed to a single day by this means; and accordingly, an emetic was the windup of every fit. After its operation, feeling very much exhausted by my day's starvation, I used to eat an egg for supper, go to bed, sleep tranquilly all night, and wake perfectly well the next morning. In a year or two I was obliged to give up this little supper after the emetic, as it showed a tendency to re-excite the asthma.

Thus I went on till I was twenty—a weekly attack lasting all day, perfect abstinence till the next morning, and an emetic at night. Sometimes I tried to do without the emetic; the only result was that I had a miserable night and a second day's asthma. Sometimes I ventured to take a little food on the day of my asthma, but I always repented it; it increased my sufferings so dreadfully that I had much better have borne the hunger. I used to endeavour to appease my cravings by sucking stick chocolate, or gelatine lozenges, or such things; but even these poor substitutes for food would often make me worse. If the cause of the asthma was cold (and this undoubtedly will produce it), and the asthma complicated with bronchitis, the emetic would sometimes fail to relieve me, and the asthma would run on that night and the next day. Under these circumstances, the attack has sometimes lasted three and even four days. But these attacks were quite different from the ordinary ones—more stuffing at the chest, more cough, more expectoration; and I do not remember them to have occurred more than two or three times in my life.

The period of my greatest suffering was undoubtedly from my fifteenth to my twentieth year; for not only were the attacks frequent, but the dyspnoea was of a very severe kind, and lasted twelve or fourteen hours at each attack, till the emetic put a stop to it at nightfall. Before I was twenty, however, and before I came to London, the disease showed signs of abatement; it lost its periodicity, the intervals became irregular and longer, so that I would go three or four months without an attack.

On coming to London fifteen years ago, my asthma at once and (I hope) finally left me, with the exception of modified attacks, which generally await me if I go into the country. Ever since I first came to town, I have been like another person. Those things of which I used to be afraid, such as suppers, cold, unwholesome food, excitement, ceased to affect me; in short, I became in every respect a perfectly healthy person. I threw away my pillows and bolsters, and lay quite flat, a thing I had never done before in my life. My appearance was so changed that my friends in the country could hardly persuade themselves I was the same person. My figure greatly improved, my shoulders became less high, my back less round. The asthmatic tendency, however, is clearly not lost, only in abeyance as long as I am in London, for the day I revisit the country that day it returns; even before I am out of the railway carriage I feel it. I feel something different to what I have since my last country visit—a certain tightness and constriction about the chest warns me of what is coming. And this is the same everywhere—north, south, east, and west—I have tried all directions. Some places are certainly worse than others (and those seem the worst whose air would be reckoned by most people the best and purest, such as elevated and bracing situations); but London appears to be the only place where I am really well. Even in London all places do not agree with me equally; if I have taken up my residence in the higher and more open parts of town or have ventured into the outskirts, I have always had little reminders that I am still an asthmatic. The most perfect air for me appears to be somewhere near the banks of the river, in the lowest and most crowded situations. During the last fifteen years, I have on more than one occasion gone as long as eighteen or twenty months without so much as an asthmatic feeling, but that has only been by abstaining from going into the country for that period. On some occasions, however, I have gone into the country with perfect impunity, and been as well there for two or three months as in London. Why, nine times out of ten, my asthma drives me back, and the tenth I am well and able to stay, I cannot even attempt to explain; it seems to me to depend on the inexplicable caprice of the disease.

Let me now endeavour to describe one of my fits as they occurred nearly every week from the age of fifteen to twenty.

I generally knew, the evening before, that I was going to have an attack by an unwonted drowsiness that overpowered me. It was no use trying to resist it; even if I succeeded in keeping myself from quite going to sleep I was so heavy and stupid I could do nothing and understand nothing. It was so conspicuous that others could see, as well as myself, when an attack was coming on. As far as I remember, I had no other premonitory sign, and I do not think my breath was in the least affected when I went to bed. About three o'clock in the morning my sleep was disturbed by a tightness of breathing that rendered it impossible for me to lie any longer. My waking would often be preceded by distressing dreams that I was being smothered or drowned, and a miserable semi-consciousness of the piping wheezing that I was making. But for some time the difficulty of breathing, though enough to prevent my sleep, was not enough to wake me thoroughly up, coming, as it did, in deep, profound mid-sleep. Half knowing what was the matter, half believing my distressing dreams, I would raise myself on my elbow, obtain a trifling relief, sink down again, and again have to raise myself. Then the dyspnœa deepening, I could not lie down at all, but rested, still half asleep, first on one elbow, then on the other, still hearing in my dreams the droning wheeze of a score of constricted broncules all over my chest. By-and-by it reached such a pitch that I was obliged to sit fairly up in bed and make a final struggle against the sleep that overwhelmed me. Soon I could not even stay in bed; with difficulty and by slow stages I would creep out of bed, and, supporting myself by leaning on every piece of furniture I found near, get to a chair and sit down in it, leaning forward on a table on which I had placed a pillow, and there I was fixed for the day. Sometimes my breath was too bad to sit, and I was obliged to stand, leaning against the high sill of a window, supporting all the weight of the upper part of my body on my elbows, and so thrusting my shoulders up to my ears. This I found the easiest position of all. Here I would stand for hours, labouring as it were for my life, looking out into the darkness till the dawn came and grew into day. In this way I have watched hundreds of sunrises, and I fancy am more familiar with early morning atmospheric effects than most people, unfortunately. After standing or sitting in this way for two or three hours, the extremity of the spasm would abate, and I would even get—leaning forward, and laying my arms on my pillow and resting the side of my face upon them—a little tolerably tranquil sleep. In the winter I was greatly embarrassed and my sufferings much increased by having to put on my clothes and light a fire. Sometimes the slightest attempt at dressing was more than I could manage, or even the fatigue and movement of letting others dress me, and I was simply wrapped in blankets till the labouring for my breath had somewhat abated and I could suffer myself to be dressed. It was often hours before this could be done, and then only in slow stages—first, putting one leg into a trowser and then resting, then another rest between the trowsers and waistcoat, and another between the dressing and the washing, and so on. The effort of breathing was such that the perspiration collected in beads on my forehead and trickled down my face, and all my clothes were damp and sticking to me. But while my head and body were so hot, my hands and feet were quite cold and blue; the cold generally extended above my knees, and accompanying it there was a deep aching pain in one or both shin bones from the knee to the inner ankle, sometimes insufferably severe. This, I think, I always had at every attack; even in summer when my legs were not particularly cold; it never went off till evening.

One early symptom of the attack which I have forgotten to mention, was a profuse secretion of urine, limpid and white, like pump-water. So early a symptom was this, that it used to disturb me even before my attack was fully established. I had no cough, the wheezing was perfectly dry, and there was no mucus in the air-tubes, or expectoration till late in the day.

My figure was quite deformed—I was bent double, and my shoulders were so high that I seemed to have no neck. I sat propped up with pillows in an easy-chair, unable sometimes to speak or move, sometimes even not enough to make dumb signs to those about me. An arm-chair, with very high arms, suited me best, because it elevated my shoulders. This was a thing that contributed more to my comfort than anything else; in fact, no position that did not elevate my shoulders could be tolerated. To be saved all trouble of supporting my body, to have my shoulders well raised without my own efforts, and the body thrown forward—these were the three essentials to an easy position. In the evening I took the emetic, and within ten minutes of taking it, as soon as the first sensation of sickness was felt, and before vomiting had taken place, the spasm was gone. The sense of relief on the giving way of the spasm was something beyond expression. The following morning I had a little expectoration, and then all was over till the next fit.

Let me now say a word or two as to *cause*. The original cause of the disease was, undoubtedly, the whooping-cough. The only thing that I had clear evidence acted as the exciting cause of the attack was food—food of certain unwholesome kinds, or overloading the stomach, or eating late in the day; above all, this last. Almost anything may be eaten, and in any quantity, provided it was taken early. But a supper was fatal, and for the last few years of the disease anything solid, taken even at tea-time, at seven o'clock. An early dinner at two o'clock was for years the last meal at which I dare eat; at tea I might *drink* a little, but if I ventured to eat even a scrap of bread and butter I was sure to be awoke the next morning at three or four o'clock with an attack. Certainly, on some occasions cold has given rise to a mongrel attack, half asthma, half bronchitis; but unless it produced bronchial inflammation, I do not think it had any tendency to produce asthma. Those who watched me thought that violent mental excitement tended to bring on an attack the following day. I should mention that sometimes slight fits (not the true periodical morning attacks) would be brought on at any time of the day by laughing, by dust, by hay effluvium, or nursing a cat.

As for *treatment*, two things alone did me any good—strong depressants, and any sudden, violent mental emotion. Of the depressants, the two that acted the most efficiently were ipecacuanha and tobacco.

The ipecacuanha I had been accustomed to take in emetic doses from my earliest childhood. Twenty grains of powder never failed to cure me in a

14

quarter of an hour. It was conceived by those who administered it to me that it acted by relieving the stomach and clearing the air-passages, but this could not have been the case, as the spasm gave way as soon as the sense of nausea was felt, and before any vomiting or expectoration had taken place; moreover, from my day's starvation, my stomach was as empty before the operation of the emetic as after. An emetic was the closing scene of each attack: how long the attack would have lasted had I not taken one I cannot say, but the spasm showed very little inclination to give way till the ipecacuanha began to take effect. I rarely took the emetic before the evening, but I now think that if I had taken it immediately on the asthma awakening me I should have cut short the spasm at once, and saved myself a day's suffering. As I had an attack nearly every week, and took an emetic at each attack, I must have taken about fifty emetics, or a thousand grains of ipecacuanha, every year for several years. From this violent treatment my stomach did not seem to suffer in the least, and at the present day my digestion is perfect.

Tobacco acted just in the same way, and evidently on the same principle, but I found it a still quicker and more potent remedy, and its effects passed off sooner. In these respects it was preferable to ipecacuanha, but it required greater care in its use, for the effects of an over-dose were very distressing, and even alarming. Its efficacy and value to me depended on my never acquiring a tolerance of it; a few whiffs of a pipe, or half a cigar, always brought on the characteristic physiological effects of the drug—faintness, giddiness, cold perspiration, and nausea, and on the supervention of these the asthma instantly vanished; in less than five seconds, I am sure, I passed from the intensest dyspnœa to perfect respiratory ease. It was not necessary that I should vomit, though I often did; my object was to carry the smoking just far enough to induce slight collapse, and no more. When I expected an attack I put a pipe by my bed over night, and the moment the asthma awoke me in the morning, lit it and smoked (and this I found sometimes a very difficult thing, having hardly breath enough to keep the pipe alight), till I felt the first sense of faintness, and then stopped. In this way I cut short the attack at its commencement; and so speedily was it all over, and so perfect the cure, that the treatment was rather preventive than curative.

On several occasions, which I need not minutely describe, violent emotion, —fear, excitement, surprise—has suddenly cured an attack. I fancy any strong mental emotion would have this effect, provided it were something sudden and unexpected.

I am an example of the amount of asthma that may be borne without inflicting any appreciable injury on the lungs; for though I was such a sufferer for twenty years, my respiratory powers are excellent. I find no difficulty in facing a hill or running a mile; my vital capacity, as shown by the spirometer, is fully what my height entitles me to, and I sleep quite low at head; under these circumstances, it is impossible there can be anything organically wrong with either lungs or heart.

If I live the rest of my days in London, there seems no reason that I may not ultimately lose every vestige of my complaint, nor does there seem any reason to think that asthma will have, in such a case as mine, any tendency to shorten life.

CASE VI.

Early history.—Effect of dust and smells.—Cure on going to Newry; relapse on return.—Treatment, dietetic and medicinal.—The three periods:—A, purely spasmodic; B, with brain pressure and fulness of blood; c, spasmodic bronchitis.—Description of a fit.—A year of perfect health in America.—Perfect and final cure by going to Van Diemen's Land.

26, Rue de Lacépède, Paris, June 4, 1858.

I was born in September, 1812. My father, who was between fifty-five and sixty at the time of my birth, was a man of sound and vigorous constitution up to the time of his last illness, which was paralysis. He died between eighty and eighty-two. My mother, who was twenty-six when I was born, was not of robust constitution or appearance, but yet well-formed, active, and healthy enough. In her family were two cases of consumption; she herself died in her sixtieth year, of the Irish famine fever. My paternal grandfather and grandmother both reached the age of eighty-four or upwards, and of their six children none died under seventy-eight. My parents had nine children, one of whom died at nine, and the other at twenty-six, the latter of consumption. The seven others are all living, and, except myself, are well-formed and healthy. Among all the relatives of whom I have spoken there was no other case of asthma but my own.

I have heard my mother say that I was a weakly infant from my birth, and that my head was too large and heavy for my slender neck to support. The asthmatic attacks, she has told me, commenced at least as early as when I was two years old. My earliest recollections about my health are of occasional fits of illness, during which I was carried about in the arms of an attendant, or more frequently *astride on the back*, and dosed with syrup of squills. Up to the age of puberty the method of relief or comfort by carrying me on the back of some person was always employed during the severe fits. Often two servant girls relieved each other the long night through in carrying me about the house, and, if the weather permitted, outside the house. The shoulders of my bearer formed a rest for my head and a clinging-place and fulcrum for my arms, as they laboured, with all the muscles of my trunk, to help the lungs in their agony. The position, too, almost erect, and yet giving external support to my frame, and leaving it no exertion to make beyond its spasmodic straining and tugging in aid of the respiration, was such as always suited me best in the attacks. I never could lie in bed, nor could I bear to be there propped up with pillows; I must get up and sit with my head forwards, my shoulders raised and curving inwards, and my hands rested on my knees, or chairs, or (as already described) the shoulders of a person carrying me. Even when I became a young man, and as tall as I am to-day, in some extremely bad fits the method of relief by placing me on a person's back, to be carried about inside or outside the house, was resorted to.

During my boyhood, up to when I was about twelve years old, I resided almost constantly at my father's house at L——, never having been fifteen miles distant from my birthplace, and hardly ever sleeping anywhere else. The attacks of asthma were, as well as I can recollect, as frequent as one in a fortnight, or even oftener. They lasted sometimes a whole night and day, sometimes longer. It was always at night I was seized, and after I had gone to sleep. I think my mother generally perceived some premonitory symptoms, such as increased colour (I was of a florid complexion) and a certain irritability of manner—a nervous desire to seem quite well, and more boisterous spirits than usual; what my mother called false spirits. She used to dose me (unknown to myself) with calomel concealed in a spoonful of jam, or of sugar, or inside some dainty cake, hoping thereby to prevent or lighten the attack. I think her impression was that the attack was hardly ever arrested when once premonitory symptoms had appeared. But she considered that strict temperance in eating, and care of my digestion, was useful in rendering the attacks less frequent. In the fits the spasmodic tugging for breath was such that it was difficult for me to swallow anything. Syrup of squills was not continued to be given after my childhood. When I was a boy of from eight to twelve years old, bleeding was sometimes resorted to either in the arm or in the foot. I remember perfectly an occasion when a bleeding (in the foot) gave me almost instantaneous and entire relief, in a fit of ordinary severity, and I think there were several occasions when it served me. During that period medicine was hardly ever given to me during the fit. I was merely carried about, nursed tenderly, my head being held as I wished, and my feet rubbed by warm hands, and every device adopted to give ease to my arms and all my body. The window of the room where I was was opened, summer or winter, and the fresh air admitted.

In my attacks, the least dust, or smoke, or smell, affected me grievously. Even in the intervals between the fits I was exceedingly sensitive to dust, smoke, or smells. I could not sleep in a room where there was scented soap, or green branches (with which in such country houses as ours the fireplaces used to be dressed in summer), or even heavy-smelling flowers— the *wall-flower* in particular, and the *violet*. My keen perceptions about dust and smoke must have made me a pest in the house. When I became fond of books (about nine or ten years old), I remarked that turning over the leaves of such as were mouldy, from damp, was a certain cause of a fit, if persisted in for many minutes.

In the intervals my respiration must have been pretty free and sound, for I was a good runner and one of the best players among the boys of our neighbourhood at the game there called *shinnie*, or *commons*, nearly the same called in the centre and south of Ireland *hurling*. During my visits to the house of an uncle, who resided near R——, I used to ascend the mountains there with ease, and I remember perfectly the ecstasy of my enjoyment of the mountain air on the top. Whether the curvature of my spine, which has since become so marked, was congenital, or whether it existed at all till about the age of puberty, I am not sure. It was about my sixteenth year that I first became conscious of it. I suspect there must have been something of it in my early boyhood, for I remember having my chest felt by the doctor, and his calling it *chicken-breast*, when I was about six or seven years old. Except asthma I was subject to no other complaint that I recollect, nor was I smaller or weaker than ordinary boys of my age.

I have said that up to my twelfth year I resided almost constantly at my father's house at L——. Most of the rooms looked north over a lawn of some four or five acres, which sloped down to a lake two and a half to three miles in circumference, with marsh or marshy meadows bordering it for a breadth of many acres on the west. The soil is heavy clay, retentive of moisture, and not artificially drained to any great extent. It lies at an elevation above the sea of between three hundred and seven hundred feet. As to my food, it was generally the rule to treat me more delicately than the other

children. It was remarked that most vegetables disagreed with me, particularly beans, *old* peas, and cabbages. Certain things that I was fond of
were unwholesome to me, perhaps because I was apt to gormandize upon
them. Many very bad attacks during my boyhood followed upon the eating
of *cheese*, particularly *new* cheese; and I remember sometimes vomiting the
cheese during the fit. The climate of Ireland is known to be very humid,
and the heavy clay soil of my native place was generally wet in the winter
and not often dry in the summer. The sun did not shine into either of the
sitting-rooms (as they looked north), and the westerly winds, which are
most prevalent in Ireland, came over the marsh.

I think I was in my twelfth year when I was sent as a boarder to Dr. H.'s
school in Newry. Newry is situated mainly in the narrow valley of a little
river, up which the tide runs from Carlingford Bay to a point above the
town. Dr. H.'s house was situated in a place scarcely rising above high-
water mark; it was three stories high. There were over twenty boarders,
and nine or ten of them slept in a room where my bed was. The space and
air would be considered quite insufficient by sanitary reformers; and I felt
the air at night quite offensive, even oppressive. I used to have dreams of
suffocation, of drowning generally, but *I never was attacked by asthma*. I
had a fine appetite, enjoyed the sports of the playground, and was perfectly
healthy. Once a fortnight or three weeks I was allowed to go home to L——
on the Saturday after school (which ended at one P.M.), returning on the
Monday. Invariably, as well as I can recollect, I was seized with a fit of
asthma the first night of my return. About midnight my mother was sure
to be attracted to my bedside by certain sounds from my breathing resembling the mewing of a cat, and I would get up and go through the stages
of a fit, from which I would be sufficiently recovered on the Monday morning for my return to Newry. I soon came to expect a fit as an inevitable
attendant upon my visit to my father's house. If I remained four, five, or
six weeks at Newry, the asthma kept away, but whenever I went home to
L——, there I was sure to find the tormentor awaiting me. I think I was
never longer than six or seven weeks without making a visit to L——,
during all my stay at Newry school, which ended with my entering Trinity
College, Dublin, in my sixteenth year. But before leaving Dr. H.'s finally,
I had several slight attacks there too, of an asthmatic kind, though none of
them as bad as at L——. These occurred in the last year of my residence
there. Most of these were so slight as merely to oblige me to get out of
bed and move away to a sitting-room, where I seated myself close to a
table, on which, after a time, I was able to rest my arms to support my
head, and thus to fall gently asleep. In the morning my breathing would
be good enough again. I may mention that it was on my removal to Dr.
H.'s that I first perceived myself able *to lie on either side* in bed. Till
then, I think I used to lie on the *right* side only.

At Dublin I stayed only eight or ten days on the occasion of my entering
college. I was to be an *externe* student. My health during the visit was
robust and my enjoyment of life seemed boundless and exhaustless. As
yet I was scarcely more than a boy, my time of puberty coming late, and I
did not reach my height till perhaps twenty-two. During the four years or
upwards of my college life, I lived nearly altogether at my father's house,
going up to Dublin about four times a year for examination, and staying
there about a week or fortnight each time. At Dublin my health was sure
to be perfect. At home the fits seemed to grow more severe, and the effect
upon my general health more injurious. They occurred pretty regularly

every fortnight or three weeks, lasting for two nights at least. I used to go to R—— on a visit now and then, and there was free from asthma. So it was with any other visits I made, as to a friend's house in Newry, to Armagh, to Belfast. Abroad I was sure to be well, but always I must expect a bad fit on the night of my return to L——. I began during this period to adopt various measures, partly by advice of doctors, partly from my own experience, in hope of preventing the attacks, or of alleviating their severity. As to regimen, it soon became plain to me that the best was strict temperance in eating (unless when I happened to be on an excursion, when I had brisk exercise and cheerful excitement), avoidance of rest in damp clothes or chilled feet, being much in the open air, being always in good temper. Naturally I was of a very cheerful disposition; but some things that do not much affect people in general were afflicting to me; for instance, the crying of infants. This, or other things no more important, depressed me so much sometimes as to bring on a fit. For food, I preferred strong coffee for breakfast, with a boiled egg and bread and butter. Chops, or steaks, or broiled fowls were best for my dinner. Salt meat I found not good for me. Potatoes, if dry and simply dressed, were digestible and safe. So were *young* peas well boiled. Carrots and parsnips were admissible, but not to be recommended. Cabbages, beans, cauliflowers, and most other garden vegetables were bad. In fact, it was best for me to eat hardly any vegetables. Riding I found exceedingly salutary; and often when miserably weak after two or even three days' suffering in the fit, I felt immediate ease on being put on horseback. Sometimes I mounted *to ride away* from an approaching fit, when I was fully aware of its approach, and sometimes the flight procured my safety; particularly as I always went to some of those houses where I had the habit of being always free from the disease. As to medical treatment in the fits, what I came to consider as the best was to take an emetic *immediately* on perceiving the accession of the fit. After the operation of the emetic I would sip at a mixture of the strongest coffee with laudanum—about thirty to fifty drops of laudanum in a large teacup of strong coffee without cream or sugar. When this treatment was adopted promptly enough, it sometimes shortened or lightened the fit. But it was difficult for me to know of the actual coming of the fit till it was already upon me. I had a strange feeling of reluctance to admit the fact of the approach of the disease even to myself, and when the symptoms were manifest to others. This strange reluctance against admitting or believing the actual coming of the fit, possessed me all the years of my asthmatic life. I have observed the same feeling in my friend Mr. M——, who became asthmatic when he was about twenty-five years old. Sometimes when I felt my digestion disordered and my head loaded with blood, symptoms which often preceded an attack, I took a dose of calomel (four to six grains) with Dover's powder (six to ten grains), and I now and then thought it beneficial. It seemed to me injudicious to take purgatives often, or indeed any drugs at all, and yet my general health grew so bad that I used to dose myself a great deal.

At the age of twenty-two I was about five feet eight inches high, nine stone to nine stone and a half in weight, a pretty good walker, and not readily tired either on foot or on horseback, and of average strength and activity for my height and weight. My complexion was florid and my temperament sanguine, though at the same time I was of very sensitive nerves and physically timid—what is styled a nervo-sanguineous temperament, I think. I was an early riser, and my habits were simple and temperate. My time was a good deal occupied in books and in sedentary idleness.

The disease had certainly gained ground against me since my boyhood. The period of my life in which I suffered most from it was from about my seventeenth to my twenty-sixth year, and during that period the violence and duration of the fits, though not their frequency, kept slightly increasing, while the intervals of health began to be marked by symptoms of constitutional derangement. In my boyhood the fit generally lasted a single night and day, seldom more than *two* nights and a day. When once it was gone I was immediately quite well—I could eat, run, enjoy myself as if nothing had ailed me, and I *did* enjoy the recoveries so greatly that they far overpaid me for the trouble of the fits. Even when I was a youth of sixteen or seventeen, I remember that the fits sometimes passed away at once so completely that I began to jump over stools and chairs, in gleeful triumph over the enemy that had just taken flight. But after my twentieth year the fits often lasted, with slight intermission or relaxation of the symptoms, for three nights and days, or more probably *three* nights and *two* days. And in the intervals of health apoplectic symptoms often appeared, such as fits of giddiness. I could not lie a minute on my back, or with my head on the same level with my trunk; the least tightness on my throat was a trouble to me; a sudden run would give me a feeling as if heart and brain were bursting their cases; I felt as if there was too much blood always in my head and neck. During my boyhood I had been (in the intervals) a good runner, and quite equal to healthy boys in general of my age at *shinnie, prison bars*, and other games that tried the soundness of respiration, and I could climb a mountain right well. Now I became *afraid* to run, because of the palpitation and feeling of oppression that any lengthened quick movement produced in me. In climbing a mountain, too, I was distressed till after profuse perspiration had relieved me. And this inability to make, *without preparation*, a quick movement of many minutes, or to ascend a steep of many furlongs rapidly, has continued with me even during those years when the asthma was utterly defeated and *hors de combat*. To be sure, in Van Diemen's Land I could run, &c., with but slight *preparation*, the wonderful dryness of the climate and my habits of life keeping me, as it were, in constant *training;* but even there I was distressed (more than other men so little encumbered with flesh) in the beginning of a mountain ascent, though nobody could pass me in running down it.

It was during that period (from my seventeenth to my twenty-sixth year) that the fits became marked and aggravated by a tendency to *coma*, which was often, during the latter part of the fit, so obstinate that my attendants had trouble in keeping me awake. I never quite lost consciousness, but I was every minute dreaming heavily and waking up again. Awake I must be kept, to make the continual efforts needed for getting breath. When the paroxysm had at length subsided, and I had got the refreshment of a sleep, there still remained, for a day or more, debility more or less, and even a tendency to asthmatic breathing at night. This latter was especially the case when there had been catarrhal symptoms at the beginning of the fit, a complication or modification which now became of frequent recurrence. I would be afraid to lie down in bed, and towards the latter part of the period, I used to sleep for many nights in succession sitting on a chair, with my head rested on pillows placed on other chairs at each side of me (I mean, resting on one of them at a time).

In the period from my twenty-sixth to my thirty-sixth year the attacks were more and more characterized by the complication with catarrh and bronchitis, while the apoplectic symptoms diminished in gravity. The fits often passed into tedious attacks of *bronchitis, with asthmatic breathing,* generally with more or less remission in the day, and lasting sometimes three, four, or five weeks. I have been more than once in my asthmatic life *six* entire weeks without going to bed; and during all the years from about my twenty-fifth to my thirty-sixth, *while living at L——,* I spent more of my nights on the three chairs with the pillows than in bed. It was ordinarily upon my *right* side that I leaned, always with head and shoulders elevated considerably; but ever since I had been sent to school at Newry I had been able to sleep occasionally on the other also.

Thus, I would describe my asthma as having gradually changed its character, or rather considerably modified it, so that the history of my case may be divided into three periods, corresponding with the three periods of boyhood, youth and early manhood, and mature age : 1st. Purely spasmodic or nervous; 2dly. The spasmodic, with pressure on the brain, over-fulness of blood, and great derangement of the circulation; 3dly. Spasmodic bronchitis. Not only, however, did those periods succeed each other by such insensible degrees that I could not say precisely when one ended and the other began, but in any of the periods there would occur cases classed by me in some other period. Thus a bad cold has sometimes resulted in a fit in the time of my youth, and then there would be coughing and expectoration at the end of the fit; or imprudence in diet, or extreme vexation and depression of spirits, may have brought on a fit in the latter years of my case or *bronchitic* period, and then there would be no expectoration or catarrhal symptoms, but a fit almost purely spasmodic.

I shall now endeavour to describe an ordinary fit of that period during which I suffered most from the disease, that is, from my seventeenth year to about my twenty-fifth. It commenced by awaking me from a slumber, generally close after midnight. I was impelled to rise out of bed instantly, and seat myself with my elbows upon my knees and my head in my hands. It was sometimes a labour for me to put on my trowsers and slippers, and a loose coat or dressing-gown, particularly the latter, on account of the raising of my arms to get them into the sleeves. Everything about me must be loose. Very often there was a disturbance of the bowels at the very first, but this seldom recurred during the fits. Excessive action of the bladder commenced early in the fit, and grew worse as the fit advanced, and this was a torment. I had to empty the bladder perhaps every half-hour, or oftener, and that at a time when the slightest exertion or movement was beyond what I could afford, all my energies being needed for the terrible toil and struggle of the respiration. The urine was quite limpid, and in considerable quantities. My mother, or my sister, or a servant, were sure to hear me, and come to attend me as soon as I could permit. I *must* get away from the bed-room, the presence of the bed seeming to me an oppression on my breathing. I moved to a sitting-room, and there (winter or summer) a fire was lit, and this must be done without smoke or dust, both of which would distress me. The skin was dry, and remained so till the crisis of the fit. The head generally ached. Except the headache, there was no other *pain,* the suffering consisting in the violent, incessant, exhausting labours of respiration. The balance seemed quite destroyed between *inspiring* and *expiring.* In spite of myself I was forced to keep tugging *in* the air with all the muscles and joints of my body, while it seemed as if it hardly went *out* again at all. A *cough,* as an expiration, was a relief, but a relief that seldom came in those fits till near the end. As the paroxysm advanced, my head became hotter, fuller, and heavier; the veins felt bursting full on my neck; my eyes were rose-coloured sometimes; my feet were icy cold. My hands, too, were sometimes cold, but not always. But the coldness of the feet was such that the rubbing with warm hands and wrapping with warm flannels, which the attendants sedulously employed, could but slightly remedy it. This coldness of my lower extremities often mounted above my knees. The blood seemed to stay in my head and chest. The pulse was generally quickened some ten to twenty beats, weak and irregular. Besides the peculiar asthmatic sound of respiration, I used to accompany almost every tug for breath with a sort of groan, which (I imagine) helped me like the *hech* of the axe-man, or served, as it best might, in place of an expiration proper. There was in the earlier stages of the fit a profuse flow of saliva (at least generally), and also a slight mucous discharge by nose and mouth, and this mucous discharge I was accustomed to feel as a relief. I could not walk but with my spine arched, so that my head was nearly on a level with my flanks—that is to say, such was the way I did always walk in the bad fits—and any movement was toilsome and difficult to me. My work was the *breathing*, and quite enough I found it. At the worst of the fit the comatose symptoms required the constant attentions of those around me. When, perhaps, two days' toiling for breath had almost exhausted my strength, and the imperfect aëration of the blood weighed heavy on the vital powers, the tendency to coma was very great. At last came the turn. Generally it appeared in the gradual subsidence of the more violent symptoms, a greater facility of keeping warmth in my feet and legs, a moistening of the skin, and a gentle slumber—quite a different thing this from the comatose slumber, which was horrid nightmare. My attendant could distinguish between them, and I myself still kept conscious enough to feel the difference. It was very often between midnight and daybreak that the favourable crisis came. In my earlier years the crisis was unmistakable; but later, from about twenty-five, there might be two or three attempts at the critical slumber before the real one came.

A word now as to the treatment generally adopted in such fits, and its effects. As soon as convenient after the fit declared itself, I took an emetic, generally sulphate of zinc in a dose of twenty to thirty grains. If this was taken early enough, I think it generally proved beneficial. But the fit advanced so fast that the emetic seldom was taken early enough to be of essential service. It seldom brought any discharge of food from the stomach, or anything but itself and saliva, and bile. After the operation of the emetic I sipped a mixture of the coffee and laudanum which I have already mentioned, fifty or sixty to a hundred drops of laudanum in a large cup of the strongest coffee; of this I sipped a teaspoonful every half-hour or so, or perhaps the whole day. As well as I remember, no other medicines served me in the fit during this period. And it was but seldom that the attack was shortened or lightened by any treatment whatever; though I had an idea that if the emetic were administered instantly on the appearance of the fit, or if possible sooner, and the coffee and laudanum employed after free evacuations of the emetic, the effects would be valuable. I remember that during my boyhood, when the fits were purely spasmodic and nervous, a patent medicine called *Wear's Asthma Tincture* several times relieved me. I think its chief ingredient was tincture of myrrh. After a year or less it lost its good effect. In my boyhood, also, I was sometimes relieved by *lavender whiskey*—that is, whiskey in which a great quantity of flower-stalks of lavender have been steeped. But this, too, lost its power after some time. During the period of those bad fits with the apoplectic symptoms I was never bled, though I remember I often felt a desire to have the temporal artery cut, or to have the nape of my neck cupped. In later years, after I had studied medicine, I sometimes felt in the fit that bleeding would relieve me; but I never had the nerve to open my own vein myself, and the doctor lived five miles away. Besides, I felt, as well as my friends, that it would take more blood than my body contained to stand bleeding once a fortnight or three weeks, which was the frequency with which the fits generally occurred in the second period, at least while I lived at L——. Almost all the "anti-spasmodics" of the *Pharmacopœia* were tried in the years between my twentieth and my thirty-fifth. None of them seemed to do me any good worth mentioning, and generally they rather added to my sufferings. Ether (sulphuric ether, I think) certainly did. I remember the violent symptoms were aggravated by a weary sickness it caused, any time I used it largely. I have remarked, too, in the case of an asthmatic friend, a serious aggravation of the fit from the exhibition of ether. It seemed to lower the vital power, and so lessen the forces needed for keeping up the struggle for breath.

Sulphate of zinc seemed the best emetic for my case. In later years, when it became rather difficult to excite vomiting, I sometimes added powder of ipecacuanha, and this combination served well enough, particularly, as I think, because the apoplectic symptoms were decreasing, and the catarrhal or bronchitic ones increasing in gravity. *Tartar emetic* proved quite inadmissible as an emetic in my fits; I think I used it but twice; but both times its relaxing effect on the muscles, and the general feebleness, or rather exhaustion, it caused were such that I felt as if I *must die*—a feeling which you probably have remarked hardly ever arises even in the most violent fits, and when bystanders suppose death inevitable. I remember that it operated on the bowels as well as on the stomach, and that in the movement which this necessitated, it was agony for me to support my weight on my limbs, and my head was lowered almost to my knees as I crept along.

I think there were cases (but seldom) when a full dose of purgative medicine prevented the fit, or postponed it. Dover's powder became a favourite medicine with me in the bronchitic period. I used to take it in doses of two or three grains (or even one to two grains), repeated every half-hour or hour for several times. If the stomach and bowels were clear, it generally proved of some advantage.

Very many other medicines and remedial measures were tried by me, but (exclusive of the grand measure of change of place) none of them were attended by results important enough to demand notice in this account of my case.

      *   *   *   *   *   *   *   *

I propose now to finish the history of my asthma by relating the cure of it, which seemed to result from change of climate, of occupation, and similar circumstances. Could I effectively perform this part of my task, I might supply valuable indications for the treatment of the disease; but in one's own personal case one is prone to omit or slur over important facts, just because of one's perfect familiarity with them.

There were two things which my experience had taught me. One was, that towns clearly agreed with me better than the country; I made frequent visits to Armagh, Belfast, Dublin, and Downpatrick, and at all these places my health was much better than at L——. The other fact was, that the fits were always worse and more frequent in summer than at any other season. A damp summer affected me worst of all. The best seasons seemed to be early spring and late autumn. Winter was not bad for *violent* fits. Dry weather suited me best. In my boyhood and early youth I had the impression that if I had the fortune to be well at the commencement of a frost, I was secure against a fit as long as the frost continued, even should that be for several weeks.

After graduating at college, about my twenty-first year, my health at L—— was so very bad, the fits recurring sometimes weekly for months together, and each fit lasting nearly three days, that I became exceedingly anxious to leave home. I rather think that about this period of my life my health was injuriously affected by the state of my spirits. All through my life I have remarked that cheerful employment, above all, such as exercises both the body and the mind, and chiefly in open air and with brisk movements, gives the greatest protection against the disease. On occasions of exciting and pleasant excursions I might eat and drink like healthy people, and with impunity. But even strict abstinence, and precautions against damp and cold and the like, could not ward off a fit if my spirits were very low.

In my twenty-third year I determined to go and study medicine at Dublin. To this I was impelled chiefly by the desire of escaping from the grievous persecutions of the disease at L——. My medical studies occupied two years; but I visited L—— in the summer for a couple of months or longer. In Dublin my health was perfect. I never had a fit or an attack worthy of the name all the time of my residence there. My constitution, too, seemed to strengthen under the influence of such continued good health. I had a fine florid complexion, and considerable vigour of body, and a person ignorant of my asthma would have supposed me the picture of health. Yet my weight (I think) never got above nine and a half or perhaps ten stone.

In my twenty-fifth year I began to keep a house of my own, and adopt the occupations of farmer and small country gentleman. The house in which I established myself was in L——, about a mile distant from my father's. It was situated on the slope of a hill. These features of the residence, together with the cheerful occupations of a farmer in easy circumstances, the feeling of responsibilities and duties that were easily and agreeably fulfilled, the early rising, open air exercise, and active habits of my new life, all operated favourably upon me. The improvement in my health consisted mainly in the lengthening of the intervals between the bad fits, but they still occurred as often as ten times a year.

In the course of the first two years of my farmer life I made tours to London, to Dublin, to Scotland, and other places. At London I have never had an attack, though at one time I spent about seven weeks there.

At the end of those two years, when I was about twenty-seven, I made a voyage to America. On the passage, which lasted sixteen days, I was free from sea-sickness, as I have been all through my life. The weather was very boisterous, the ship crowded, and my sleeping accommodation very bad. However, I had no fit on board. On arriving at New York I was perfectly well, and so I continued to be for the week I spent there. I then proceeded, by the Hudson and railroad, and lake steamers, to Hamilton, at the western extremity of Lake Ontario, and thence by stage to London, some eighty miles to the westward. Great part of the journey was made over *corduroy roads* (which may you never travel over in a springless wagon, as I did!). My health was good enough till I reached the end of

my long journey—my sister's log-cabin in the backwoods.   There, the
night after my arrival, commenced one of the most violent fits I ever suffered.   It passed away completely after a couple of days, and my health
remained perfectly good, at least entirely free from asthma, for all the time
that I spent in America afterwards, which was ten months.   I attributed
this fit to the accumulated effects of all the fatigues of my long voyage, but
most of all to the tortures of the corduroy road, which surely was as bad as
ordinary rack practice in the dungeons of the Inquisition.   It is likely that
the season of my arrival in the Canadian backwoods was peculiarly favourable, and also the weather which prevailed that year.   It was the end of
September, the beginning of the Indian summer, which was remarkably fine
that year.   The temperature was deliciously mild, the air calm and dry; the
sunlight, coming from a cloudless sky, was tempered by the peculiar dry haze
of that season; there was neither rain, nor fog, nor damp of any kind.   It
was a luxury to me to breathe, the air felt so pure and light, and my lungs
in such fine working order.   The Indian summer lasted till the first or second
week in December, when it was succeeded at once by a winter of snow and
frost.   Bright sun, hard frost, and the calm clear weather of winter lasted
till the beginning of March, when there were alternations of thaw, and
frost, and rain; and at last the spring suddenly appeared one lovely morning, with newly-arrived singing birds in her train.   In the spring there were
showers and rainy days, but yet the asthma never made a sign.   Summer
came fast after the spring, and there were terrible thunderstorms; the heat
became almost intolerable, and the vegetation was ranker than the Irish.
But still the asthma kept away from me.   In the course of the spring and
summer I made some long tours down the lakes and the St. Lawrence as
far as Montreal, and by New York, Philadelphia, Washington, across the
Alleghanies into Ohio, and to the Lakes Ontario and Detroit.   The weather
during my tour in the States was the hottest I had ever experienced, and I
felt a good deal of inconvenience from it, and even some feverish illness.
But there was no symptom of asthma.

I returned to Ireland the following year (1840), and resumed my former
life.   Again my asthma returned, but the character of the fits was modified,
as I have described in a former part of this paper: they often degenerated
into *bronchitis, with spasmodic breathing*, and sometimes lasted, or rather
lingered, for two or three weeks.   When I fell into a lingering state of
disorder, such as prevented me for weeks together from going to bed, I
used to get away to Dublin, on arriving in which city I was quite well
at once.

Such was my state of health when, in the summer of 1848, I bade adieu
to home and went to live in Dublin.   My occupation there was of the
most exciting and absorbing kind (patriotic struggling as a writer and editor
—*i. e., Anglicé*, seditious and treasonable proceedings).   In the fourth
week of my residence I was imprisoned, and was kept in one or other of
two jails for eleven months.   During that time I suffered from fever and
dysentery, which reduced me to extremity.   At the end of that period I
was taken from jail and sent on board ship to be transported to Australia.
A feeling of pride and indignation had grown strong enough in me to
counteract the depression of spirits which had attended my first knowledge
of the desperate condition of my country.   It may seem wild, but I mention it as what I still believe a reality—*I must have died then, but that I was
determined not to die so.*   But all this time I had no fit of asthma.

We reached Sydney in ninety-three days from the Cove.   After lying in

Sydney harbour for ten days or a fortnight, I was sent to Hobart Town (eight hundred miles), where I arrived about November 1st, 1849, and I was sent ashore the day after. All the time I was at sea my health was excellent. I can remember the delight of breathing the air in the latitude of Madeira, the luxury it felt to me. Not only was I free from asthma and symptoms of asthma, but in all respects I was quite well and sound. In Van Diemen's Land I was sent to a distance of forty-five miles from the sea at Hobart Town, and about 1200 feet above the level of the sea. The country there is a forest of gum trees, in which the undergrowth is kept down by the browsing of the flocks and herds. It is a mountainous country, with some great lakes, on a plateau of vast extent, which occupies the centre of the island. The sun was very fierce, and the heat of the summer weather often very great (generally in the middle of the day as much as ninety degrees Fahr. in the shade); but this heat was not nearly so sensible to me as a far lower degree would be in Ireland. The extreme dryness of the air, and something peculiar in its electrical condition, may account for the fact. I lived a very active life at first, walking and riding many miles every day. Often I would ride fifty miles a-day, besides walking a good many more, rowing a boat, &c. My health was superb. Not only did asthma totally disappear, but coughs and colds, and everything like the smallest derangement of any part of the organs of respiration. I grew active, and strong, and hardy. My weight increased to ten and a half stones, though I was taking violent exercise nearly every day.

I remained in Van Diemen's Land from November, 1849, to July, 1854. After the first year the seasons were never so dry, the excitement of novelty died away, I grew subject to fits of depression, and my health was not so perfect as during the first year; but there was never the least symptom of asthma for all the five years of my stay in Australia. I think I had not even a bad cold but once.

I left Australia in July, 1854, voyaging by Ceylon, the Red Sea, and Egypt, to France. I suffered greatly from the heat, but no asthma. I lived at Paris from October, 1854, to June, 1856. I had some severe colds on the chest, but still no asthma. In June, 1856, I went back to Ireland and remained there till October following; still I remained free from asthma. I returned to France in October, and spent the winter and spring at Pau, under depressing circumstances. There I was revisited by my old enemy in two or three unmistakable fits, besides frequent slight affections of the breathing. A change of chamber, however, and some easy precautions, drove him away, and for the last four months of my sojourn there I was free. In Paris, from the end of May, 1857, till the beginning of September, I had no asthma. In September I went to Ireland, where I remained till December. Travelling through the country I had an unmistakable fit (of only one night) at Killarney.

Except about two regular fits at Pau, and several slighter attacks, and one fit and a few threatenings in Ireland, I have had no asthma since the year 1848, i. e., ten years.

CASE VII.

Spontaneous occurrence at the age of eighteen.—Gradual increasing intensity of the disease.—Hæmoptysis.—Extreme asthmatic deformity.—Death.

William Burr, æt. 30, an emaciated man, speaking short, with the most marked asthmatic deformity I have ever seen.[1] He was quite well up to twelve years ago, when he met with an accident—fell down from a loft on his back, on some flagstones. From this he did not seem to suffer at the time; he appeared pretty well the day after the fall, went to his work, that of a groom, as usual, and did not think any more about it. A month after this, early in August, and in very hot thundery weather, having gone to bed perfectly well, he awoke in the night about twelve o'clock, "all of a perspiration," and as if he had been running fast, "and could not breathe," with a load at his chest and a wheezing in his throat. He got out of bed and sat on the side of it, and obtained a little ease, and then was able to return to bed again and go to sleep. He awoke in the morning, at six o'clock, as well as usual, and went to his work and thought no more about the difficulty of breathing he had experienced in the night. He had no cold at this time, there was no cough and no expectoration. A month or six weeks after this, about twelve o'clock in the day, when he was dressing a horse, being in all respects in his usual health, he was seized with difficulty of breathing, which became so severe in twenty minutes, that he was obliged to leave off his work altogether. When the dyspnœa was at its height he was suddenly seized with coughing, and found that what came up into his mouth was hot, and on spitting it out discovered it to be blood; the difficulty of breathing and the blood-spitting lasted about three hours and then went off together—as soon as the breath got easy the hæmoptysis ceased. The cough was very slight, the blood was about half an ounce in quantity, not pure, but mixed with mucus. The disappearance of the dyspnœa at the end of three hours was complete. He felt weak, however, and did no work for a week, and on returning to his duties found that on attempting any brisk exercise, or the laborious occupation to which he had been accustomed, his breath became short, so that he was obliged after a fortnight to give up his situation. As on former occasions, he had neither expectoration, cough, nor symptoms of cold.

He then went to a silk mill, where his work involved no exertion; on going to work, however, morning and evening, his breath would sometimes trouble him and oblige him to stand and rest, which he generally did in a stooping position resting his hands upon his thighs. At this time he was able to play with other youths, and romp and run as well as ever. One night, after he had been at the mill about six months, he was seized about twelve o'clock with an attack of the same nature as the first; he got up and sat in a chair resting his head forward in his mother's lap (who, alarmed at his condition, had come to his assistance), and in this position he went to

---

[1] This is the case that I referred to at p. 113; a photograph which I had taken of the subject of it, and which was to have shown to what a pitch asthmatic spinal curvature may reach, was unfortunately lost. The deformity was most extraordinary, and equalled that which one commonly sees as the result of organic spinal disease, although it had the distinctive asthmatic characters referred to at p. 112, and beyond a doubt was not in any way due to primary organic disease of the spinal column. It was as if the back had set in that stooping deformed shape which we not uncommonly see in the intensest asthmatic paroxysm.

sleep; in about an hour he was able to return to his bed, and when he got up in the morning at six o'clock, he felt no traces of his attack, and went to work as usual.

He went on then for a twelvemonth, working every day, and during the day feeling no dyspnœa, but frequently a little night and morning, obliging him to walk to and from his work slower than the rest; and then, at the usual time of the night, twelve o'clock, he was seized with an unusually severe attack, which did not go off as before, but left him with an unusual amount of dyspnœa and incapacity for exertion throughout the day. About one o'clock on this day, breathing tolerably easy while he was still, he went a short distance with a message, and, though only creeping, very much increased the difficulty of his breathing; this obliged him to stand still, and while thus resting himself he began spitting, and again found that what he expected was blood. This time he spat nearly a pint; it poured out of his mouth and nose, making quite a puddle in the road, and he was carried home in a very weak state. He was unable to resume his work for a month, and during this time whenever he spat there was a little blood with the mucus. After this the blood only appeared when the breath was unusually difficult, as on violent exertion, or in the mornings, or on the occasion of an attack, and after lasting on and off in this way for two years entirely ceased, and for the last eight or nine years he has seen none. From the time of this severe attack with hæmoptysis he never returned to his regular work at the mill, but did little odd jobs, knife and boot cleaning, &c.; his morning dyspnœa increased and became quite regular, and sometimes of an evening, too; but he slept well, and had no very violent nocturnal attack for a twelvemonth. He now found food increase his dyspnœa, and often for a month together he would have a slight attack every day after dinner, lasting for two or three hours (that is, during the time that digestion was going on), so that he has sometimes gone without his dinner to avoid the attack; then, for three or six months, perhaps, he would be free from these after-dinner attacks, and then they would come on again. Sometimes they would come on after supper, but he rarely ate supper, because he found that if he did so he was worse the next morning. Sometimes his breath would be very bad of an afternoon, and then clear up in the evening, and he would have a good night, sometimes he would be quite well throughout the day and bad at night; but always the same for many days and weeks together—the habitude, the diurnal rhythm, always strongly marked. For some years he went on in this way by day, with occasional intense attacks at night, occurring at from six to twelve months' interval, always coming on, and waking him from his first sleep, about twelve o'clock, and going off at about three or four. Sometimes the attack was not so severe as to oblige him to get out of bed, but he would turn round and kneel up in bed towards his pillow, with his hands resting on his knees, and in this way, in an hour or two, get sufficient ease to lie down. Sometimes, with leaning forward on his elbows on the bed, or on other pieces of furniture, his elbows would be quite sore and the skin rubbed off. After some years, however, now about three years ago, the attacks ceased to leave him in the morning but lasted on through the day, at first only a little in excess of the ordinary time, going off in the forenoon, then lasting the entire day, then not leaving him at all, but keeping him up a second night; sometimes it would come on in the morning, and last a day, a night and a day, then two nights and two days, then three nights and two days, and so on; and as the attacks became longer, they became more and more intense, and the intervals shorter.

The points most worthy of remark in this case are—

1. The sudden and apparently causeless access of the disease at the age of eighteen, a most unusual thing. There were none of the ordinary causes of young asthma—infantile bronchitis, measles, whooping-cough, nor of old asthma—chronic bronchitis, or heart-disease, nor any evidence of asthmatic tendency or nervous temperament.

2. The *hæmoptysis*, not by any means a common event in asthma, and which, it will be observed, never occurred except as an accompaniment of the asthmatic paroxysms, and in a quantity proportionate to the intensity of the dyspnœa.

3. The invariable occurrence of the paroxysm at twelve o'clock at night, during the first sleep, with one single exception, when it occurred at twelve o'clock in the day.

4. The influence which thunder and hot sultry weather seemed to have in exalting the asthmatic tendency, a circumstance, however, not singular, but which I have seen in other cases.

5. It also well illustrates the gradual progress that asthma makes, in unfavourable cases, from bad to worse. At first the recovery from the attacks is perfect, no trace is left behind; then appears an incapacity for brisk exercise or violent exertion, with otherwise perfect breathing; then slight night and morning dyspnœa in the intervals of the attacks; then the severe and long attack, after which the dyspnœa never leaves him; then regular severe morning exacerbations; then the attacks cease to leave him at the usual time in the early morning, but last till noon, then till night, then till next day, and so on, till they last three days and nights; then his deformity appears and increases; till now he is bent double, creeping and helpless, a permanent wheezer, his attacks frequent, severe, and long.[1]

CASE VIII.

History of gradual establishment of disease.—Provocatives.—Well marked influence of London air, absolute and relative.—Efficacy of nitre-paper.

E. P., æt. 30. Had always had excellent health, and was in perfect health at the time, when, having overwalked herself, and reclined for an hour or so on a couch near an open window, she apparently caught cold, and was seized in the course of three hours (about nine o'clock, before going to bed) with difficulty of breathing, a sense of constriction at the chest, and headache. The idea entertained was that she had caught cold, and that the attack was incipient bronchitis. The only remedies applied were, putting her feet in warm water, a little mustard to her chest, some warm gruel, and being put to bed. Gradually, towards morning, the breathing began to get easier, profuse frothy expectoration gave increased relief, and she was able to lie down as the day came on. In the forenoon

[1] This case terminated fatally, in the country, about two years after these notes were taken, and nine months after my seeking the patient. I may mention that there was considerable organic change in the lung (emphysema, and thickened and contracted bronchial tube), and that nothing afforded any relief except the inhalation of the fumes of burning nitre-paper.

she got some sleep, and as the day advanced felt much as usual, except a little wheezy and fatigued. The following day she was as well as ever. This attack was in September. For three months she continued perfectly well. About the first week in January she experienced a second attack, brought on apparently by taking *beer after soup.* The attack came on soon after dinner; it was much milder than the first, but it was the occurrence of this second attack that first suggested the idea that the first attack was asthma. The breathing was relieved by bedtime, and she had a good night, but bolstered up. Some time in February, being out at a party, she caught cold, and suffered an attack of asthma, followed by bronchitis, which confined her to the house for ten days; she was then very careful of herself all the spring. Then, from an error in diet—milk and beer producing fla-. tulence—she suffered another attack; and throughout the summer similar errors in diet brought on occasional attacks, which gradually increased, both in frequency and severity, as the winter months drew on. She had a very bad winter. Every antispasmodic remedy that could be thought of was tried, but with little benefit: she was looked upon as a confirmed asthmatic. In the great majority of cases the attacks were brought on by errors in diet —anything that fermented in the stomach. She knew beforehand that if she took any of these things she would have a paroxysm: any effervescing or fermenting substance, particularly beer, always produced one. Exposure to fogs, damp, or smoke, would make her a little wheezy, but as long as her diet was carefully regulated this speedily went off. In this spring she had a very long and severe attack, and consulted Dr. C——, who recommended lobelia and Indian hemp, from which she derived benefit for the time; they checked the attack, but left her in so uncomfortable a state that it was only as a last resource she would take them. As the summer came on she began to try change of air, and soon discovered that the sea air was prejudicial, greatly increasing the severity of the paroxysms.

Soon afterwards she came to London, expecting to derive benefit from residence there, in consequence of a case having come under her knowledge in which a gentleman, suffering from most severe asthma, had been completely cured by residence in London. On arriving in town, she took up her abode in Lombard Street, that she might be in the densest part of the city, for that, from the history of the case she was acquainted with, was the part in which she expected to receive the greatest benefit. Her expectations were fully realized—she regained her health and strength; and from being so weak as to be quite debarred from walking, she was soon able to walk, with perfect ease, an hour at a time. She then made a tour in the west of England—Leamington, Reading, Bath, Clifton, and the Channel Islands, but throughout this tour she was attacked with asthma, and got no permanent freedom from her complaint till she came back to London, where she immediately became quite well, as on the former occasion. She waited till her health was recruited by her residence in the city, and then returned to Scotland. She immediately became worse than ever, and passed a winter of most severe suffering. It was then determined that she should come and live permanently in London as the only thing that afforded a chance of the restoration of her health, and she again returned to the City, with the same result as before—perfect cure, restoration to health and comfort in all respects. Soon after this she moved three miles further west to the neighbourhood of Cavendish Square, and there, although she enjoyed an almost perfect immunity from attacks, she was not so perfectly well as in the city; and she used frequently to go into the city for short visits, for

15

what she called a "dose of health." After being a twelve-month here in a state of very much improved health, she removed to the neighbourhood of Bayswater, and there her asthma began to reappear, and she had occasional attacks of the old spasmodic type. She was still, however, much better than anywhere out of London. Sometimes she would visit the seaside or the country in expectation that the change would be useful, but she was always the worse for it. Thus we may say there were four degrees in which she was affected by local influences—she was better in any part of London than in the country, but in its westerly suburbs she was decidedly asthmatic; in the city she was perfectly well, and in the intermediate situation between these last two her condition was intermediate; the fact being that the more completely urban the air was the better it agreed with her.

In this case every remedy was tried that could be thought of, but, with a single exception, with no beneficial result. That single exception was nitre-paper. She had been advised, by way of experiment, though little expecting benefit, to give it a trial, and to her surprise, on the first occasion, of her using it, experienced great relief; in her after-trials the relief was still more complete, because she managed it better than she had at first, and was more familiar with its manipulation. From that time she found it an unfailing remedy. It effects were rapid and complete, and never varied. There was, however, one exception to its efficacy, and that was whenever the asthmatic attack was brought on and accompanied by bronchitis; in that case the relief it gave was trifling—it was, indeed, hardly any good; the fact was, that it only relieved the bronchial spasm, only put a stop to the asthmatic portion of the dyspnœa, while the bronchitic portion persisted; and moreover, there was, in the inflamed condition of the bronchial mucous membrane, a permanent exciting cause that probably restored the bronchial spasm as soon as relieved. At first the paper was used only every month or so, as the attacks were rare; but as the disease became more severe, the attacks occurred more frequently, and at last the paper had to be resorted to every day. Always at night, before going to bed, she burnt it in her room; indeed, without it she could not have got any sleep, or even gone to bed. It invariably had a marked sedative effect—sent her off to sleep in a few minutes, and gave rise to such an overpowering drowsiness that she was obliged to be watched, lest she might fall forward or drop the burning paper on her dress. She would give warning when she felt her drowsiness coming over her, in order that the burning paper might be taken from her, and that she might put herself in a position from which she could not fall, as she had not power to save herself. Even by day, and when not previously sleepy, it would put her to sleep, as well as cure her asthma, in ten minutes; but if at all sleepy, as in the evening, she would be quietly asleep in a third of that time. Now, we know that many remedies that relieve asthma are immediately followed by sleep, in consequence of their removing that laborious dyspnœa, which is the cause at once of the wakefulness and the weariness. But that this was clearly not the way in which the nitre fumes acted, but that they acted as a positive sedative, was shown by the fact that if her asthma awoke her at night from sleep, and prevented her sleeping, the burning of the paper had the same speedy sedative effect. As soon as her asthma woke her, she would strike a light and burn her paper (which she always kept by her bedside), and get immediate relief; and so quickly and suddenly would the sleeping come on, that, though quite independent of her husband in the commencement of her operations, she was always obliged to wake him that he might take the paper of her when the drowsiness overcame her. In three minutes after lighting the paper she would be sound asleep; sometimes her husband could hardly take the paper quick enough, so sudden were its sedative effects. Now, here she was awoke from sleep to relapse again into sleep in two or three minutes; there had been no accumulated want of sleep, no weariness from protracted laborious dyspnœa. So uncertain was the time at which an attack might occur, and so certain was the effect of the nitre-paper, that this patient never went anywhere without taking some of it with her in her pocket. If an attack came on at any time, she would fly to it. Sometimes, when making a morning call, she would find her asthma approaching; she would bear the increasing dyspnœa as long as she could, and then, when she could bear it no longer, she would ask to be allowed to retire to some room to use her remedy, and in ten minutes return to her friends as well as ever.

CASE IX.

History of case.—Inoperativeness of all remedies.—Perfect cure by stramonium.—
Method of administration.

When a boy, I was subject to wheezing and shortness of breath upon any slight cold, which wore off as I grew up, and for many years I forgot it; but when in China, in the year 1799, I was seized with a severe paroxysm of spasmodic asthma, accompanied with hepatitis, since which time I have been frequently, and of late years I may say constantly, afflicted with asthma. The paroxysm commences with the usual symptoms of cold, together with purging and much evacuation of urine, succeeded by intolerable flatus in the stomach and bowels, frequent convulsive cough, constant wheezing, with painful dyspnœa, being unable to fill the chest with air; any sudden exertion, speaking above a word or two together, or attempting to walk up a hill or up stairs, bring on, at these times, suffocation; much frothy tenacious saliva is discharged from the throat, with some congealed phlegm from the bronchiæ, and in the mornings what is expectorated is often streaked with blood, and sometimes a little pure blood is coughed up. The paroxysm runs its course in from three to five days, when the flatus subsides and expectoration becomes free and easy, being, instead of frothy tenacious saliva, and the jelly or white of egg-like substance, common phlegm, with a little good-looking pus. Health, appetite, and spirits quickly return. For the last three years I have never had an interval of above ten or twelve days free from this distressing complaint. I cannot assign any cause for its commencement, and it goes off as unaccountably. With respect to the cure of this disease, I have been unwearied in my applications to effect it; all my medical friends, both in India and England, have, at one time or another, prescribed for me, and I have not neglected to resort to all the books that came within my reach which treated on this subject—but all in vain. A few grains of calomel (submurias hydrarg.) I have found, by experience, is the only medicine that is of service to me, taken on the accession of the fit; it purges and accelerates the evacuation of urine. Diuresis and catharsis being the first symptoms of an attack, I was led to encourage this natural propensity by taking the calomel, and I soon found it of benefit, by shortening the duration of the paroxysm.

Dr. Bree's valuable publication encouraged me to persevere with his plan

of cure for upwards of two years, to which I as strictly adhered as my situation would allow; but, I am sorry to say, without any other benefit than
that arising from taking the infusion of coffee during the paroxysm, which
expelled the flatus and prevented sleep.   Always experiencing most misery
after a few hours' sleep, I was glad to keep awake, especially as I did not
find any difference in the duration of the paroxysm whether I slept or not
—on this account the coffee was invaluable to me; but still the disease
remained uncured, and, in despair, I resorted to the smoke of the stramonium,
more with a view towards experiment, than from any hopes of good to be
derived from it.   The effect, however, was wonderful—even to me almost
incredible; the very first time I smoked, the irritation and constant cough
ceased, and the flatus was expelled, and I expectorated from the bronchia
pieces of clear congealed phlegm, from half an inch to about an inch in
length, and the thickness of a crow's quill, which enabled me to fill the
chest with air.   The sensation I experienced the first two or three mornings
was no less singular.   On the first morning I was called up about two
hours before my usual time of rising to go to Camberwell.   I got ready
quickly, not thinking of my complaint, but the moment I stepped into the
street, I found I had not power to walk, though perfectly free from pain or
any other sensible indisposition.   I merely felt exhausted, and so feeble as to
want support.   Coffee was got ready, and I ate my accustomed breakfast,
which restored me at once, and I walked to Camberwell in an hour, the
distance being about four miles.   I must remark, that when I commenced
smoking the stramonium, the paroxysm was declining.   It had been the
most severe I ever remember to have experienced, and it is the last I have
had, though I have frequently taken cold since, but with no other inconvenience than a little shortness of breath and wheezing, which went off on
taking my pipe in the evening.   I have now been four months free from my
complaint, and I have every reason to believe that I shall feel no more from
it, though I shall continue smoking the stramonium at intervals, for a length
of time to come.   The way in which I employ this remedy is thus: I fill a
common tobacco-pipe with the stramonium cut in small pieces, and inhale
the smoke as much as possible into the lungs, which causes heat and pain
about the fauces and throat, and I am obliged to breathe once or twice before
I can inhale it again, when I draw in the smoke; and so on, alternately,
until the herb is consumed, which occupies about half an hour once a day.
The saliva I swallow.

I think it right to observe, that I find considerable difficulty in procuring
the stramonium unmixed with other herbs.

Mr. Harris, wholesale druggist, of St. Paul's Churchyard, was good enough
to supply me with a little, and on this being consumed, I sent my young
gentleman for a fresh supply, but, by mistake, he went to a Mr. Harris,
patent and quack medicine vendor, and bookseller, also in St. Paul's Churchyard, and brought me a packet with a printed paper attached, specifying it
to be " Stramonium, or asthmatic herb tobacco, prepared from the recipe of
surgeon Fisher," &c. &c., and notwithstanding this was as different as possible from what I had before been using with so much benefit, I was induced
to try it; but after smoking it as directed, for three days, I was sensible the
complaint was returning; and I verily believe in another day or two I should
have been laid up with a severe spasmodic paroxysm of asthma, had I not
got supplied with the genuine stramonium, and from that day to this I have
enjoyed perfect health.

I am happy to add, that since I have experienced so much benefit from the smoke of the stramonium myself, I have recommended it in two cases of spasmodic asthma with the best effect.

CASE X.

Disease apparently congenital.—1. Ordinary asthma. Exciting cause. Symptoms. Remedies.—2. Hay-asthma. History of the case. Description of a paroxysm.— 3. Cat-asthma. Asthmatic symptoms. General and local symptoms. Nature of the affection.

I have every reason to believe that I have been subject to an asthmatic affection from the time of my birth, and that my asthma is constitutional or congenital; the recollection of my earliest years is associated with much suffering from it. As well as my memory serves me, at the youngest period of life it was at the worst, and has gradually diminished up to the present time. In childhood I do not know that I was ever entirely free from it, that is to say, I could never take a deep breath without a wheezing sound, but now, except when suffering from attacks, I am free from the least trace of it; notwithstanding it was then, as it is now, almost entirely under the influence of exciting causes.

Exciting causes.—These are numerous, dissimilar, and some subtle and unaccountable; they are chiefly these: Cold, change of air, a recumbent posture, laughing, coughing, sneezing, bodily exercise, hay-fever, and, what is decidedly remarkable, the proximity of a common domestic cat. Several of these causes are secondary to others, and cannot be easily distinguished; for instance, I do not know that a recumbent posture would, or moderate exercise would ever produce a paroxysm without a present tendency from the effect of cold, an unfavourable air, &c. The two last in the above catalogue of causes I shall consider separately—hay-fever and the cat-asthma; the first of these is entitled to this distinction because it is invariably accompanied by other symptoms, asthma being only one among many peculiarities equally conspicuous; and the last on account of its singularity.

I shall now describe my common asthma, that is, my asthma exclusive of that produced by hay-fever, or the proximity of a cat.

I was an exceedingly delicate child—pale, thin, weak, sickly-looking, and cadaverous. Besides asthma, a foe ever present or near, I was subject to sore throat, bronchitis, swollen glands in the neck, enlarged tonsils, Eustachian tube deafness, headaches, and habitual wakefulness at night, a variable appetite, and an inability to stoop my head low, from a feeling of sickness which it invariably produced; I was debarred from the natural and healthful sports of childhood, for I could neither run nor laugh heartily without danger of a suffocating paroxysm of temporary asthma. At the age of twelve or thereabouts, I went to reside at a school at Salisbury, where the inland air, and probably the regular mode of living, produced a total disappearance of all these symptoms of delicate health, and I became stout and strong, and my appearance remarkably healthy and robust. During this time I do not remember to have had one paroxysm of asthma, or that my sleep was at any time disturbed by it, nor on my return home for the vacations, on finally leaving school do I remember any recurrence of it. But two or three years after I had left Salisbury, my general health still remaining excellent, I remember I was perpetually distressed and burdened with *tightness of breathing* (to use an expression that seems to imply the sensation), to a degree and with a frequency sufficient to destroy my comfort. Thus, in my early life, my health was bad and my asthma severe; at Salisbury my health was excellent and my asthma was gone; subsequently, my health remaining good, my asthma returned. So stands the case as bearing upon the question whether a good or bad state of general health has an influence on the asthmatic tendency, and the inference to be drawn from the facts, considering the possible influence of other exciting causes, is involved in much uncertainty.

In my case the most prominent and frequent of all the exciting causes is, what is commonly called *taking cold*, and this acts either directly, when the asthma becomes the immediate consequence, or remotely through the intervention of inflammation or congestion of the lungs, when the asthma comes on later. As it regards the first, if I walk in the garden when the air is damp and chilly, in ten minutes my breathing becomes sensibly affected. At night, if my dress is not securely closed in front, or the bed-clothes well adjusted about my neck and shoulders, a certain degree of asthma presently ensues. It has sometimes happened that I have fallen asleep without having made these necessary arrangements, and the consequence has been, that I have awoke with a fit of suffocation, which, after the removal of the cause, has subsided in the ordinary way. The asthma consequent on cold on the chest (bronchitis) is of a most painful and distressing kind; unlike that produced by cold directly, it often lasts for days. In my childhood I suffered grievously from it; I can remember, when I was very little, spending hours at a time on a footstool, with my head on a chair, as the best means of obtaining rest, together with ability to breathe. But it has frequently happened, at all events of late years, that I have had very severe colds, attended with soreness of chest and expectoration, without any concurrent asthma.

Another of the primary causes of asthma with me is change of air. That this produces my asthma I know from the fact that attacks have often occurred for the first few days or weeks after arriving at a place where, during a former residence—and, subsequently, when the effect of the change had passed off—I was as free from all trace of the complaint as I have ever been.

The remaining exciting causes—a recumbent posture, laughing, coughing, sneezing, bodily exercise—I call secondary causes, as I cannot be sure I have ever suffered from any one of them without being at the time in a condition of tendency to asthma from some primary cause. So great is the influence of laughing to induce asthma that I have always been obliged, especially in childhood, to avoid it as much as possible on account of its distressing consequences. Coughing, though a symptom of the complaint, is also a source of aggravation, and, when there is no appearance of asthma, is sufficient to call it into existence. A violent fit of sneezing in the summer will produce asthma, otherwise not. I have always suffered from the effects of bodily exercise especially in childhood; but even at my present age I cannot run a considerable distance, or jump a child, or skip with a skipping-rope, without the occurrence of some asthma.

Symptoms.—Not the least interesting part of this subject is the form of my asthma—its conditions and symptoms—which I shall endeavour to describe. The difficulty of breathing that characterizes it may exist either as a paroxysm of suffocation or a continuous feeling of tightness and impediment: this last may continue for days or weeks, with some variation in degree, and prevails during damp seasons, and the influence of hay-fever. The paroxysm is attended with a wheezing sound, more or less audible, but this only occurs when the paroxysm is about to diminish ; at the commencement and throughout the worst there is no sound which can be perceptible to any one but myself, as on listening, I can only hear a faint long sigh, such as I should imagine would be produced by blowing through a sieve. At this time the visible signs are, a distressed expression of face, open mouth, elevated shoulders, and somewhat of heaving or gasping—all these in proportion to the degree of spasm. Presently a change ensues, the wheezing sound commences, the attack then becomes more distressing to observers, but less so to the patient. Apparently a looseness of the mucus follows the commencement of sound, which mucus continues to present itself at the top of the trachea, and to be disposed of in the ordinary way, even after the sound which gradually becomes fainter, has ceased altogether. The lungs then resume their former normal condition ; but an occasional deposit of mucus, and a necessity of clearing the throat, will occur at intervals for some time after, but not long, if the spasm is produced by some sudden and violent exciting cause, and does not indicate an asthmatic condition. The *continuous* form of asthma which I have noticed is but a mild and continuous phase of the other, but is always indicative of a liability to spasm from any secondary cause. It is unattended with sound, except on making a deep expiration, which, if performed, is immediately followed by a cough, or inclination to cough ; but during the whole of the period the mucus continues to be abundant, impeding the voice, and requiring to be perpetually removed. This deposition of mucus is one of the most characteristic features of the complaint. I believe no asthma, however slight, exists without this concomitant (of course I am understood, here and throughout, to be recording only my own experience), for which reason I am always careful to avoid laughing before singing ; for though the asthma thereby produced may not be perceptible, the subsequent impediment by the production of mucus indicates some previous asthmatic affection.

There are two peculiarities to which I have not yet referred—the asthmatic headache, and an itching sensation about the chin, the middle part of the chest, and at the back between the shoulders. This headache is never present except in a violent paroxysm, with which it subsides, commencing after the difficulty of breathing has existed for some little time. Such headaches do not accompany all violent paroxysms of asthma, but are of rare occurrence ; still they are so peculiar and characteristic as to be entitled to rank among the symptoms of asthma. They are unlike any other headaches, unaccompanied by nausea, and consist of an acute pain over the brows and in the front part of the head, and a feeling of fulness ; they are greatly aggravated by coughing, during which the pain becomes intense. The other peculiarity is as characteristic, but more remarkable ; this belongs chiefly to the asthmatic paroxysms, but to which, unlike the headache, it is not entirely confined. I refer to the itching sensation about the chin, the middle part of the chest, and at the back between the shoulders. This itching does not resemble ordinary itching, being of a peculiar irritating character ; when very bad it might almost be called *stinging*, and it is impossible to allay it by rubbing or scratching, or to determine the exact part which itches. If the chest be rubbed all over, the itching seems to fly to the back about the region of the backbone between the shoulders, or to the chin ; the same occurs with the chin and the back ; whenever an attempt is made to remove the itching by rubbing or scratching, if it moves at all, it appears in one or other of the three localities mentioned, and so till the end of the spasm, or till that symptom subsides. The most ordinary is the itching on the chin, and though so little benefit is derived from it, it is impossible to avoid scratching; the nails go up instinctively, and persevere in a vain application of the usual means of alleviation. I shall have occasion to refer to this symptom in reference to the hay-fever and cat-asthma.

Remedies.—Of remedies I have not much to say, as I have seldom used any; to speak paradoxically, the best remedies are the avoiding the causes. As taking cold is so frequent a cause of asthma, I have found it of the greatest importance that that should be prevented, and when a cold is the occasion of asthma, the obvious means of alleviation are those which tend to cure the cold. It is essential to me to keep the feet dry, and it is of great advantage to keep the extremities warm, especially during the presence of asthma. As a recumbent position is not the most convenient for breathing, besides being sometimes a direct cause of asthma, I sit upright during the paroxysm, or, in case of fatigue, lean forward, resting my head on a table, or on something placed upon it of a convenient height. I have never been obliged to have recourse to emetics for asthma: I have taken antimony with very great advantage as regards the difficulty of breathing. As well as I can remember, all the symptoms of asthma disappeared, but the effect of the medicine was so distressing and so depressing that the remedy was never repeated. I tried smoking tobacco for some little time, and discarded it for the same reason; the alleviation that it afforded was only in proportion to a sensation of faintness and nausea, and a horrible feeling; consequently, smoking was speedily abandoned as a source of comfort. If I had persevered till habit had overcome the painful effects of the poison, I believe smoking the tobacco would have had no effect at all, and would have ceased to be a remedy. I have occasionally had recourse to mild doses of ipecacuanha, and have found it a most comfortable and useful medicine.

There is an instinct in suffering which suggests the immediate requirements of the sufferer, and the natural means of palliation. For instance, in asthma, the next desire after a favourable position of the body is fresh air, cool air, and plenty of it. Frequently when I have been walking in the country, and have been conscious of the presence of some asthma (perhaps principally during the past season), and have been visiting some of the cottagers in their warm close rooms, I have been obliged to escape, from a feeling of actual suffocation, to the open air. For the same reason we see asthmatics with their mouths open, with the aspect of fish ejected from their natural element.

I have now described my case as respects the common asthma, including exciting causes, symptoms, and remedies. It only remains to relate the peculiarities of my asthma as it presents itself during hay-fever, and in consequence of the proximity of a cat; which two subjects for the sake of convenience, I shall detail separately, and as distinct from the common asthma, though in reality it is but one asthma, and every attack, from whatever cause, and with whatever accompaniments, is consequent on an asthmatic constitution.

HAY-ASTHMA.

My hay-asthma differs from the common asthma only in its origin and its accompaniments; it is necessary, therefore, I should describe the malady as a whole, detailing all the symptoms and peculiarities of what is commonly called hay-fever.

It seems reasonable to suppose that I must have been liable to hay-fever, at the ordinary season, during the whole course of my life, but till within the last few years I was never aware of its presence, or of the existence of such a malady. From the frequency of my asthma, and common colds in early life, it is probable that the recurrence of asthma at a particular season, and the other symptoms of hay-fever were overlooked, and that when I became less generally subject to asthma, the tendency to hay-fever remaining, that complaint more distinctly declared itself; or it may be that of late years I have become constitutionally liable to hay-fever—either more susceptible of the influence, whatever it may be, or have acquired a constitution capable of evolving the symptoms.

The period of the commencement of the hay-fever, and the length of its continuance are very variable, being never exactly the same two years following; for one or two seasons, not long since, it did not make its appearance at all, or was so slight as to be scarcely perceptible. Speaking generally, I begin to perceive it about the middle of May, and it ceases about the middle of July; but I have observed that this depends somewhat upon the forwardness of the season, and the progress of vegetation.

That which distinguishes my case (as I suppose) from the ordinary cases of hay-fever, is that the asthma is the most conspicuous feature. During the period of hay-fever there is always a liability to spasm from an exposure to the influence, or there may be, for a part or the whole of the period, a slight but continuous asthma, and a liability to paroxysms from any secondary cause. I have suffered most from paroxysms while taking country walks, walking through grass meadows, and especially in one particular garden surrounded by fields. The prevalence of the influence in this locality is very remarkable, as there is nothing peculiar in the neighbouring soil or its products. I know one other locality where the influence is still more excessive; here there is abundance of flowering grass and rushes, the region is flat, the soil marshy, and in the neighbourhood there is a great variety of indigenous vegetation. If the influence arises from the grass, it is not necessary it should be cut and dried, that is to say, the proximity of *hay* is not essential.

The paroxysm generally commences with sneezing, which continues as long as the operation of the influence which produces the spasm. The sneezing appears to be the most readily produced of any of the symptoms, and results directly from the influence; it is of a peculiarly irritating character, and greatly aggravates the asthma; it is followed and accompanied by a stinging, itching feeling in the nose, an irritability all over the skin of the face, a watery condition of the eyes, and consequently of the nose. I have frequently returned from a walk with my handkerchief as if it had been dipped in clear water; the eyes become injected, the *carunculæ lachrymales* more or less swollen, and the face wears somewhat the same appearance as during a severe cold. When the paroxysm has continued for about an hour there ensues a feeling of disarrangement about the upper part of the throat and palate and back of the nose, as though the whole of that region were mashed up together, so to speak, and had become swollen and undefined. This condition is frequently accompanied by an itching sensation in the Eustachian tubes, which induces a desire to move the back of the tongue, or to thrust the fingers into the ears, so as to allay the itching, but as the part affected cannot be reached, the itching can scarcely ever be alleviated. If this condition of the throat and palate continue for some time, perhaps about an hour, there ensues a feeling of soreness in the throat and chest, as in the case of a common cold. There is, during the whole of this period, a feeling of general irritability; on such occasions the tickling of a hair, the blowing of the wind, any inconvenience or disarrangement of dress, the hitching of brambles, all interference, weight, or incumbrance, become quite intolerable. But the most conspicuous symptom is the asthma, which must always continue longer than the sneezing, since sneezing on such occasions always produces it, and when it has reached the worst it takes some time to subside. The asthma during these paroxysms is violent, with a feeling of tightness and suffocation; it is accompanied with a wheezing sound, and is followed by much mucus. These paroxysms of hay-asthma always exhibit the peculiar phenomenon of the itching of the chin; this itching, unlike the other symptoms of the hay-fever, is attendant only on the asthma, and belongs exclusively to it.[1] After all the symptoms have mostly subsided, which, if the paroxysm occur in the evening, seldom happens entirely before sleep, the throat remains sore, at least in appearance, being red and vascular; the edge of the palate is very red; and the parts contiguous somewhat swollen and undefined, and there is considerable mucous exudation. Always after these attacks, there remains for some little time a liability to asthma from every slight cause, and an inclination to the short asthmatic cough. The asthma may recur on lying down in bed and disturb the early sleep, but this with me is not of common occurrence. During a good night's rest all is set to rights, and every symptom disappears, except those appearances which, were I not aware of the circumstances, would lead me to suppose I was recovering from one of those severe but short colds to which I am subject in the summer time;—the face is somewhat pale, the eyes stiff and injected, with considerable enlargement of the *carunculæ*, which are somewhat encumbered with that kind of inspissated mucus which nurses call "sleeping dust." The throat is sore, and there is a degree of stiffness and swelling about the palate and tonsils, and the lymphatic glands beneath the jaw frequently appear swollen and distinct, and feel about the size of acorns. If the paroxysm on the previous evening has been long and severe, there is a feeling of languor and debility, but this and all other indications disappear as the day advances.

I have had attacks of hay-fever more frequently in the evening than at any other part of the day,[2] but I believe that this results solely from the circumstance that evening is the time for walking in the summer.

The remedies for these paroxysms which I have tried, if remedies they may be called, are very simple. The best treatment is to use the means which inclination dictates, and then to wait with patience till the symptoms subside. If an attack occurred in the evening, having provided myself with a perfectly dry handkerchief, and being comfortably and warmly dressed, I should sit quite still, half-reclining in a chair, in a room with the doors and windows closed, and so remain in stillness and rest, avoid-

---

[1] This differs from the experience of a lady, an acquaintance of mine, who is a victim of hay-fever, and who, although her hay-fever symptoms are quite free from any admixture of asthma, suffers grievously from this itching of the chin and between the shoulders, so that, to use her own expressions, "she could tear the inside of her chin out."

[2] This is not always the case with hay-fever; the morning is often the worst time. In the case of the lady referred to in the previous note, an attack invariably comes on from five to seven A. M. The source of these early attacks appears to be the first bright light of the summer sun.

ing, if possible, coughing and scratching the chin, till I felt able to attend to some quiet employment, and then wait for sleep to complete the cure. If the attack occurred in the daytime, I should in addition be careful to exclude light and noise. Light is particularly disagreeable and hurtful during attacks, but apart from this it is always comfortable on such occasions to shut the eyes.

This includes all I have to say respecting acute hay-asthma. The other phase of hay-fever is that slight continuous asthma which prevails frequently during the first half of summer, together with a frequent itching of the chin. This chin-itching is so conspicuous a feature in hay-asthma, that it may be considered a characteristic symptom, although it is by no means confined to that form of asthma which is produced by hay effluvium.

CAT-ASTHMA.

This singular phenomenon is, I imagine, almost peculiar to myself: I never heard of a similar instance, except in the case of one individual, a near relative of mine, who is subject to the same affection, only in a less degree. The cause of this asthma is the proximity of a common domestic cat; the symptoms are very similar to those of hay-fever, and, as in the case of hay-fever, are occasioned by some sudden influence inappreciable by the senses. I cannot recollect at what time I first became subject to the cat-asthma, but I believe the liability has existed from the earliest period of life. I believe some asthma would present itself if I were sitting by the fire and the cat sleeping on the hearth-rug; but the effect is much greater when the cat is at the distance of one or two feet, or still closer; it is still further increased by the raising of the fur and moving and rubbing about, as is the habit of cats when they are pleased, also by stroking their fur; but most of all when they are in the lap just under the face. The influence seems to be stronger in kittens from two months old and upwards than in full-grown cats. Having been almost always accustomed to cats, I have had abundant opportunity of testing the peculiarities of this singular phenomenon.

With respect to the symptoms, I have only to say they closely resemble those of hay-fever, with only such difference as might be expected from the near proximity of the cause, from its defined and local nature, and also for the facility for its entire and immediate removal. The paroxysm is consequently generally more violent than that of hay-fever, and the symptoms are not allowed to go through their regular course. The asthmatic spasm is immediate and violent, accompanied with sneezing and a burning and watery condition of the eyes and nose, and excessive itching of the chin, which may also extend to the chest and between the shoulders; the eyes are injected, and instinctively avoid the light, and the caruncles are more or less enlarged. I believe if the cause were suffered to continue, all or most of the other symptoms of hay-fever would ensue, only with a more excessive and conspicuous asthma. After the removal of the cause, the symptoms I have described begin immediately to subside, and if the paroxysm is not very severe, the cure is effected in five or ten minutes, leaving, as in all other cases of asthmatic spasm, a tendency to mucus at the top of the windpipe, which being repeatedly removed in the ordinary way, the last symptom disappears, and the lungs and throat resume their normal condition.

This includes all I have to say respecting the cat-asthma; but I shall here notice the evidence of the more general influence of cats on my system—of the existence of what I am disposed to call cat-poison. I mention this partly because of its singularity, and partly because the symptoms arising from this general influence are often co-existent with those of cat-asthma, and are only occasioned by a different application of the same cause as produces, by its application to the respiratory surface, the asthmatic spasm.

The symptoms of this poisoning are consequent on touch or puncture. The eyes, lips, and cheeks are susceptible of the effect of touch, but a puncture of the claw affects equally any part of the surface of the body. The eyes are more readily affected than the lips, and the lips than the cheeks. I have often known the eyes and lips most painfully affected by being touched by the fingers after handling a cat. That such a result may be produced by such a means proves very strikingly the power and subtlety of the influence. The eyes would at all times be affected by this means, but I do not think the lips would, unless there were some little crack or flaw in the skin, from cold or any other cause. The effect on the eye of rubbing it just after touching a cat is to produce a hot, stinging irritation of it, a profuse flow of tears and injection of the whole eye, a tender, painful swelling of the *carunculæ* (the sensation is that of painfulness and itching combined), and intolerance of light. If one eye only is touched the other merely exhibits the ordinary effect of sympathy. The result on the lips is an enlargement of the whole lip, and sometimes a sort of lump or protuberance at the part principally affected, together with a feeling of heat and irritation. The cheek is not influenced by this secondary touch, but is affected by the slightest touch of the fur of the animal. If the cat rubs against the face the cheek immediately becomes hot, a little swollen, and of a suffused red; sometimes there appears a defined little protuberance, something like nettle-rash, which I imagine is produced by the puncture of a hair.

• The wound from a claw, whatever be its form, is always surrounded by a white, hard elevation or wheal, very much resembling the appearance consequent on the sting of the nettle. The pain, which is very much greater than attends ordinary scratches, is accompanied by a feeling of irritation and itching, like the pain of the scratch and a nettle-sting combined.

I must not omit to observe that I have never discovered any trace of such influence in any other animal, with one slight exception; a deep scratch on my arms with the claw of a rabbit has, in two or three instances, produced the same sensation and appearance as those above described, only less clearly developed.

The saliva of a cat is perfectly innocent, and a bite with the tooth in no way differs from ordinary wounds of the same character; in a word, I believe the influence is, in its source, exclusively cutaneous.

CASE XI.

Asthma from bronchitis in adult life.—Capricious and curious effects of locality.—
Physical signs.—Inoperativeness of all remedies.

—— H., Esq., living near Kidderminster, applied to me in July, 1859, on account of spasmodic asthma. He was quite well up to last October, when he caught a severe cold on his chest, with soreness beneath the sternum, cough, and expectoration, but he did not lay up, nor did he seek medical advice. Finding in the following January that he was getting worse, he applied to his medical attendant, who told him that he had been, and was then, suffering from bronchitis. He experienced, I think, but little benefit from treatment. It was not till February that the asthma showed itself. It came on first in nightly paroxysms, waking him from one to two o'clock in the morning. Finding this new symptom increasing upon him, he consulted Dr. ——, of Birmingham, who told him it was spasmodic asthma. Dr. —— did him little, if any good. He then went to St. Leonards, and put himself under Dr. ——; for some time he got no better, and had his attacks every night; but one day, he says, something snapped in his left side, and he almost immediately began to mend. Dr. —— told him it was a pleuritic adhesion that had given way, and ordered the infriction of mercurial and iodine ointment. For the rest of the time that he was at St. Leonards he was almost entirely well, and fancied himself quite cured. He then went to Malvern, and had not been there ten minutes before his asthma seized him, and he had a very bad attack; as long as he was there his asthma continued, and he therefore very promptly left. After this he came to London to consult Dr. ——, and put up at Wood's Hotel, Furnival's Inn, Holborn, and there was perfectly well. On returning home he was as bad as ever; and coming to Reading was advised, by a medical friend there, to come to town to consult me. Mr. H—— is a fine, strongly built, and muscular man, remarkably well "fleshed-up." Chest movements good; percussion everywhere clear without any emphysematous hyper-resonance; no emphysematous configuration of the chest or back. On auscultating the chest, I find—1, respiration accelerated about twenty-five a minute, I should think; 2, expiration a little prolonged, post-expiratory rest almost lost; 3, respiratory murmur not loud anywhere, but at the apices, and below and behind, decidedly deficient; 4, on forced respiration these parts are found to be the seat of very slight emphysematous crackling, the latter also of a little rhonchus and sibilus; forced respiration everywhere else gives the normal puerile sound.

The patient goes to bed well every night, at one or two o'clock he wakes up with, or rather is awoke by, severe dyspnœa, and obliged to assume the erect position. After an hour or two the difficulty of breathing gradually subsides, and before it is time to rise he is able to fall back and get a little sleep; but he finds that even these little snatches make him worse, and that he wakes from them with his breathing not so free as when he lay back. He gets up to breakfast, but it is not till ten or eleven o'clock that his breath becomes perfectly free. When I saw him, ten o'clock, that time had not quite arrived. The attack generally goes off with a little expectoration. For some time, for some weeks, I think, he had, besides these nocturnal attacks, a little attack every evening at eight o'clock.

He has taken the following remedies without any benefit: Indian hemp, lobelia, extract of stramonium, camphor, ether, squill, ipecac, and chlorodyne; also the fumes of nitre paper. The thing that he says has done him the most good is a draught containing antimony (not in nauseating doses), ammonia, and ether. He has not tried tobacco, antimony, or ipecacuanha ad nauseam, stramonium smoking, nor chloroform.

I ordered him to smoke tobacco to collapse, the moment his asthma came on him, the more likely to be easily induced as he has never habituated himself to smoking. Also to try smoking stramonium. Also to get some of Corbyn's ipecacuanha lozenges, and nauseate himself with them when the attack comes on. Also to hold chloroform over his head as a reserve.

This is a case, as it has not been of long standing, and has inflicted no notable organic mischief on the lungs, of the cure of which I should be sanguine. It is one of the cases having an organic origin, being clearly due to the bronchitis. There is no history of asthma or lung disease in his family He never had any symptoms of it before.

The situation of his house is evidently high and dry. The air, therefore, from which I should expect the greatest good to him, would be low and moist. Either a mild, relaxing marine air, such as Torquay, Ventnor, Hastings, or London near the river, such as Bridge Street, Blackfriars. Such advice I accordingly gave him.

August 20th. This patient has come to me to-day much worse than when I saw him last, and with a very bad account of himself in the interval. He has been to Ventnor, Southampton, and various other places on the south coast, and has not, I think, had one good night. On the contrary, his nights have been awfully bad, and his attacks have generally come on from six to eight in the evening. The dyspnœa also only imperfectly leaves him by day, so that he is constantly troubled with it, and now, as he is talking, I can clearly recognize it. He spits a great deal more—an evidence and a measure of the increased embarrassment of breathing, and the consequent pulmonary congestion. He has lost flesh, too, and looks paler and seedy ; in fact, he is suffering greatly from want of sleep. As he infers that his recent experience is against a mild and relaxing place agreeing with him, he is anxious to try a bracing one. Accordingly, with my approbation, he is going to North Wales. As he has tried three of Corbyn's ipecacuanha lozenges without any success, I have recommended him to take four or six. I have also advised him to try smoking strong shag tobacco, with the view of producing some nausea.

A week or two after writing the above I heard from this patient that on his way to Wales he had stopped at Leamington, and there had found himself so perfectly well that he had prolonged his stay. He had not had the slightest return of his symptoms. The hotel at which he was staying, " the Castle," was one at which he had on a previous occasion enjoyed excellent nights, when he could not sleep in other parts of Leamington : and, what is still more curious, it was at this very hotel and in the same part of it that another asthmatic patient, who was invariably ill when he left London, had passed, to his surprise, three excellent nights ; in fact, been as well as in town. How long Mr. H—— stayed at Leamington, or what has been the subsequent history of his case I have not been informed.

B.

TABULATED CASES.

ANALYSIS OF TABLES.

In the following tables is contained an analysis of forty-four cases of asthma. The notes of these cases I have tabularly arrangèd, in order to show their points of coincidence and contrast, and facilitate the estimate of their collective results. Of ten more cases I have imperfect tables, but I have not inserted them from their being in some points defective. About half of these cases have come under my personal observation; for the notes of the rest I am indebted to my medical friends in London and the country.[1] I may mention that all those who have so kindly helped me are men on whose opinions and observations I can entirely rely, and that I have been very particular to embody the notes of no cases except those of the true spasmodic form of the disease.

The èvents in the history of asthma that my tabulated notes record are—

1. Name, age, sex.
2. Appearance, especially in relation to asthmatic physique.
3. Occupation.
4. Residence, past and present.
5. Age at first appearance of the disease.
6. Cause. Under this head I have stated—a, the original cause of the disease; b, the provocatives of the attacks.
7. Frequency of attacks.
8. Time of day (or night) at which the attack occurs.
9. Premonitory symptoms.
10. Whether the disease is unmixed or complicated with other chest-diseases.

---

[1] The way in which I have collected these notes is this: I have issued to my medical friends, with the request that they would fill them up for me with any cases under their observation, slips of paper ruled so as to have, one under the other, compartments for the different events of asthma mentioned in my tables. These they have filled up and returned to me, and have thus furnished me with complete abstracts of cases in the very shape in which I required them, and fit, without any change, for incorporation with my own cases similarly recorded. I would recommend such a plan to any who may be studying any particular disease, and who wish to enlarge their data beyond the sphere of their own observation. I have found, as the result of the plan I have adopted, that I have not only acquired a wider basis for facts with which I was previously acquainted, but have learnt many points in the clinical history of the disease which were essentially new to me.

11. Of what standing the case has been.

12. Whether inherited or not, and family history.

13. Associate diseases (such, for example, as nervous affections, dyspepsia, &c., frequently co-existing with asthma).

14. Effects of remedies.

The first point illustrated by my cases, to which I would call attention, is the question of age. On this point my tables furnish information in three aspects :—

    a. The actual ages of the individuals at the time the notes of their cases were taken.

    b. The age at which the disease made its first appearance.

    c. The length of time the asthma had existed.

I will examine my tables on these three points in order.

    a. The actual ages at the time of taking the cases.—I have records of age in forty-eight cases. The relative numbers in the successive decades of life are as follows :—

Under 10	.	.	0		
From 10 to 20	.	.	4		
" 20 " 30	.	.	15		
" 30 " 40	.	.	9	48	Average age of living asthmatic 38
" 40 " 50	.	.	10		
" 50 " 60	.	.	5		
" 60 " 70	.	.	3		
" 70 " 80	.	.	2		

Thus we see that none were under ten years of age; that the largest number in any one decade was in that from twenty to thirty—fifteen out of forty-eight—*i. e.*, within one of the third of the whole number; and that in each succeeding ten years the numbers became fewer and fewer. The youngest case was twelve years old, the oldest seventy-eight. Now, these numbers prove two facts: first, that very young people may be asthmatic; and secondly, that asthmatics reach a great age, and, therefore, that the disease has but a slight tendency to shorten life. These two facts are, however, much more strikingly illustrated by the testimony of my tables with regard to the other two aspects of age in asthma, viz., the time of life of its first access, and the length of time that the disease has existed.

    b. The time of life of first access I have considered in the chapter on the Clinical History of Asthma (p. 84), to which I refer the reader.

    c. The third point with regard to age that my tables teach is the *standing of the disease*—the length of time it has existed. In four cases in which it had declared itself in the first year of life—in which, therefore, the asthma was as old as the individuals—the ages at the time of taking the cases were twenty-seven, thirty-five, thirty-seven, and forty-seven. Another patient, aged forty-five, had been asthmatic from two years old. One aged sufferer of seventy-one had had his complaint from thirty-seven, that is for thirty-four years; another, aged seventy-eight, from his thirty-third year, that is for forty-five years. The longest duration of the disease I have met with is forty-seven years, and that was in one of the four cases I have just mentioned, in which it had existed from the earliest infancy. Nothing can show, to my mind, more clearly than this, the little tendency that asthma has to shorten life. And this is a fact that is generally known, and so popularly believed, that the possession of asthma is vulgarly spoken of (like the possession of an annuity) as a pledge of longevity.

It is, however, of the pure nervous asthma—in which the respiratory organs are sound, and the breathing healthy, in the intervals of the attacks—that this protracted duration of the disease and feeble tendency to shorten life can alone be predicated. Organic asthma is a very different thing. I do not think that a life affected with bronchitic or cardiac asthma would average worth two years' purchase. It would be well for Insurance Offices if they recognized this distinction. But they make no difference—asthma is asthma to them. I know one office in which all cases of asthma are refused; and in others, in which they are admitted, there is but one asthma-scale of increased premium. The result is, that some cases pay far too little and some far too much, and that many offices lose what would prove to them valuable lives.

The average duration of asthma, as furnished by my notes, is twenty-two years. But this must necessarily be below the mark, for it merely represents the average time the disease had lasted, from its commencement to the time the notes of the cases were taken. In only one of those cases that came under my observation was there any threatening of an approaching fatal termination: all the others, except some of the oldest, were as likely to live twenty years as not. The only way, manifestly, of forming a correct estimate of the average duration of asthma would be to calculate from its first commencement to the time of death.

Sex.—For the influence of sex on liability to asthma I must refer the reader to Chapter IV., p. 88, the data there given being furnished by my tabulated cases.

Appearance.—In almost all my cases there is something scored against the asthmatic under the head of appearance. Some of the descriptions are as follows: " High-shouldered, thin"—" very thin, cartilages of ribs drawn in"—" very thin, and short for his age"—" sallow, emaciated, countenance anxious"—" tall, slight, not unhealthy-looking"—" emaciated, high-shouldered, round-backed"—" tall, leucophlegmatic"—" thin, countenance indicative of suffering"—" asthmatic physique strongly marked"—" thin, with distressed look"—" thin, high-shouldered, anxious"—" pale, thin, narrow-chested"—" pale, thin, and stoops"—" thin, pale, rather dusky"—" emaciated, and very high-shouldered"—" thin, dusky, eyes watering"—" marked asthmatic deformity"—" skin and bones"—" figure asthmatic"—" diminutive, emaciated, cyanosed." In truth, the asthmatic is generally a miserable-looking wretch—round back, cyanosed, veiny, and thin, with a face marked with the lines of suffering, and a premature senility. If the asthma has come on young, he is *generally* below the average height. Some asthmatics, however, as my tables show, have nothing whatever the matter with their appearance, and would be taken for perfectly healthy people.

Occupation.—On analyzing the forty-seven cases in which " occupation" is specified, I find thirty-two were males and fifteen females. I find that of the thirty-two males twenty-two were gentlemen—men of private fortune, clergymen, professional men, military men, and merchants; and ten were tradesmen, artisans, or labourers. Thus more than half the male asthmatics were gentlemen. Of the fifteen women, nine, or two-fifths, were ladies. The upper-middle and upper classes would seem then to contribute twice as many cases of spasmodic asthma as the lower (thirty-one to sixteen); and this conclusion seems the more certain and striking when we remember the numerical inferiority of the upper classes, and that they ought therefore to

16

furnish fewer cases of asthma, even supposing they were equally liable to it. But would this conclusion be correct? is it really as it seems? This appears to me to be just one of those cases where the numerical method may fail, where it may give the fact, but not the interpretation thereof, and where the immediate and apparent conclusion may be the wrong one. The reason why the upper classes furnish so large a proportion of the cases may be that asthma, in the rich, is sure to come under medical cognizance, in the poor not. I have known some poor asthmatics who, from the chronicity and apparent incurableness of their disease, and the tolerableness of their health in the intervals, never think of consulting a doctor about it. The rich do not sit down so patiently under their maladies, but seek relief wherever they can hope to get it; so all their cases come under our observation, while of the poor many I believe pass unrecorded. It may well be, however, that the upper classes *really are* more liable to asthma than the lower, and that this depends on the tendency of the state of hyper-civilization in which we live (and to the effects of which the upper classes are most exposed) to generate a morbidly sensitive nervous organization. It may be, too, that those diseases which, when severe, so frequently lay the foundation of asthma—measles, whooping-cough, infantile bronchitis—when falling on the children of the poor cut them off at once; while those of the rich, from the medical and sanitary advantages they possess, and the tenderness and care with which they are nursed and guarded, pull through them, and survive as asthmatics. The rearing of an asthmatic child is a difficult task, and I have no doubt many of the poor perish in the process.

As far as my tables go it would seem that particular occupation has no influence in affecting liability to the pure nervous form of the disease; and in this respect we see a strong contrast between uncomplicated and complicated asthma, the liability to the latter being greatly influenced by occupation and the external circumstances of life that it involves. Asthma which is a mere appendage to bronchitis, for instance, is of course induced by the causes of bronchitis, such as exposure to wet and cold, and out-door employment in inclement seasons; and cardiac asthma by occupations that involve excessive and sustained effort, and exposure to those depressing influences that generate fatty and ossific change. To organic asthma, therefore, depending on lung or heart-disease, we find the lower classes much more liable than the upper; and if I had recorded cases of this kind, the proportionate numbers of the rich and poor in my tables would have been very different. If I were asked what occupations, in my experience, tended most to induce bronchitic asthma, I should say those of costermongers, cabmen, and Covent Garden porters.

Residence.—The column under the head "residence" shows that every conceivable variety of locality may be the residence of asthmatics—every part of the United Kingdom, the Continent, America, Egypt, and Spain, the Cape, India, Australia; the crowded city, the open country; high dry situations, and low damp ones; inland, and the sea-coast; in a relaxing, and a bracing air; on chalk, gravel, and clay soils. I have instances of asthmatics in all of them. It also shows that the disease may continue during prolonged residence in one locality and under perpetual change of place. But the influence of residence is far better illustrated by the teachings of another column, that of *the Effects of Remedies*, where in a great number of cases it will be found stated that residence in certain specified localities has effected a cure. For the results of my cases in illustration of the therapeutical influence of locality, I must refer the reader to Chapter XIII., which is devoted to the examination and discussion of this subject.

One case (Case V.) furnishes one interesting point. It is the case of a native Hindoostanee lady, aged 40, who came under my care about a year and a half ago, and who gave me, in relating her symptoms, a very clear history of a well-marked case of pure spasmodic asthma from which she had suffered (in her native country) for twenty years. It shows that the phenomena of the disease are not modified by climate, and that they are identical in the Hindoo and European constitutions. One new feature in her asthma she did notice, however—the tendency of hay and flowering grass to induce it; she had some very severe attacks brought on in this way, in fact, regular hay-asthma. From this she had never suffered in her native country, and had been at a loss to explain the phenomenon until I offered her its solution. I have known similar instances. A late Governor of the Bombay Presidency had suffered from hay-asthma all his life, till he went to India. During the whole of his residence there, twenty years, he was perfectly free from it. But no sooner did he return to England than his old symptoms reappeared. A lady of my acquaintance who suffered greatly from hay-asthma, went to the Cape. During the seasons there in which she had been accustomed to expect the visitations of her complaint, she had not a trace of it; but on coming back to England it reappeared in the old way. I think she has twice spent some years at the Cape, and both times with the same result. It would seem, then, that the particular species of grass, the emanations from which give rise to the symptoms, must be indigenous to this country, or at least to Europe; for hay-asthma seems to be as abundant on the Continent as in this country.

Causes of Asthma.—Under the head of causes of asthma, I have adopted a division, which I think a perfectly natural one, into the original cause of the asthmatic tendency (*i. e.*, the essential cause of the disease), and the provocatives of the attacks. Under the first division—the essential cause of the disease—I find in the forty-six cases in which it is recorded, that in twenty-two it is assigned to some bronchial affection. Of these twenty-two three are whooping-cough bronchitis, and nineteen catarrhal bronchitis; this, in a large number of cases, has been infantile bronchitis, or that of early childhood, in many was very slight and seemed to be nothing more than a common cold on the chest, and in almost all was so completely recovered from, that the cases afterwards presented the character of pure spasmodic asthma, and not that of bronchitic asthma. In some cases the original chest affection was so slight that it was not recognised, and the cause of the asthma was called "cold," or "cold and damp;" but we cannot conceive how these agents should affect, and permanently affect, the physiology of the bronchial tubes, except by affecting their mucous membrane, and the one and only way in which cold and damp affect the bronchial mucous membrane we know to be by more or less inflaming it. All cases, therefore, assigned to cold I have set down as bronchitic, although the bronchitis may originally have been so slight as not to be recognized.

In sixteen out of forty-six cases the cause of the asthma appears to consist in a constitutional proclivity to the disease, requiring for its development no appreciable cause. Some of these cases are set down in my notes as "cause unknown," or "constitutional tendency," or "congenital," but I believe they are all one and the same, and depend on a peculiar morbid irritability of the nervous system of the lungs, which is a part of the individual. Many of these cases appeared very early in life, quite in infancy, and in the majority of them distinct inheritance could be traced. Nothing could prove more than this their constitutional character. Indeed, in most cases where asthma appears to be hereditary it will be found to be this apparently spontaneous kind. And that we can easily understand;—the more intense the tendency to the disease, the slighter will be the circumstance (if any) that is necessary to elicit it.

. In two cases the disease is assigned to suddenly suspended eruption—in one case smallpox, in another infantile eczema. Now this, remembering the intimate association of the skin and bronchial mucous membrane, as shown by the materials they eliminate, the bronchitis of severe burns, &c., I think possible.

In two cases the disease was supposed to be induced by grief and trouble. This, remembering its nervous nature, I also think possible.

In one case it appeared immediately after typhus-fever—in one was supposed to be caused by liver complaint—in one by sudden hard work and sobriety after habitual drinking, and in one came on suddenly on going to Ashby, as if that air had caused it. In these four cases I consider the causation apocryphal.

Now, what do these cases teach ? Disregarding the isolated cases, I think they teach two things :—

a. That in twenty-two cases out of forty-six, that is nearly half, the asthma was due to something organically and vascularly affecting (though perhaps slightly and temporarily) the bronchial mucous membrane.

b. That in sixteen cases out of forty-six, that is in more than a third, it appeared to depend on a constitutional idiosyncrasy, in some cases congenital, in some cases inherited—that the cause was intrinsic not extrinsic.

The implied pathological teaching of these facts I have fully discussed in Chapter VI.

In the second class of causes—the immediate excitants of the attacks—my tables show that asthma exhibits the most extraordinary variety. If I were to mention all the provocatives of the asthmatic paroxysm, I should mention almost as many as there are cases in my tables. But I think they may be divided, with few exceptions into three classes: respired irritants ; alimentary irritants, or circumstances affecting the digestion ; and circumstances affecting the nervous system. Among respired irritants, materials affecting the air breathed, I find : "Dust, hay effluvium"—" any air but Richmond"—" all airs but London"—"a hot, ill-ventilated room"—" smell or presence of mustard in any form, smell of a poulterer's shop, fresh skins" —" cold, damp, dust, mustiness"—"lighting a lucifer match, *cat influence*" —"east wind"—"ipecacuanha effluvium"—" grass pollen, dust generally" —"particular smells, dust, and smoke." Among the provocatives of the attacks acting through the digestive organs, I find mentioned in my tables : —"A late full meal"—"deranged stomach"—"a late dinner or supper"— " pie-crust, eggs, any sweets, heavy malt liquor"—"pastry or indigestible food"—"a glass of hock"—"a glass of port wine, immediately"—"any food of a fermenting or gaseous kind"—"eating beans, old peas, or cheese." In two cases "milk" would always bring on an attack, in two "coffee" is mentioned, in three "malt liquor." Among the nervous excitants of asthma, I find, "anything that troubles the mind"—"nervous excitement" —" severe exertion"—"mental depression"—"any sudden fear or alarm."

There are two provocatives of asthma enumerated under the immediate excitants of the attacks that I hardly know where to place : "Hot weather," and "laughing." Whether they act on the nervous system or directly on the respiratory organs, I cannot tell; but many people are much worse in hot weather, some only troubled with their complaint then, and many asthmatics I know who dare not laugh for fear of bringing on an attack, especially after a meal or in the hay season.

Frequency of Attacks.—Of the forty-four cases, eleven are specified as irregular, having no periodicity, the remaining thirty-three were periodic; the proportion therefore of periodic to non-periodic asthma is exactly three to one. The intervals at which asthma may occur may be divided into *natural* and *arbitrary*. In ten of the cases at which the period is mentioned the interval is arbitrary, in twenty-nine it is natural; the proportion, therefore, of natural to arbitrary periodicity in asthma is nearly three to one. What I call natural periods are the diurnal, the weekly, the monthly, and the annual. Of the twenty-nine naturally periodic cases, in sixteen the period was nightly, in three weekly, in four monthly, and in six annual. Of the three weekly cases all, curiously, occurred on a Monday morning. Of the six annual cases all were summer or autumn asthma, four summer and two autumn; one of them was true hay-asthma. In asthma annually periodic, a summer instead of a winter periodicity distinguishes the purely spasmodic from the bronchitic form of the disease—a very important diagnostic point. Of the ten cases in which the periodicity was arbitrary, in one case the asthma occurred every six days, in three every fortnight, in one thrice a month, in one once in three weeks, and in four every two months. In some cases the periodicity may be said to be double—a period within a period; thus, in the annually recurring cases, the summer or autumnal batch of asthma has commonly a diurnal periodicity throughout the time of its continuance. In some the periodicity may be said to be complex, to be regularly irregular; thus in Case 4 "a severe attack occurred once a month all the year round, and in the summer a slight attack every night in addition;" in Case 21 "nightly in July and August, once a month the rest of the year;" in Case 34 "every night slightly, and once a month severely." In some of the cases the periodicity may be said to be an *advancing* one—the intervals getting shorter; in some a *receding* one—the periods lengthening.

Time of Attack.—The evidence of my cases as to the time that asthma chooses for its accession is as follows: In the forty-two cases in which it is stated (in two there being no record), the time of the attack was constant in thirty-five and variable in seven, *i. e.*, constant in five cases out of six. Of the thirty-five cases in which the time of attack was constant, it occurred in the early morning in twenty-eight, and in the evening in seven, *i. e.*, in the morning in four cases out of five. In other words, morning asthma is four times as common as evening asthma, and a stated time for the appearance of the attack five times as common as a variable one. These results may perhaps be more clear if tabularly expressed, thus :—

Stated . 42 { Variable . 7 . . 7
{ Constant . 35 { Morning . 28
{ Evening . 7
Not stated . 2 2

My tables show that of the twenty-eight morning cases, in twenty-five the attack commenced from midnight to four o'clock; three occurred later than four o'clock, of these, one was from four to five, one from five to six, and one from three to seven. From two to three o'clock A. M. is clearly by far the commonest time for asthma to appear. I may remark that, as a rule, the cases of asthma in which the time of attack is irregular, are cases in which the disease is irregular, and not typically marked, in other respects.

Premonitory Symptoms.—My tables show that premonitory symptoms were wanting in twelve cases out of forty-four; they were present in the rest, that is, in nearly three-fourths of the cases. But from these I think seven must in fairness be taken, as the premonitory symptoms in these appeared to be nothing more than the first traces of the invasion of the attack. In eighteen cases the premonitory symptoms were nervous; of these eighteen, the symptoms in four consisted of "unusual drowsiness overnight," in three of "headache," in seven something affecting the spirits and mental condition, such as—"a sense of unusual security," "a sense of unusual health," "a conviction of the approach of the attack," "boisterous spirits," "irritability of manner," "fidgetiness," "feeling dull, low, and miserable, without a cause," in one "neuralgic aching of bones," in another "profuse diuresis," in another "giddiness." In five the premonitory symptoms were referable to the stomach, such as flatulent distension, a sense of fulness, tightness of dress, dyspepsia, gastralgia, nausea.

The details in the column headed "*Unmixed or complicated with other lung disease,*" are such as hardly admit of intelligent and profitable analysis; and coming from various sources, and requiring for their accuracy the most critical auscultation, they are, in my opinion, the least reliable portion of the tables.

For the teaching of the column relating to "*Family history,*" I must refer the reader to Chapter IV., especially the paragraphs treating of the hereditariness of asthma.

An analysis of the last column is simply impossible; it would be little less than rewriting the chapters on Treatment.

Number. Name. Sex. Age. Appearance. Occupation.	Residence, past and present.	Age at first appearance.	Cause. α Original cause of disease. β Provocatives of attacks.	Frequency of attacks.	Time of attack.	Premonitory symptoms.	Unmixed or complicated with other lung disease.	Of what standing.	Associated diseases and family history.	Effects of remedies.
1. B. D., m., æt. 29. Middle height, high shouldered, thin. *Solicitor.*	Ringwood till 18, London till 21, Fordingbridge the last five years.	2 yrs.	α Apparently arising from the sudden disappearance of a chronic scaly eruption. β A hot ill-ventilated room always induces an attack.	Every few weeks in summer and autumn, less frequently in spring and winter.	Generally in the evening.	None but gradually increasing dyspnœa.	No complications.	27 years.	No associated diseases. Not inherited. Of very healthy family.	The three years he was in London he had no attack. Tobacco and stramonium do no good. Expectorants, antispasmodics, and stimulants have been tried; small repeated doses of ipecacuanha have relieved most, but treatment by *avoidance* is best; exercise in open air, early hours, *but little food.*
2. D. M., m., æt. 35. Very thin, cartilages of ribs drawn in. Improved since recovery. *Professional.*	Near the sea till 30, since then in London.	8 mo.	α Whooping-cough at three months old. β A full heavy meal, especially towards night or before sleep. Certain foods. All airs but London. Change of air.	At first rare. Then for 12 years once a week; then more seldom. For fifteen years almost ceased.	Morning from 3 to 4 o'clock.	Oppressive drowsiness felt the night before. A profuse pale diuresis in the early part of the night.	The slightest trace of emphysema.	Whole life; 35 years.	Since the asthma has disappeared, he has been troubled occasionally with violent fits of colic. Asthma not in any way inherited; but sister very asthmatic, and brother much troubled with hay-asthma.	London air has permanently cured him. An emetic of ipecacuanha would always cure an attack, or smoking tobacco *ad nauseam.* Neither opium, lobelia, hyoscyamus, ether, stramonium, expectorants, nor tonics ever did him any good. Nitre-paper of great benefit.
3. E. D., m., æt. 57. Fair, in medium flesh and rather high-shouldered. *Mediocre.*	1, Kirby Moorside, a rich valley; 2, Whitby; 3, London; 4, Oxford; 5, London again.	1 mo.	α Congenital peculiarity. β In by far the greatest number of cases atmospheric.	Irregular. Always on change of place.	3 A.M.	None; unless, perhaps, a feeling of unusual security.	Unmixed.	Life-long.	Neuralgia. Paroxysmal sternutation. Grandfather bowed down by asthma for some years before his death, æt. 46.	An emetic of ipecacuanha, ʒj, or ʒss, has generally done good, often removed the attack, and left the patient, after a short sleep, perfectly well. Calomel, when it acted as an emetic, had an equally beneficial effect.

Number. Name. Sex. Age. Appearance. Occupation.	Residence, past and present.	Age at first appearance.	Cause. α Original cause of disease. β Provocatives of attacks.	Frequency of attacks.	Time of attack.	Premonitory symptoms.	Unmixed or complicated with other lung disease.	Of what standing.	Associated diseases and family history.	Effects of remedies.
4. G. J., m., æt. 16. Very thin, and short for his age.	Richmond.	3 yrs.	α Pertussis at 3 years. β Any air but Richmond. Excitement, hot weather, deranged stomach.	In summer every night slightly. Severe attack once a month.	From 1 to 3 A.M.	Oppression of the chest. Headache.	Slightly emphysema.	13 years.	No associated diseases. Not inherited. Phthisical on mother's side.	Nitre-paper does most good. Occasionally morphia, and chloroform, inhaled in small doses, have done good. Stramonium, lobelia, or tobacco in any form, do no good.
5. Mary A., f., æt. 44. A native Hindoostanee lady. Moderately stout and healthy looking.	In India up to four months ago. Since at Enfield.	24 yrs.	α None known. β Oppressive heat, dust, hay effluvium, & late dinner, supper, indigestible food.	Irregular; 2 weeks to 6 months; 3 years the longest interval.	About 9 o'clock in the evening.	Lethargy, slight sense of oppression and constriction about the chest.	Remarkably free from any lung complication. No emphysema. and very little bronchial congestion.	20 years.	Dyspepsia; subject to acid eructations, heart-burn. Not inherited. No family history of any lung affection.	The only one tried before I saw her was some unknown powder, prescribed by a native doctor-astrologer, of which she was to take 5 yrs. three times a day. It neither purged or vomited her, but who thinks did her good. Ordered—Corbyn's loz. Stram. Nitre-paper. London air. Result not known.
6. Maria R., f., æt. 22. Sallow, emaciated, countenance anxious. Gentlewoman.	Neighbourhood of London.	14 dys.	α Unknown. β Smell or presence of mustard in any form. Smell of a poulterer's shop, that is, feathers and fresh skins Stomach derangement, eggs or milk. S. W. wind. Wet.	Various; generally 3 in a month.	Various.	Dyspnœa, headache, giddiness.	Loud rhonchus and sibling over both lungs. Emphysema.	Lifelong.	Occasional attacks of bronchitis, after which the lungs are much relieved (!) Not inherited. Phthisical on mother's side.	Expectorants and sedatives do most good, with ether Any attempt to use mustard as a counter-irritant brings on intense dyspnœa. Feels best in dry frosty weather.

Patient	Residence	Exciting causes	Frequency	Time	Premonitory symptoms	Physical signs	Duration	Associated disease / inheritance	Remedies and remarks
7. Thomas S., m., æt. 47. Thin. *Farmer.*	School till 17; London till 19; since in country.	a Smallpox driven in on the lungs.(?)	Formerly very frequent, scarcely free for weeks.	From 2 to 4 in the morning.	Often none. Frequently feeling much better than usual the day before an attack.	Simply a very severe case of spasmodic asthma.	33 years.	Attack generally accompanied by disordered liver. No inheritance. Father gouty. Relatives sickly.	Principal remedy, smoking pure tobacco, attending strictly to diet, avoiding everything that disagrees, and choosing a locality that suits. "Different rooms even make a difference to me. By these rules I have cured myself."
8. William C., m., æt. 29. Full-Faced, thick upper lip. *Butcher.*	Twickenham and Richmond.	a Unknown; seemed to come on gradually with cough. β Rest; full stomach; lying on the right side.	Every Monday morning after the Sunday's rest.	Midnight, or soon after.	Tickling in the throat, nausea, perspiration. Sometimes none.	Emphysema of both lungs. Chest too resonant; barrel shaped. Heart's sounds indistinct.	17 years.	No associated disease. Grandfather now suffers from asthma. Father died of phthisis.	Tartar emetic in full doses acts best; symptoms immediately subside on the supervention of nausea and vomiting. Lobelia not good; leaving off suppers has had a very beneficial effect. An emetic of zinc. sulph. once cured.
9. Thomas H., m., æt. 30. Leuco-phlegmatic. *Farmer.*	South Devon.	a Cold and bronchitis. β Damp and the usual objectionable articles of diet.	Uncertain.	Variable.	Incipient tightness of chest.	Bronchitis.	9 years.	Hepatic congestion in spasms. Not inherited. Father bronchitic.	Lobelia and squill cures the attacks. Chlorodine certainly gave temporary relief. Has been less subject to his attacks since he has smoked tobacco daily.
10. Grace M., f., æt. 45. Tall, slight, not unhealthy. *Gentlewoman.*	South Devon, and abroad in northern latitudes.	a Grief, trouble, and cold. β Cold, damp, dust, mustiness, jolting in a carriage. Anything that troubles the mind.	From once a week to once a month.	Evening, lasting sometimes 3 days.	Dulness, a feeling of weight in the head, and impressed with the belief of the approach of the attack.	Bronchitis.	8 years.	Nervous spasms and hysteria. No inheritance. Mother bronchitic.	Nitre-paper always benefits. Colchicum and stramonium give speedy relief. Swallowing a piece of bread or meat often stops the return of the spasm. Fanning with a feather at a distance gives great relief.
11. George E., m., æt. 43. Emaciated, high-shouldered, round-backed. *Solicitor.*	Plymouth and London, where asthma came on.	a Occurrence apparently spontaneous. β Errors in diet; vegetables, fruit, pie-crust, any sweets, pickles, heavy malt liquor.	Diurnal. Every afternoon from 3 to 4. Dining sparely, from 1 to 2.	Afternoon, sometimes evening.	Dyspeptic symptoms, sense of distension, flatulence.	Slight congestive bronchitis, and emphysema.	22 years.	Highly nervous temperament. Father suffered from asthma; died at 57. Paternal uncle dreadful sufferer from it. Paternal grandmother decidedly. Second paternal uncle slightly.	Of late years always better in London. The strong fresh air of Dartmoor very beneficial. Strong mental excitement, or pre-occupation, or anything unexpected will dissipate an attack. Half gr. extr. stram. has given relief. Great relief from strong coffee; slighter from an evening cigar.

Number. Name. Sex. Age. Appearance. Occupation.	Residence, past and present.	Age at first appearance.	Cause. α Original cause of disease. β Provocatives of attacks.	Frequency of attacks.	Time of attack.	Premonitory symptoms.	Unmixed or complicated with other lung disease.	Of what standing.	Associated diseases and family history.	Effects of remedies.
12 Edward P., m., æt. 29. Tall, leuco-phlegmatic. *Clergyman.*	North-Wales; Sudbury, in Suffolk.	6	α Exposure to wet. β Digestive derangement,—certain airs—e.g., cannot live in London.	At first every two months. Now three times in two years.	Various.	Coryza sometimes.	Seems often mixed with congestion of the liver.	23 years.	No associated disease. Inherited from father and grandfather. Father's sister died of it.	Remedies directed to the relief of the chest useless. Calomel has sometimes done good. Boating and gymnastic exercises afforded much relief. Certain air very beneficial, as Oxford and Sudbury.
13 Annie J. L., æt. 37. Appearance nothing special. *Gentlewoman.*	South coast, low, mild situation; London.	In-fancy.	α Supposed bronchial catarrh. β Nervous excitement, coffee, laughing, light-ing a lucifer, cal influence.	Quite irregular, according to exciting causes.	No rule.	In the ordinary asthma none. In hay-asthma sneezing.	Associated with bronchitis in childhood. At present no complaint	Life-long.	Bronchial susceptibility. Very nervous temperament. Not inherited. Two brothers with both ordinary and hay-asthma.	Sitting up or standing relieves the spasm. The nausea of tobacco-smoking and ipecacuanha immediately cure; mucus rises to the top of the trachea, is expectorated, and so the spasm passes off.
14 John P., m., æt. 61. Thin, countenance indicates suffering. *Incapable of work.*	Downton, valley surrounded by chalk hills.	31 yrs.	α Bronchitis from unusual exposure to cold in an inundation. β Change of weather; any other excitants not stated.	Every fortnight.		Feeling of having taken a "fresh cold," increased expectoration and cough.	Considerable bronchitis.	30 years.	Health in other respects perfect. Several indirect branches of the family have been asthmatic, but neither parent.	Orthodox remedies worthless. Seven years ago tried Lacock's wafers, and soon greatly improved. During the second year had but one attack, and that in a thunder-storm; since then, five years, *entirely free.* Sleeps low, walks well, can do anything.
15 Penelope K. W., L., æt. 31. Tall, stout, and pale. *Gentlewoman.*	Downton; low, gravel, surrounded by chalk.	4 yrs.	α An ordinary child's cold. β Certain localities will immediately induce; also any disturbance of the digestion.	Once in three weeks; latterly much rarer.	Generally evening.	Fulness and tightness, rendering it necessary to loosen her clothing.	No lung complication apparently.	17 years.	Paroxysms of extraordinary generation of flatus, giving rise to "flatulent hiccup." Mother slightly asthmatic; maternal great-grandmother a martyr to it.	Ordinary remedies useless except inhalation of the fumes of nitre-paper, which have always relieved the attack, except when complicated with bronchitis. In certain localities she is quite well.

Patient	Residence & age	Cause	Period	Time	Symptoms	Complication	Duration	Associated disease	Remarks
16. Charles B., m., æt. 23. Tall, well-formed, thin. *Grocer's Assistant.*	Belgrave Gate, Leicester. 20 yrs.	α Unknown. Went to Ashby for 8 months, and was attacked there. β Severe exertion, malt liquor, pastry, or indigestible food.	Every 2 or 3 months; but slight dyspnœa more frequently.	Irregular.	Generally shivering and "aching of the bones."	Uncomplicated.	3 years.	No associated diseases. No hereditary tendency, parents living, family healthy.	Have seen him twice or thrice; the attacks last from 24 to 36 hours, but not severely; an emetic has been useful, and a combination of T. opii, ether chlor., and M. camph., seemed beneficial. Nitre-paper fumigation apparently useless.
17. Y. Z., m., æt. 49. Short, slight, fair. *Surgeon.*	Stokesby, Middlesbro' and within ten miles. 46½ yrs.	α Original cause unknown. β Atmospherical influence.	Every 6 days, but breathing never free.	Uncertain.	A mere increase of the usual dyspnœa in walking, &c.	Unmixed.	4 mos.	Indigestion. No inheritance.	"After all remedies had failed, I experienced immediate relief on driving three miles into the country towards Stokesby; I therefore went to reside at Stokesby, and three weeks cured me. If again attacked, I shall do the same."
18. William H., m., æt. 45. Appearance perfectly healthy. *Private Gentleman.*	Near Kidderminster, high, dry situation, on red sandstone. 44 yrs.	α Bronchitis. β Certain airs, as Malvern, Kidderminster, Ventnor, &c.	Every night for weeks.	From 1 to 2 A.M.	None.	Slight bronchitis; trace of emphysema.	8 mos.	No associated diseases. No history of any lung disease in his family.	Indian hemp, lobelia, extr. strm., camphor, ether, squill, Ipecacuanha, chlorodyne, nitre-paper, all useless. Perfectly well at Wood's Hotel, Holborn, and the "Castle," Leamington; not tried tobac., ant., or Ipecac. *ad nauseam*, stramonium-smoking, or chlorof.
19. A. B., m., æt. 71. Broad-chested, well-made man. *Military.*	India 19 years, since a yrs. Guernsey. 37 yrs.	α Liver complaint. β Disordered stomach, damp situations with much vegetation, a glass of hock.	In the autumn almost daily.	Generally after first sleep.	Tickling in the throat, and then coughing.	Uncomplicated.	34 years.	Liver and stomach disease. No inheritance.	Always well in London and Bath. Nitre-paper gives immediate relief; strong coffee and a cigar the same, but less. Has cut short an attack by going a mile to the sea-side. Apparently permanently cured himself by walking 20 miles a day.
20. Anne M., f., æt. 67. *Widow.*	Near Peterboro' and Cambridge. 62 yrs.	α Followed typhus fever. β Excitants of attacks not mentioned.	Every 2 or 3 weeks, becoming more frequent.	Towards night.	Pain between the shoulders and feverishness.	Unmixed.	15 years.	No associated diseases. One sister died of consumption, father of renal disease, mother in childbirth.	Emetics were formerly used with great relief. Has found now that small nauseating doses of ant. pot. tart. give more relief than anything else.

Number. Name. Sex. Age. Appearance. Occupation.	Residence. past and present.	Age at first appearance.	Cause. α Original cause of disease. β Provocatives of attacks.	Frequency of attacks.	Time of attack.	Premonitory symptoms.	Unmixed or complicated with other lung diseases.	Of what standing.	Associated diseases and family history.	Effects of remedies.
21. George S., m., æt. 27. Asthmatic physique strongly marked. *Tailor.*	Formerly Hackney road, lately Cross street, Regent st., since which not so well.	22 yrs.	α Hardwork, late hours, fatigue, trouble at loss of wife. β Hot weather of summer, worse in July and August: heavy supper.	Nightly in July and August. Every month during the rest of the year.	Four hrs. after going to bed.	None.	Congestion of bronchial tubes.	5 years.	Dyspepsia; pain in scrobiculus, heat, and weight after eating; heartburn, irregular appetite. No inheritance.	Ether is the only thing that has done him any good: 20 drops 3 times a day whenever he felt his breath bad. The relief was almost immediate.
22. George P., m., æt. 43. Thin, with distressed look. *Shoemaker.*	Ealing 20 years; London 12 years; Southampton 11 years.	13 yrs.	α Apparently sober. sudden soberness and hard work after a course of hard drinking. β The hot weather of summer.	An attack every morning during the summer. None in the winter.	4 o'clock in the morning.	Feels very dull, low, and miserable, with nothing really the matter, for 2 or 3 days before an attack.	Unmixed.	30 years.	No associated diseases. Not inherited. Family healthy.	Had about a dozen physicians in London, and several medical men in Southampton. The following has done most good —Acid nit. gtt. xxx, tr. scill. ʒij, vin. ipec. ʒij, ext. conii ʒij, aquæ ʒvj.—Cochl. ampl. ij 4ta quaque hora.
23. Thomas S., m., æt. 57. Thin, high-shouldered, anxious. *Private Gentleman.*	Doughty st., Foundling.	56 yrs.	α Catarrh. β Dyspepsia.	Every night.	1 A.M.	None; awakes with the attack.	Unmixed.	1 year.	Nervous, depressed. and irritable. Had some dyspepsia 6 or 7 years ago. Father died asthmatic at 47.	Morphia, chloroform, ♏xxv in mist. acaciæ om. nocte, stramonium-smoking, lobelia, quinine, iron, arsenic, pepsine, ipecacuanha, purgatives, change of air, all useless. Most good from attending to digestion and regulating diet.
24. William S., m., æt. 22. Pale, thin, narrow-chested. *Banker's Clerk.*	Wiltshire: within the last year Lymington.	1 yr.	α Unknown. β Not mentioned.	Once in four weeks.	Various.	Nothing definite.	Narrow chest, chronic cough, slight mucous expectoration.	21 years.	Constitution delicate. Grandfather had asthma after yellow fever. Uncle asthmatic, but not father.	Since living in Lymington the paroxysms are much mitigated. Never laid up from business here, but in Wiltshire for days together. Once spent three months in London without an attack.

			Exciting causes.	Frequency of attacks.	Time of attack.	Premonitory symptoms.	Chest condition.	Duration.	Associated disease and family history.	Treatment and remarks.
25. Marianne F., f., æt. 26. Tall, stout, healthy-looking. *Washerwoman.*	Always lived in London.	26 yrs.	α Getting wet; the symptoms of cold were but slightly marked—nothing like bronchitis. β Sleep and recumbency.	Every night.	1 A.M.	None.	A little emphysema about the spices. Expectoration prolonged r. 23 sitting.	2 mos.	Purpura from poor living, dyspepsia, constipation. Father confirmed asthmatic; mother died of phthisis.	Nitre-paper always cures the attacks.
26. James R., m., æt. 25. Pale, thin, and stoops. *Private Gentleman.*	Lymington.	In child h'd	α Uncertain, probably cold. β Not mentioned	Once or twice a week.	Early morning.	A restless night precedes the paroxysm.	Chronic bronchitis; heavy mucous expectoration; mucous rales.	From childhood.	General feebleness of constitution. Inherited from father.	Mitigated by a combination of conium and squills.
27. George T., m., æt. 47. *Shoemaker.*	Milford, Hampshire.	frm infancy.	α Infantile cold. β Not stated.	Once in 3 or 4 months.	2 or 3 A.M.	Thoracic tightness.	Some slight bronchitis; loose frequent cough.	Life-long.	No associated diseases. Father died of phthisis; mother healthy at 83.	Blotting-paper saturated in a solution of saltpetre, and burnt in his room, enables him to breathe easily.
28. John R., m., æt. 49. *Brickmaker.*	Lymington.	39 yrs.	α Chill in water and clay. β Not stated.	Every month.	2 A.M.	Slight catarrh and suffocation.	Habitual cough.	10 years.	Œdema of the ankles. No asthma in family; mother still living at 80.	Squill, colchicum, nitre, and soda, three or four times in the day; and calomel and colocynth at night, give most relief.
29. Eliza H., f., æt. 27. Thin, pale, rather dusky. *Gentlewoman.*	London and neighbourhood till 24, well; since locomotive; in Wales very bad.	12 yrs.	α Whooping-cough at 12 years old. β Bronchitis; cannot say cold positively; late dinner or supper; dyspepsia or constipation.	At first every winter; since May (5 mos.) 7 attacks.	Generally in evening.	None.	No appreciable lung disease.	15 years.	Deficient menstruation, constipated bowels. Father a confirmed asthmatic; brother with hay-asthma.	Had tried ipecacuanha, ether, valerianate of zinc, with no benefit. Was prescribed a slight regular aloetic purge, tonics, an early dinner, and nothing after it, plain spare diet, avoidance of unwholesomes. Cure complete.
30. Henry H., m., æt. 55. Emaciated and very high-shouldered. *Merchant.*	Poole, mild and relaxing air.	About 30 yrs.	α Supposed standing about in a field in the month of November. β Not mentioned	Formerly nightly; latterly once or twice a week.	2 o'clock A.M.	Drowsiness.	Considerable bronchial congestion and emphysema.	25 years.	No associated diseases. No trace of asthma in the family.	The only remedy which is efficacious is nitre-paper burnt in his bedroom overnight, which nearly secures his being well in the morning.

Number. Name. Sex. Age. Appearance. Occupation.	Residence, past and present.	Age at first appearance.	Cause. α Original cause of disease. β Provocatives of attacks.	Frequency of attacks.	Time of attack.	Promonitory symptoms.	Unmixed or complicated with other lung disease.	Of what standing.	Associated diseases and family history.	Effects of remedies.
31. Elizabeth D., f., æt. 37. Appearance nothing peculiar. *Cook.*	Montague st., Russell sq., London.	37 yrs.	α Catarrhal bronchitis. β None appreciable.	Every night at 3, or every morning as soon as up.	3 or 7 A.M.	None.	Slight remnants of bronchitis.	2 mos.	Always has been dyspeptic. No asthma or chest disease in the family.	At first the attacks were nightly at 2 or 3 A.M. Since leaving off suppers they had entirely ceased. Two of Corbyn's ipecacuanha lozenges gave her some relief.
32. Wm. W., m., æt. 78. Has aged greatly of late. *Private Gentleman.*	Lostwithiel, in Cornwall, dry situation.	33 yrs.	α Not to be ascertained. β Errors in diet, east wind.	No attack for 45 years till 8 months ago; since then two a week.	Between 12 and 2 at night.	Indigestion; pain in the region of the stomach.	Heart weak and dilated; pulse at times intermittent.	45 years.	Nervous and dyspeptic; legs swell. Not inherited.	He has derived the most benefit from ipecacuanha and tartar-emetic; lobelia, squills, and the three ethers, sulphuric, nitrous, and chloric, have not given him any relief.
33. Mary B., f., æt. 62. Thin, dusky, eyes watery. *Shirtmaker.*	Clement's la., Strand.	52 yrs.	α An attack of bronchitis. β Principally catarrhal; the attacks are nightly, but a supper makes them earlier and more severe.	Every morning regularly; never omitted since their establishment.	4 to 5 A.M.	None can be noticed, from the attacks being diurnal.	Heart perfectly right; no dry, or moist sounds; respiration 16; therefore uncomplicated.	5 mos.	No associated disease. No thoracic disease in the family.	Nitre-paper the only thing tried, and that successful.
34. Wm B., m., æt. 20. Marked arithmatic deformity. *Incapable of Work.*	Rickmansworth. Hertfordshire.	18 yrs.	α Occurrence spontaneous. β Suppers, cold, change of air.	Every night slightly; every 2 or 3 months severely.	Midnight.	None.	Passive bronchial congestion; collapse posteriorly; emphysema in front.	12 years.	Health in other respects good. Very nervous temperament. Not inherited. Family delicate, but no special lung diseases.	Abstinence late in the day, stramonium-smoking, and inhaling the fumes of burning nitre-paper are the only things that do him any good.

35. Elizabeth P., f., æt. 36. Skin and bones. *Gentlewoman.*	Scotland and London.	30 yrs.	α Fatigue and cold. β Malt liquor; any food of a fermenting or gaseous kind; sweets; any air but London.	Every month, or oftener. In bad airs every night	About 3 A.M.	Not stated.	Some bronchitis, partial collapse, and some emphysema.	Health otherwise faultless. Of a quick, susceptible nervous system. Not inherited.	5 years.	Cured by London air. Better at Bayswater than in the country; better still in Cavendish square; perfectly well in the city. Nitre-paper was the only remedy that did her any good; its effect was complete and immediate. It would cure the severest paroxysm in 1 or 2 minutes.
36. James A., m., æt. 24. Remarkably healthy. *Professional.*	Poole, Dorsetshire, and London.	8 yrs.	α Haymaking when a little boy. β Grass-pollen; bright sunlight in June and July; dust generally; laughing, especially after eating.	Every summer, daily, from about May 20th to July 10th.	Sneezing by day, asthma by night	The sneezing precedes the asthma, and its amount very much determines the degree of the asthma.	Unmixed.	None. I think inherited. Grandfather a great sneezer; brother has hay-asthma and asthma; sister the latter.	26 years.	Exclusion of light mitigates the sneezing and eye symptoms. Tobacco-smoking greatly relieves. Light food, with weak brandy and water instead of wine, very much lessens the asthmatic tendency. Beer bad, wine better, brandy and water best.
37. John M., m., æt. 43. Asthmatic spinal curvature, slight, but healthy-looking. *Gentleman Farmer.*	At L—, in Ireland, Dublin, Van Diemen's Land, and France.	In 2d yr.	α Apparently constitutional. β Particular smells, dust, and smoke; eating beans, old peas, cheese, &c.; mental depression. Worse in summer, especially if damp.	Every week at worst; every month at best; in cities never.	Soon after midnight.	Increased colour, irritability of manner, a nervous desire to seem quite well, unusually boisterous spirits.	Probably some little pulmonary collapse and emphysema.	Morbidly sensitive to smells, dust, and smoke. Highly nervous. Asthma not inherited. Family robust.	43 years.	Being carried about on an attendant's back always relieved in an attack. Strict temperance in eating diminished their frequency. Bleeding in foot once instantaneously relieved (emotional?). Certain airs, such as Dublin, Armagh, Belfast, London, perfectly cured—in fact, all cities. Voyage to Van Diemen's Land permanently eradicated the disease. Opium and strong coffee the best remedy.
38. George P., m., æt. 39. Asthmatic figure. *Merchant.*	Seaport town in Dorsetshire.	4	α None ever recognized. β Suppers, malt liquors, and cold, dust, smells, as of violets, wallflowers, &c.	Every two months; worse in autumn.	2 or 3 A.M.	A slight amount of dyspnœa on going to bed.	A very slight, if any, organic mischief.	Health in all other respects perfectly good. Grandmother and several grand-aunts and uncles asthmatic.	35 years.	None of the ordinary remedies have done any good. Total abstinence from food during an attack mitigates and shortens it. Smoking appears to relieve, by promoting expectoration.

Number. Name. Sex. Age. Appearance. Occupation.	Residence, past and present.	Age at first appearance.	Cause. α Original cause of disease. β Provocatives of attacks.	Frequency of attacks.	Time of attack.	Premonitory symptoms.	Unmixed or complicated with other lung disease.	Of what standing.	Associated diseases and family history.	Effects of remedies.
39. Rebecca W., f., æt. 12. Diminutive, emaciated, cyanosed.	A low street in Westminster.	quite an infant.	α Original cause not known. β Cold, fog, wet, misty mornings.	Every morning; formerly rarer.	From 4 to 6 A.M.	Unusual drowsiness overnight.	Slight chronic bronchitis and emphysema.	All her life, 12 years.	Health otherwise good. Not inherited.	Great benefit from nitre-paper and leaving off suppers.
40. Anne C., f., æt. 47. Perfectly healthy appearance. *Poor Married Woman.*	St. Martin's lane.	47 yrs.	α Thinks it was a severe cold. β Cannot tell, as she has her attacks every night.	Every morning.	About 1 A.M.	None.	Slight bronchitis.	3 mos.	Health otherwise good. Not inherited. Two brothers and a sister, and nearly all her relatives, died of consumption.	Not stated.
41. James R., m., æt. 26. Emaciated.	Lymington.	from Infancy.	α Not known. β Not known.	Exacerbations every night; never quite free.	3 to 4 A.M.	Fidgetiness.	Always wheezes.	Life-long.	Chronic bronchitis. Asthma inherited from his father.	Not stated.
42. Jane G., f., æt. 66. Appearance healthy.	Scotland, London, Lymington.	53 yrs.	α Not known. β Not known.	Irregular once; now in 2, 3, or 6 weeks.	Early morning.	Catarrh, with gradually developing asthma.	Some dilatation of the heart, irregular pulse.	13 or 14 years.	No associated diseases. Not inherited.	Purgatives, especially calomel, seem to be the only thing that has been tried.
43. Eliza B., f., æt. 54. Rather plethoric. *Gentlewoman.*	Bath, Cheltenham, India (here quite well), the Cape 6 mos. (ill all the time).	24 yrs.	α Cold. β Fog, damp, neighbourhood of trees, sea-air, bad smells, dust.	Formerly lasted for weeks or months, then free for 6 or 8 mos.; of late years nearly well.	12 o'clock at night.	Tightness of breath before going to bed.	Lungs and heart apparently sound.	30 years.	Highly nervous temperament. Father and his sisters asthmatic; also mother's aunts.	Coffee was once of great benefit, but lost its effect. Then two glasses of hot port wine were found to relieve at once, and have continued equally efficacious.
44. Wm. B., m., æt. 18. Extremely thin and pale. *Clerk.*	Lancaster.	6 yrs.	α Inherited. β Excited by cold and eating too freely. *Always brought on by taking milk.*	Every two or three months.		Headache and a sensation of fulness in the throat.	Not known to be complicated.	12 years.	Suffering from spermatorrhœa, but improving, nervous and hypochondriacal. Inherited; several members of his family asthmatic.	A blister or other counter-irritant to the chest soon relieves. A rhubarb pill two or three times a week useful. He had no attack for 6 or 8 months.

INDEX.

THE END.

LANE MEDICAL LIBRARY

To avoid fine, this book should be returned on
or before the date last stamped below.

MAY 19 1920

OCT 1 1954

APR 8 1955

MAY 14 1979

CPSIA information can be obtained at www.ICGtesting.com

232223LV00003BA/34/P